Encyclopedia of Diet Fads, Second Edition

Encyclopedia of Diet Fads, Second Edition

Understanding Science and Society

Marjolijn Bijlefeld and Sharon K. Zoumbaris

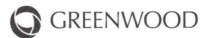 GREENWOOD

AN IMPRINT OF ABC-CLIO, LLC
Santa Barbara, California • Denver, Colorado • Oxford, England

Library of Congress Cataloging-in-Publication Data

Bijlefeld, Marjolijn, 1960–
    Encyclopedia of diet fads : understanding science and society / Marjolijn Bijlefeld and Sharon K. Zoumbaris. — Second edition.
        pages cm
    Includes bibliographical references and index.
    ISBN 978-1-61069-759-0 (hard copy : alk. paper) —
ISBN 978-1-61069-760-6 (ebook)   1. Reducing diets—Encyclopedias.
2. Weight loss—Encyclopedias.   I. Zoumbaris, Sharon K., 1955–   II. Title.
    RM222.2.B535   2015
    613.2'503—dc23   2014024609

ISBN: 978-1-61069-759-0
EISBN: 978-1-61069-760-6

19   18   17   16   15   1   2   3   4   5

This book is also available on the World Wide Web as an eBook.
Visit www.abc-clio.com for details.

Greenwood
An Imprint of ABC-CLIO, LLC

ABC-CLIO, LLC
130 Cremona Drive, P.O. Box 1911
Santa Barbara, California 93116-1911

This book is printed on acid-free paper ∞

Manufactured in the United States of America

Contents

Introduction

Dukan, Paleo, Master Cleanse, Subway, P90X, Baby Food, Biggest Loser—fad diets appear like clockwork, each with its own set of rules. What will Americans do to lose weight? Just about anything, it seems. When we first wrote this book, there was a variety of quick and easy fixes that had flooded the market. Now, a decade later, there are even more. Many of these products or devices are costly; some are not safe; and some are simply outrageous. Consider a bristle brush to scrub fat away or magic weight-loss earrings, or try pretending you live in the country of France.

Dietitians and physicians will say there is only one fundamental combination to help most people lose weight: eat less and exercise more. Some other time-honored suggestions for real success include eating regular meals instead of skipping meals, especially breakfast. Keeping a food journal and writing down the day's food total is another helpful behavior. And all of these are free. Through its Dietary Guidelines for Americans, the DASH diet, and the restyled MyPlate, the government recommends an assortment of healthy food choices that include vegetables, fruits, grains, fat-free or low-fat milk products, fish, lean meat, poultry, and beans.

Americans also have more access to information now than they did even a decade ago. The Internet and a variety of apps for smartphones make it possible to look up fat and calorie content in foods in seconds. Many restaurants and most fast-food restaurants provide nutrition information on their menu items. And the government has recommended the first major overhaul to the Nutrition Facts labels that appear on packaged foods.

This updated volume introduces a wide variety of weight-loss means and methods, new and old. Some entries describe a particular diet; some describe a support group or service; and some entries focus on the people who have changed the way

Americans eat. It combines advice from nutritionists and physicians, weight-loss gurus, and government and private agencies whose role it is to oversee the ever-growing weight-loss industry.

No doubt, there will be disagreements about the effectiveness of a certain diet plan. One person may swear by a high-protein diet like Paleo, whereas another may swear by a plan that restricts or permits only certain foods. Entries may contain a description of the diet plan and arguments from those who say it is unsafe.

While weight loss may not seem like a topic of debate or tremendous confusion, yet here are distinct and seemingly opposing voices. An August 13, 2013, article in *Psychology Today* cited a study that found that 52 percent of Americans found it easier to do their taxes than to figure out how to eat healthfully. That might help explain the draw of diets, especially those that promise incredible results in days or with no real effort required of the dieter. But these diets have shown little overall weight-loss success for many Americans. However, there is some good news. There is new evidence that obesity rates among preschool children have started to drop. Are those numbers a sign that programs, like the high-profile Let's Move initiative from First Lady Michelle Obama, are making a difference? Time will tell whether this downturn is the beginning of a trend or simply a little dip in the ongoing increase in obesity rates.

Who or what is at fault in the first place? Researchers are now looking at antibiotics and our high consumption of these drugs as a possible cause for some of our increasing girth. Consider that for decades, agriculture used antibiotics to pack the pounds on everything from chickens to beef cattle. There were early experiments in the 1950s to see if antibiotics could stimulate growth in young children. Yes, they did. Now, as the medical community works to stop the overuse of antibiotics, which has led to a growth in antibiotic-resistant bacteria, scientists are wondering if people have been "fattened up" not just by diet and lifestyle, but also by exposure to so many drugs.

While scientists continue those studies, what comes next? For most people, small steps can add up. Moderation in food consumption, by cutting down on sweets, fats, and carbohydrates, may do the trick. An increase in the level of daily physical activity will not only burn additional calories, but it can also provide some energy—a positive cycle. In the long run, this combination results in long-lasting weight maintenance, not just a quick-fix weight loss.

In all cases, before starting a diet to lose weight aggressively, consult a doctor. An extreme or a rapid weight loss can have severe consequences. And realize, too, that losing weight is just one part of healthy living. Maintaining a good weight and a diet that provides enough energy to feel good and be active is a lifelong goal.

EARLY HISTORY OF DIETING AND FAD DIETS

In dieting, as in life, everybody wants a quick answer, a quick meal, and a quick success. The elusive promise of quick weight loss is the driving force behind the popularity of best-selling books, powders, liquids, pills, and programs. Each year these new fad diets appear on the scene—everything from high-protein, low-carbohydrate plans to fasting and liquid meals. And Americans—teens included—desperate to lose weight for decades embraced them enthusiastically. However, that trend is now slowly changing as research suggests fewer Americans are on a diet. Some 23 percent of women in 2012 were dieting compared to the 35 percent on diets in 1992. While numbers for obesity have slowed, overall childhood obesity has more than doubled in children and quadrupled in adolescents in the past 30 years, according to the Centers for Disease Control and Prevention (CDC).

These sobering statistics go a long way toward explaining why the lure of quick, easy weight-loss schemes is so hard to resist. Unfortunately, fad diets aren't healthy and don't work for the long haul. Consider this: 95 percent of all dieters will regain their lost weight in one to five years; 35 percent of "normal dieters" progress to pathological dieting or full-blown eating disorders; and Americans spend more than $60 billion annually to try and lose pounds, on everything from weight-loss programs and diet-related products to gym memberships.

Not only are diet theories and products nothing new, they date back to centuries to a time when people had no scientific understanding of digestion and food assimilation. And while today's consumers make their decisions based on improved research and understanding of how the body works, they still fall victim to fad diets that focus on one true aspect of nutrition, which is then exaggerated to an extreme. For women in particular, the lure of fast, effortless weight loss is strongly tied to the demands of fashion and beauty.

Thinness as a beauty ideal surfaced in the early 1800s with the emerging Victorian woman. This thin, genteel, docile creature replaced the idealized voluptuous women painted in the 16th and 17th centuries by artists like Rembrandt and Rubens. And as thinness became the defining feature of beauty in the United States, an 18-inch waist became the Holy Grail of physical perfection. Unfortunately, this measurement was so out of line with normal body dimensions that to achieve it, most women resorted to a practice called tightlacing, a procedure immortalized in Margaret Mitchell's *Gone with the Wind*. This extreme corset tightening eventually caused headaches, fainting spells, and uterine and spinal disorders.

In the 1830s, as literacy increased, technology advanced, and the publishing industry expanded, American women became the target of medical-advice books as well as beauty manuals, all of which encouraged thinness. Still, there were critics like writer Harriet Beecher Stowe who vigorously lamented the increasing problems associated with dieting and the national preoccupation with thinness. Lois Banner in *American Beauty* quoted Beecher Stowe's opinion of the misuse of dieting by American women: "We in America have got so far out of the way of a womanhood that has any vigor of outline or opulence of physical proportions, that, when we see a woman made as a woman ought to be, she strikes us as a monster. Our willowy girls are afraid of nothing so much as growing stout; and if a young lady begins to round into proportions like the women in Titian's or Gorgione's picture, she is distressed above measure, and begins to make secret inquiries into reducing diet, and to cling desperately to the strongest corset."

A decade earlier the popular English poet Lord Byron influenced beauty and diet practices and standards in America as well as in Europe. According to scholars, Byron was known for his tendency to gain weight. By 1822 the poet had starved himself into what biographers call an unnatural thinness. In fact, Banner in *American Beauty* traces the popularity of drinking vinegar to lose weight to Byron, whose favorite weight-loss regimen was to subsist for some days on vinegar and water. A liquid cleanse remains popular today like the Master Cleanse, which uses lemons and maple syrup. But Byron's most lasting contribution to the popularity of fad diets came from his statement that the sight of a woman eating was disgusting. Biographer Leslie A. Marchand attributed this quote to the poet in *Byron: A Portrait*. "A woman," he wrote, "should never be seen eating or drinking, unless it be lobster salad and champagne, the only truly feminine and becoming viands." Following this remark, fashion historians say women in Europe and the United States took up systematic fasting. Indeed, thanks to Byron and other cultural factors, dieting was commonplace by 1900.

Others who influenced society's early love affair with diets included Englishman William Banting, credited with writing the first diet book. Born in 1797, by age 40 the 5-foot-5-inch Banting was extremely obese. He consulted doctor after doctor but nothing helped and his growing girth was ruining his life. By age 60 he was unable to stoop and tie his shoes and he walked backward down the stairs to lessen the stress on his joints. Finally, in 1863 at age 66, he consulted Dr. William Harvey, a surgeon known for his starch- and sugar-free diet treatment for diabetes. Banting immediately lost weight by eating only lean meats and dry toast and eventually went from a high of 202 pounds to a comfortable 156 pounds. Eager to share his success with the world, Banting wrote his diet book, a testimonial titled *A Letter on Corpulence*. Following its publication, *banting* or *to bant*, meaning to diet, became a household word in England and in America. At his death in 1878, more than 58,000 copies of his diet book had been sold, and a total of 12 editions had been published between 1863 and 1902.

Meanwhile, in America in 1837, talk of diet and health nearly incited a riot in Boston. Sylvester Graham, an evangelical New England preacher and speaker, faced an angry mob one evening as he attempted to lecture on food and hygiene reform. Graham was a controversial figure whose Spartan views on diet and drinking had strongly divided the Boston crowd. Critics of Grahamism included the writer Ralph Waldo Emerson, who mocked Graham as "the prophet of bran bread and pumpkins." While Graham was also called the father of all modern diet crazes, he is most widely remembered as the namesake of the graham cracker. His career as a lecturer grew out of his earlier study of human physiology, diet, and nutrition, a choice largely influenced by his 1830 appointment as general agent for the Pennsylvania Temperance Society. During this time Graham developed the "Graham system," as he liked to call it, based on the French vitalist school of medicine. He believed nutrition had moral as well as physical qualities and any desire for food or drink, except for stark hunger and thirst, was depraved. Gluttony was a debilitating expression of an unhealthy urge and Graham was determined to launch an all-out war on debauchery and gluttony.

Graham was one of the first American health reformers to reach a mass audience via lectures. He traveled a circuit through Massachusetts, Rhode Island, Maine, New York, New Jersey, and Pennsylvania. In his talks he recommended a strictly vegetarian diet but did allow for a small daily ration of roasted beef or boiled mutton for those who wanted some meat. He did not believe in cooking vegetables or in warm food in general, since he considered heat a stimulant. And he was particularly adamant about the evils of commercially baked white bread, made from highly refined flour. Graham argued that any good wife and mother must feed her family homemade, coarse bread, served stale after 24 hours. Long after Graham's death in 1851 his followers, called "Grahamites," whose ranks included John Harvey Kellogg of cornflake fame, would continue to advocate vegetarianism, temperance, and bran bread. Many of the most ardent Grahamites were women who were attracted to his recommendations on diet, health care, and dress reform, which criticized disfiguring corsets and advocated loose, comfortable clothing. And while knowledge about nutrition would not be discovered until the early 20th century, Graham was also ahead of his time in understanding the importance of fiber in the diet. Even though the modern version of Graham crackers are a far cry from the coarse, whole wheat bread Graham championed in his time, he was clearly an early voice in preaching that you are what you eat.

Sylvester Graham died in 1851 but his influence on the American diet was only beginning. Per capita meat consumption began to decline as Americans shed their fears of fresh fruit and vegetables and began to eat more balanced meals. Graham had moved public opinion away from gluttony and poor digestion toward slenderness and eating to produce good health. Although Graham died in the 19th century, his way of thinking significantly influenced another man who founded a 20th-century version of Grahamism. Like Graham, Bernard Adolphus McFadden, born in 1868 near Mill Spring, Missouri, believed there was a specific way to eat and live that would produce ultimate health and longevity. He was a man who practiced what he preached and historians believe his philosophy, known as physical culture, is largely at the root of today's health and fitness consciousness in America.

The core belief of McFadden's philosophy was that people got sick because of poor diet, lack of proper exercise, stale air, lack of sunshine, tobacco, alcohol, and drugs. Like Graham, McFadden believed meat should play a minor part in the diet. He preferred fruits, vegetables, and whole grains and, like Graham, he also thought white bread was the worst food a person could eat. He advocated fasting on a regular basis and believed it was a cure for all ailments. Another important component of his physical culture regime was regular exercise, such as walking, and he encouraged women not to wear corsets or any kind of restrictive clothing. In 1892, he changed his last name to "Macfadden," in an attempt to glamorize his name.

Macfadden's ultimate philosophy of health was shaped by his early years as a sickly child. By the time he was 11, both his parents were dead—his father of alcoholism and his mother of tuberculosis. He finally overcame his poor health when relatives in Illinois took him in. Working on their farm turned him into a strong, healthy teenager. At 5-feet-6-inches tall he was not a big man but he had incredible stamina and energy and developed his 145 pounds into a powerful upper body and a strong chest. Macfadden was so convinced he was right about health and nutrition that he campaigned to be the country's first secretary of health in the cabinet of President Franklin D. Roosevelt. When that failed, he campaigned for the Republican nomination for president in 1936, promoting himself through his publications and funding campaign expenses with money from his business. The results were disastrous: stockholders ousted him from his publishing company, he failed to win the nomination, and he lost a great deal of money.

Macfadden's eventual undoing came from his need to carry his ideas to an extreme. In 1955 he developed a urinary tract blockage. Since he believed fasting was a cure for all ailments, he attempted to treat his final illness by fasting but instead became severely emaciated. By the time he reached a hospital, doctors could do nothing to save him. He died on October 12, 1955.

At the same time that American men and women were trimming their waistlines through programs like Macfadden's physical culture, medical doctors were telling patients that obesity was bad for their health. This advice added authority to the new insurance industry ideal height-and-weight charts. Many insurance companies had been charging larger premiums for heavy clients since the 1830s, but as more middle-class families bought policies and as medical examinations became mandatory, Americans now looked to these ideal tables as the most important indicator of their overall health. Self-styled obesity experts quickly followed, and those entrepreneurs helped shape the lucrative diet business with a hastily created array of prescription and patent medicines guaranteed to dissolve and expel unwanted fat.

These early digestive cures included Berledets, made of boric acid, cornstarch, milk, and sugar, and Human Ease, a combination of sodium bicarbonate and lard. Sassafras tea was a chief ingredient in Densmore's Corpulency Cure, while mineral water made up the bulk of Lucile Kimball's powder, along with a little soap and Epsom salt. Arsenic, used for years to stimulate the flow of digestive juices, was turned into an obesity tablet by mixing it with strychnine, caffeine, and phytolacca. Hillel Schwartz describes in *Never Satisfied* how Phytoline, made from phytolacca or pokeberry, a well-known emetic and purgative, was created and marketed as a fat-dissolving preparation. In 1936, another manufactured drug, dinitrophenol, was sold as a weight-loss medicine. Dinitrophenol, a derivative of benzene, was commonly used in the synthesis of different color dyes. At low dosages it would speed up metabolism. Unfortunately, dieters quickly experienced serious side effects: rashes, loss of the sense of taste, and blindness from cataracts. Some who exceeded the recommended dosages of dinitrophenol died from hyperpyremia, a condition where the body literally burns itself up, according to Carl Malmberg in *Diet and Die*. Finally the government in 1938 banned dinitrophenol. The American Medical Association's (AMA) *Nostrums and Quackery* series, first published in 1912, detailed these and some of the other most blatant examples of the various fake obesity cures.

Early diet books were also growing in popularity, such as Dr. Lulu Hunt Peter's *Diet and Health* or Vance Thompson's *Eat and Grow Thin,* which reached its 112th printing in 1931. The early 1930s also saw the introduction of another new weight-loss product, the diet drink. One of the best-known reducing drinks was Dr. Stoll's Diet Aid, sold through beauty parlors in the 1930s. A combination of milk chocolate, starch, and an extract of roasted whole wheat and bran, users mixed it by the teaspoon into a cup of water as a diet substitute for breakfast and lunch. Twenty years later in 1959, doctors at the Rockefeller Institute, studying metabolic changes, mixed together evaporated milk, corn oil, dextrose, and water and created another low-calorie diet drink whose balance of protein, fat, and carbohydrate closely resembled breast milk. Metrecal, a product of the Mead Johnson Company, famous for its Pablum baby food, reawakened the public's interest in diet drinks. Today Nestlé, another distributor of infant formulas, markets Metrecal under the brand name Carnation Slender.

Even at the height of the Depression, the diet industry was flourishing, soon to grow by leaps and bounds with the introduction of amphetamines in the late 1930s. First used clinically in the mid-1930s to treat narcolepsy, a rare disorder resulting in an uncontrollable tendency to sleep, amphetamines skyrocketed in use when doctors began prescribing them for appetite suppression and the treatment of depression. At the time, pharmacologists were actually looking for a synthetic substitute for the expensive ephedrine, which had been used to treat asthma. Under the trade names Benzedrine, Methedrine, and Dexedrine, amphetamines, with their clear effect on appetite and weight loss, became the new darling of the diet industry. Amphetamines stimulate the central nervous system by increasing heart rates and blood pressure while reducing fatigue. However, people who use amphetamines on a regular basis build up a tolerance to them until dieters need higher doses to achieve the same effects. So widespread use by dieters in the 1930s created related problems of drug dependency and addiction. As early as 1943, the AMA publicly opposed the use of amphetamines for the treatment of obesity because of problems of dependence, but doctors continued to recommend them for dieters. Five years later, doctors began recommending Dexedrine as the drug of choice for weight loss and justified it by adding a prescription for barbiturates to calm the amphetamine jitters.

Post-World War II Americans began joining dieting groups. Take Off Pounds Sensibly (TOPS) was the first of the group programs and boasted a membership of 30,000 by the late 1950s. Overeaters Anonymous was started in 1960, Weight Watchers in 1961, and the Diet Workshop in 1965.

Calories Don't Count was the catchy title of a diet book written in 1960 by Dr. Herman Taller, a Rumanian-born physician who practiced obstetrics in Brooklyn. He told people they could eat as many protein and fatty foods as they wanted, but he recommended that dieters severely cut back on carbohydrates. His diet also prescribed six capsules a day of safflower oil. While book sales jumped to more than a million copies in less than a year, in 1962 Taller was fined $7,000 for violating the federal Food, Drug, and Cosmetic Act, and was sharply criticized by the U.S. Food and Drug Administration (FDA). FDA commissioner George Larrick, quoted in the July 13, 1962, issue of *Time*, said, "This best-selling book was deliberately created and used to promote these worthless safflower oil capsules for the treatment of obesity, cardiovascular diseases and other serious conditions. One of its main purposes was to promote the sale of a commercial product in which Dr. Taller had a financial interest." Larrick went on to say that there is no easy, simple substitute for weight loss, but added that in the end calories do count.

And so to lose unwanted pounds, desperate dieters continue to look for answers from NutriSystem, herbal capsules, skin patches to liposuction, and acai berries. Yet, ironically, in most cases the pounds come back once the fad diet ends. In this newest edition we find the dieting public has embraced a whole new crop of schemes and fads no matter how far-fetched. Yet, the real solution has always been available. Simply eat more fruits, vegetables, and whole grain food, fewer junk and fast foods, and, most important, exercise.

FURTHER READING

Adams, Samuel Hopkins. *The Great American Fraud*. Denver: Nostalgic American Research Foundation, Inc., 1978.

Avena, Nicole. "The American Diet: Do You Really Know What You're Eating." *Psychology Today*, August 19, 2013.

Banner, Lois W. *American Beauty*. New York: Alfred A. Knopf, 1983.

"Benzedrine and Dieting." *Newsweek*, September 8, 1947, 48–49.

"Calories Do Count." *Time*, July 13, 1962, 56–57.

Cambridge World History of Food. New York: Cambridge University Press, 2000.

Centers for Disease Control and Prevention. "Trends in the Prevalence of Extreme Obesity among US Preschool-Aged Children Living in Low-Income Families, 1998–2010." *JAMA* 308, no. 24 (2012): 2563–65.

Kennedy, Pagan. "The Fat Drug." *The New York Times*, March 8, 2014, http://www.nytimes.com/2014/03/09/opinion/sunday/the-fat-drug.html (accessed 9/23/14)

Malmberg, Carl. *Diet and Die*. New York: Hillman-Curl, Inc., 1935.

Ogden, C. L., Carroll, M. D., Kit, B. K., and Flegal, K. M. "Prevalence of Childhood and Adult Obesity in the United States, 2011–2012." *Journal of the American Medical Association* 311, no. 8 (2014): 806–14.

Pillsbury, Richard. *No Foreign Food: The American Diet in Time and Place*. Boulder, CO: Westview Press, 1998.

Roberts, Paul. "The New Food Anxiety." *Psychology Today*, March–April 1998, 30–40.

Schwartz, Hillel. *Never Satisfied: A Cultural History of Diets, Fantasies and Fat*. New York: Macmillan, 1986.

Encyclopedia
of Diet Fads

Acai Berry Diet

Think of super foods and the acai berry tops the list, both alphabetically and nutritionally. The acai, pronounced ah-sah-EE, compares favorably with other very nutritious fruits like blueberries and pomegranate in the amount of healthy antioxidants they contain. Antioxidants are the molecules that combat cell-damaging free radicals. Research has shown that diets rich in fruit, vegetables, and other plant foods are associated with less damage from free radicals.

Acai berries were introduced to the United States in 2001 and they now show up in every kind of food and drink imaginable. They are cholesterol-free, low in saturated fats, and high in fiber. Researchers have studied the effects of the fruit and suggest it may help ward off diseases like cancer and heart disease. So it is no surprise that the acai berry is now also an ingredient in various diet and detox programs.

The berry is a rich source of nutrients but nutritionists warn dieters that no one single food can provide a "magic pill" for weight loss. Individuals lose weight when they eat fewer calories than they burn and when they adopt a lifestyle that includes healthy, fresh foods, and exercise or physical activity.

While there is no one single "acai berry diet" or specific detox plan using acai, there are plenty of products available in stores and online that feature acai as a main ingredient and also promote weight loss.

Web sites selling acai products are especially plentiful and claim dieters will burn fat better, cut down on cravings, boost metabolism, and cleanse their system by removing toxins using acai. Some ads even suggest acai will increase weight loss above dieting and exercise alone and will contribute to a loss of up to 20 pounds in one week.

The pretty purple berry does have a unique characteristic that few fruits offer; it contains monounsaturated fats (MUFAS). The MUFAS in the acai satisfy hunger when included in a calorie-controlled diet, much like in the avocado. MUFAS are also found in nuts, seeds, dark chocolate, olives, flax, and olive oils. One problem with the berries is that they do not travel well and when used commercially there is usually very little pure acai in the product. Nutritionists warn that when buying acai products, it is important to read the label, as many of the drinks contain a lot of added sugar. One smoothie was found to have 48 grams of sugar in each bottle with lots of that coming from the apple, banana, grape, and plum juices added to make it palatable. In fact, blueberries, blackberries, and raspberries may be more practical and economical choices since they are more readily available, and more reasonably priced. Acai products are usually quite expensive.

The Center for Science in the Public Interest, known for its work as a nutrition watchdog group, issued a warning in 2009 to U.S. consumers about companies offering free trials of acai diet products. It cautioned customers to be aware that free samples can sometimes result in monthly charges. Several nutritionists suggest that a healthy diet alternative with plenty of antioxidant benefits can also be created using the DASH (Dietary Approaches to Stop Hypertension) diet. The DASH diet calls for an abundance of fresh fruits and vegetables along with low-fat dairy products, lean proteins, and whole grains and, if followed correctly, will supply a healthy amount of antioxidants. So while acai gets plenty of hype as a "superfruit," it is just as easy for consumers to get antioxidants from more mainstream fruits like oranges and raspberries. And for those hoping to lose a few pounds, consumer groups suggest checking the ingredients of any acai diet product to make sure it does not contain stimulants or laxatives. Knowing the caloric and nutritional value of what you put into your mouth is one of the healthiest choices you can make.

See also: DASH Diet.

FURTHER READING

"Acai Smoothie." *Muscle & Fitness/Hers,* November–December 2010, 11(6), 19.
Alexander, Brian. "Fountain of Youth or Fraud?" *Self* 32, no. 8 (August 2010): 91.
"Consumers Warned of Web-Based Acai Scams." The Center for Science in the Public Interest, March 23, 2009. http://www.cspinet.org/new/200903231.html.
Hildebrandt, Stephanie. "A Dose of Berry Wellness: The Health Benefits of Berries Resonate with Consumers." *Beverage Industry,* October 1, 2012.
Zelman, Kathleen M. "Acai: Weight Loss Wonder Fruit?" WebMD. http://www.webmd.com/diet/features/acai-weight-loss-wonder-fruit.

Aerobic Activity

During aerobic activities, oxygen breaks down carbohydrates and converts them into lasting energy. Aerobic exercise is ideal for burning fat. Examples of good aerobic activities include running, swimming, and aerobics classes, which combine fast-paced stretching, strength, and endurance exercises—all activities that make your muscles use oxygen. Aerobic exercises are repetitive—bicycling, swimming, jogging, brisk walking, basketball, skating, dancing, and jumping rope.

What do aerobic exercises do for you? By strengthening your heart, aerobic exercises get fresh blood pumped more rapidly to muscle groups. That helps tone those muscle groups because they can keep moving longer. Aerobic workouts break down carbohydrates, fats, and proteins so they are the ideal workouts for losing fat.

To make the most of aerobic exercises, work out for at least 15 to 30 minutes at your target heart rate. If you can't go that long, break it down into 10-minute intervals, but aim for 30 minutes a day, three or four days a week. Have rest days in between so that your body can recover and to prevent injuries. As your body gets stronger, increase the level of intensity or the time of the activity. Do it gradually, though. Don't expect to jog 30 minutes one month and an hour-and–a-half the next. Instead, try covering more ground in that 30 minutes, or extend the slow jog to 40 minutes or so.

The Centers for Disease Control and Prevention recommends the following:

2 hours and 30 minutes (150 minutes) of moderate-intensity aerobic activity (such as brisk walking) every week *and* muscle-strengthening activities that strengthen all the major muscle groups on two or more days a week

or

1 hour and 15 minutes (75 minutes) of vigorous-intensity aerobic activity (jogging or running) every week *and* muscle strengthening activities on two or more days a week

or

an equivalent mix of moderate- and vigorous-intensity aerobic activity *and* muscle-strengthening activities on at least two days each week.

During aerobic activity, it's important to monitor your heart rate. This can be done by wearing a heart monitor while you're exercising, using the heart monitor function on treadmills and other exercise equipment often found in gyms, or stopping to measure your pulse periodically during exercise. If your heart rate is below your target, increase the intensity of the workout. If it's above, take it down a notch.

There are several formulas to determine a target heart rate, but the simplest one is to subtract your age from 220 to calculate your maximum heart rate. So if you're 20, your maximum heart rate would be 200. Then a target heart is a percentage of that. A sedentary person just starting an aerobic program should use 50 percent as a target heart rate, recommends the American Heart Association. As you get stronger, you can increase your target heart rate, topping out at 85 percent.

A 20-year-old would have a predicted maximum heart rate of 200 (220–20), so the target heart range would be 100 (50 percent) to 170 (85 percent). A 30-year-old would have a target heart of 190 (220–30), with a target heart rate between 95 and 162.

See also: Target Heart Rate.

FURTHER READING

Hope, Jenny. "How a Brisk Walk Boosts a Woman's Brain: Aerobic Exercise Can Increase Size of Area Involved in Learning and Memory." *Daily Mail*, April 8, 2014. http://www.dailymail.co.uk/health/article-2600226/How-brisk-walk-boosts-womans-brain-Aerobic-exercise-increase-size-area-involved-learning-memory.html.
"How Much Physical Activity Do Adults Need?" Centers for Disease Control and Prevention. http://www.cdc.gov/physicalactivity/everyone/guidelines/adults.html.
http://www.cdc.gov/physicalactivity/everyone/measuring/index.html.

Amphetamines

Amphetamines belong to a group of medicines called central nervous system (CNS) stimulants. They act on the CNS—the brain and the spinal cord—increasing heart rate and blood pressure while reducing appetite and fatigue. Dieters have used amphetamines to treat obesity for many years, in both prescription and over-the-counter forms. However, medical use of amphetamines is now restricted primarily to treating narcolepsy, a sleep disorder, and attention-deficit hyperactivity disorder (ADHD). Adderall and Ritalin are stimulant drugs in the amphetamine family widely prescribed for the treatment of ADHD and hyperactivity. In treating ADHD, these medicines are part of a total program that includes social, educational, and psychological components. There are also nonstimulant prescription drugs for the treatment of ADHD.

When initially taken, amphetamines produce feelings of well-being, increased competence, and alertness. Their effects are similar to those of cocaine, but their onset is slower and their duration is longer. High doses of amphetamines can cause tremors, sweating, heart palpitations, or anxiety. Exhaustion and depression follow when the drug wears off. In general, chronic abuse produces a psychosis that resembles schizophrenia and is characterized by paranoia, picking at the skin, preoccupation with one's own thoughts, and auditory and visual hallucinations. Violent and erratic behavior is frequently seen among chronic abusers of amphetamines. Amphetamines have a high potential for abuse, since regular use can lead to greater physical tolerance, requiring higher doses to achieve the same effect. This causes psychological dependency, characterized by a craving for the drug and a belief that one cannot function without it. Doctors caution dieters that without long-term changes in exercise and eating habits, using amphetamines is not a long-term weight-loss solution and is not an appropriate substitute for good nutrition and a healthy lifestyle.

See also: Dimethylamylamine HCl (DMAA).

FURTHER READING

"Obesity." In *Gale Encyclopedia of Medicine*. Detroit: Gale Group, 2002.

Anaerobic Activity

Anaerobic energy is created by burning carbohydrates, not oxygen. Anaerobic exercises are characterized by maximum bursts of energy, of short duration, to build muscle strength. They include weight lifting and sprinting, for example. Muscle-strengthening activities let you work on specific groups of muscles by using resistance. These exercises can be performed with free weights, weight machines, or even the resistance created by the weight of your own body—push-ups, chin-ups, or sprinting. Before doing a muscle-building routine, make sure you warm up with stretches to prevent painful cramping that can result from lactic acid buildup in muscle tissue. Stretching at the end of the workout is also important.

See also: Aerobic Activity.

FURTHER READING

"How Anerobic Threshold Exercises Increase Weight Loss." *Fit Day.* http://www.fitday .com/fitness-articles/fitness/weight-loss/how-anaerobic-threshold-exercises-increase-weight-loss.html#b.

Steinberg, Steve. "The Anaerobic Alternative." *Men's Journal,* April 2013. http://www .mensjournal.com/health-fitness/exercise/the-anaerobic-alternative-20130404.

Anemia

Anemia is a condition in which a deficiency in the size or number of red blood cells or the amount of hemoglobin they contain limits the exchange of oxygen and carbon dioxide between the blood and the tissue cells. It results from a variety of conditions such as hemorrhage, genetic abnormalities, chronic disease states, or drug toxicity.

Small children and teenagers have a higher iron requirement than at other times in their lives. The human body needs iron for energy production: too little iron leaves you tired and at risk for iron-deficiency anemia. Iron is especially important for teenage girls who are menstruating, since iron is essential for the expansion of blood volume. The highest incidence of iron deficiency occurs in adolescent girls.

Iron is a trace mineral found in red meat, liver, fish, green leafy vegetables, enriched bread, and some dried fruits such as prunes, apricots, and raisins. Some people consume most of their iron requirements by eating meats, but the incidence of iron-deficiency anemia in vegetarians is not significantly different from that in omnivores, according to the American Society of Clinical Nutrition. Foods high in iron include spinach, broccoli, raisins, chickpeas, pinto beans, whole grains, and blackstrap molasses. In fact, calorie for calorie, spinach has 14 times the iron of sirloin steak. However, as with calcium, absorption of iron is also affected by diet, and iron from plant foods is not as easily absorbed as iron from animal foods. For that reason vegetarians and people who need to boost their iron levels should eat foods rich in vitamin C to help increase the absorption of iron in the body. Citrus fruits and juices, tomatoes, and broccoli are all good sources of vitamin C.

Recommended iron intake for boys aged 14–18 is 11 milligrams per day, decreasing to 8 milligrams per day after age 19. For girls aged 14–18, the recommended iron intake is 15 milligrams per day and increases to 18 milligrams per day for women aged 19–50. Blood loss, such as that which occurs during menstrual cycles, is a major cause of iron deficiency, which can be corrected either by eating more foods that are higher in iron content or by taking iron supplements. Coffee, tea, wheat bran, eggs, and soy inhibit iron absorption. Medications such as antacids, for example, can also interfere with iron absorption.

Iron demands also peak for pregnant women. The requirement of iron intake for pregnant women is 27 milligrams per day and decreases to 9 or 10 milligrams for lactating women.

See also: Dietary Guidelines for Americans; Vitamins.

FURTHER READING

"Iron and Iron Deficiency." Centers for Disease Control and Prevention. http://www.cdc.gov/nutrition/everyone/basics/vitamins/iron.html.
Robbins, Carolyn. "Nutrition & RDA for Iron." *SFGate*. http://healthyeating.sfgate.com/nutrition-rda-iron-7177.html.
"Understanding Anemia—Symptoms." WebMD.com. http://www.webmd.com/a-to-z-guides/understanding-anemia-symptoms.

Anorexia Nervosa

Anorexia is *not* a diet plan. It is an eating disorder—a pathological fear of weight gain. Anorexia and other eating disorders can be considered mental health issues, and mental health services have been greatly expanded under the Affordable Care Act. The National Association of Anorexia Nervosa and Associated Disorders estimates that up to 24 million people of all ages and genders suffer from an eating disorder—anorexia nervosa, bulimia, and binge-eating disorder—and 86 percent of them report that the problem developed by the time they reached the age of 20. Intentional starving often begins around the time of puberty and involves extreme weight loss, defined as at least 15 percent below one's normal body weight. For regularly menstruating adolescent girls and women, skipping three menstrual cycles (except pregnancy) is another medical indicator of a serious problem. Even though someone with anorexia may look emaciated, she may still be convinced that she's too heavy. Anorexia is the third most common chronic illness among adolescents, and 95 percent of those who have eating disorders are between the ages of 12 and 28.

The vast majority of people affected by these eating disorders are adolescent and young adult women. Males and older women can also develop eating disorders, but young women are often most influenced by idealistic—and generally unachievable—standards of beauty. In a survey by the Centers for Disease Control and Prevention, more than one-third of the high school girls surveyed thought they were overweight. That compares to 15 percent of the boys who answered the same way.

According to the National Institutes of Health, approximately 1 percent of adolescent girls develop anorexia nervosa and another 2 to 3 percent develop bulimia nervosa. As girls approach adulthood, the numbers increase. Studies indicate that by the time they reach college age, somewhere between 4.5 and 18 percent of women have a history of bulimia. The National Center for Health Statistics estimates that about 9,000 people admitted to hospitals were diagnosed with bulimia in 1994 and about 8,000 were diagnosed with anorexia. Males account for only 5 to 10 percent of bulimia and anorexia cases. While people of all races develop the disorders, the vast majority of those diagnosed are white.

Both anorexia nervosa and bulimia are destructive conditions and can lead to serious damage, even death. One in ten cases of anorexia nervosa leads to death from starvation, cardiac arrest, other medical complications, or suicide. About 1,000 women die of anorexia each year, according to the American Anorexia/ Bulimia Association. The National Center for Health Statistics noted that anorexia nervosa was the underlying cause of death noted on 101 death certificates in 1994 and was mentioned as one of multiple causes of death on another 2,657 death certificates. In the same year, bulimia was the underlying cause of death on two death certificates and mentioned as one of several causes on 64 others. According to the Harvard Eating Disorders Center, anorexia has the highest mortality rate among eating disorders.

See also: Bulimia Nervosa; Eating Disorders.

FURTHER READING

Chang, Samantha. "More Men and Teens Suffer from the Eating Disorders Anorexia and Bulimia." *Examiner.com*, February 23, 2014. http://www.examiner.com/article/increase-eating-disorders-among-men-women-and-teens-a-cause-for-alarm.

Mellin, L., S. McNutt, Y. Hu, G. B. Schreiber, P. Crawford, and E. Obarzanek. "A Longitudinal Study of the Dietary Practices of Black and White Girls 9 and 10 Years Old at Enrollment: The NHLBI Growth and Health Study." *Journal of Adolescent Health* 20, no. 1 (1991): 23–37.

Antioxidants

Many claims have been made about the health benefits of antioxidants. These are substances that counteract the harmful free radicals created by oxidation.

Oxidation, for example, can rust cars. Some oxidation in the body is good because it produces energy and kills bacterial invaders. But, in excess, it can damage tissues. Antioxidants are found naturally in many foods, primarily fruits and vegetables. They are also available as supplements, but whether or not they are helpful is still a matter of debate. There are claims that antioxidants in large quantities can help prevent or reduce the effects of a variety of diseases, including cardiovascular disease, diabetes, Alzheimer's, and various forms of cancer. Vitamins with antioxidant properties include vitamins E, C, and A as beta-carotene. Some minerals such as selenium, lutein, and lycopene are also considered to have antioxidant properties.

Research on the effect of antioxidants is continuing. In 2014, for example, two studies found that the carotenoid lycopene, found in tomatoes, pink grapefruit, and watermelon, may decrease the risk of prostate cancer.

On April 10, 2000, a panel at the Institute of Medicine of the National Academies of Science reported that megadoses of antioxidants haven't yet been proven to be helpful and might in fact be dangerous. According to the press release announcing the findings, "A direct connection between the intake of antioxidants and the prevention of chronic disease has yet to be adequately established," said Norman I. Krinsky, chair of the study's Panel on Dietary Antioxidants and Related Compounds, and a professor of biochemistry at Tufts University School of Medicine, Boston. "We do know, however, that dietary antioxidants can in some cases prevent or counteract cell damage that stems from exposure to oxidants, which are agents that affect a cell's molecular composition. But much more research is needed to determine whether dietary antioxidants can actually stave off chronic disease."

As such, the panel established the following recommendations for dietary supplementation of antioxidants. It increased recommended intake levels of vitamin C to 75 milligrams per day for women and 90 milligrams per day for men. Smokers, who are more likely to be impacted from the cell-damaging biological processes and deplete more vitamin C, need an additional 35 milligrams per day. The report set the upper intake level for vitamin C, from both food and supplements, at 2,000 milligrams per day for adults, saying intakes above this amount may cause diarrhea. Food sources for vitamin C include citrus fruit, potatoes, strawberries, broccoli, and leafy green vegetables.

Vitamin E recommendations were also increased, and men and women are now advised to consume 15 milligrams of vitamin E from food. Food sources for this vitamin are vegetable oils, nuts, seeds, liver, and leafy green vegetables. Synthetic vitamin E from vitamin supplements should not exceed 1,000 milligrams of alpha-tocopherol per day for adults. Alpha-tocopherol is the only type of vitamin E that human blood can maintain and transfer to cells when needed. People who consume more than this amount place themselves at greater risk of hemorrhagic damage because the nutrient can act as an anticoagulant, according to the report.

The report also recommended that men and women need 55 micrograms of selenium per day. Food sources include seafood, liver, meat, and grains. The upper level of selenium, including natural and supplement sources, should be less than 400 micrograms per day. More could result in selenosis, a toxic reaction that can cause hair loss and nail sloughing.

The report did not set a recommended daily intake or upper intake level for beta-carotene and other carotenoids, which are found naturally in dark-green and deep-yellow vegetables. However, it cautioned against high doses, recommending supplementation only for the prevention and control of vitamin A deficiency.

The report stressed that a balanced and varied diet will provide adequate amounts of these vitamins and minerals without requiring supplements. The American Heart Association concurs in a February 1999 Science Advisory, "Antioxidant Consumption and Risk of Coronary Heart Disease: Emphasis on Vitamin C, Vitamin E, and Beta-Carotene," which concluded, "The most prudent and scientifically supportable recommendation for the general population is to consume a balanced diet with emphasis on antioxidant-rich fruits and vegetables and whole grains. This advice, which is consistent with the current dietary guidelines of the American Heart Association, considers the role of the total diet in influencing disease risk. Although diet alone may not provide the levels of vitamin E intake that have been associated with the lowest risk in a few observational studies, the absence of efficacy and safety data from randomized trials precludes the establishment of population-wide recommendations regarding vitamin E supplementation."

See also: Dietary Guidelines for Americans; Vitamins.

FURTHER READING

"Antioxidants: Beyond the Hype." The Nutrition Source. Harvard School of Public Health. http://www.hsph.harvard.edu/nutritionsource/antioxidants/.

Charnow, Jody. "Lycopene May Decrease Prostat Cancer Risk." *Renal and Urology News*, February 28, 2104. http://www.renalandurologynews.com/lycopene-may-decrease-prostate-cancer-risk/article/335907/.

Dietary Reference Intakes for Vitamin C, Vitamin E, Selenium, and Carotenoids. Institute of Medicine of the National Academies, August 3, 2000. http://www.iom.edu/Reports/2000/Dietary-Reference-Intakes-for-Vitamin-C-Vitamin-E-Selenium-and-Carotenoids.aspx.

Appetite Suppressants by Prescription

The popularity of prescription appetite suppressants goes up and down like a roller coaster. The drugs work largely by increasing levels of serotonin, which is a brain chemical that controls feelings of fullness. Widespread use of prescription diet pills first began several decades ago with the introduction of amphetamines. In those early days the pills' potential was as great as their abuse by users because they called for increasing doses to be effective. In fact, by the 1970s a crisis of amphetamine abuse had emerged, as people began injecting these drugs intravenously and they were sold on the street as "speed." Doctors responded to the problem by limiting prescriptions, and the drug fell into disfavor as an obesity treatment.

Appetite suppressants made a comeback in the 1990s with the famous combination of drugs fenfluramine and phentermine. Millions of prescriptions for fen-phen, as it was popularly called, were written before it was pulled from the market in 1997 when the U.S. Food and Drug Administration (FDA) received reports of dangerous side effects; some 30 percent of patients taking the weight-loss pills had developed a fatal form of heart-valve disease. At the same time Redux, or dexfenfluramine, was also withdrawn by the FDA when cases of a rare but fatal type of pulmonary hypertension or lung condition known as PPH developed in those taking the drug for more than three months.

Once again prescription appetite-suppressant sales slumped. But the market demonstrated another upturn with the arrival of the diet drug Xenical, which is also available in a lower-strength, nonprescription diet supplement, Alli. In contrast to the other prescription appetite suppressants, Xenical ignores brain chemicals and instead interferes with the absorption of fats in the digestive system. The drug works by blocking an enzyme needed to digest fat and prevents about 30 percent of ingested dietary fat from being absorbed by the body. That undigested fat shows up in the stools, and side effects include bloating, flatulence, oily stool diarrhea, and fecal incontinence. And because Xenical can deplete fat-soluble vitamins, doctors say users must take a multivitamin.

In 2012, the FDA approved its first two new weight-loss drugs in more than a decade. They were Belviq (lorcaserin), which promotes the feeling of fullness, and Qsymia, a combination of an appetite suppressant and an anticonvulsant.

Health care professionals say they do not recommend the use of appetite-suppressing drugs to anyone who is not clinically obese, since there are side effects and risks to taking the medications. The typical requirement is that a patient must have a body mass index (BMI) of 30 or higher, or a BMI of 27, with an obesity-related condition, such as high blood pressure or Type 2 diabetes. These medicines are available only with a doctor's prescription and must be used in conjunction with a reduced-calorie diet and increased exercise. And while they are useful during the first few weeks of a weight-loss program, their appetite-reducing effects tend to decrease over time, just as the other, earlier prescription choices did, creating the potential for abuse. Doctors note that many dieters also do not realize that once they stop taking the appetite suppressants, the body may need time to adjust. During this transition period, anyone who experiences extreme tiredness or weakness, mental depression, nausea or vomiting, stomach cramps or pain, or trouble with sleeping or nightmares should contact a physician. When deciding to use an appetite suppressant, health care professionals suggest weighing the risks of taking the medicine against the good it may do.

See also: Amphetamines; Belviq; Fen-Phen; Qsymia; Xenical.

FURTHER READING

"Obesity." In *Gale Encyclopedia of Medicine*. Detroit: Gale Group, 2002.

Artificial Sweeteners

Sugar has 15 calories per teaspoon. For anyone trying to lose weight, sugar-sweetened snacks and drinks can present a real problem. Yet few people are willing to give up sweets entirely. As a result, artificial sweeteners that provide the taste of sweetness without the caloric punch are popular. These sweeteners are hundreds of times sweeter than sugar. In other words, a little goes a long way. There are five kinds of artificial sweeteners on the market: saccharin, aspartame, acesulfame potassium, sucralose, and neotame.

Artificial sweeteners are known as nonnutritive sweeteners. They provide no energy, as other caloric foods do. There are also nutritive sweeteners, such as honey, molasses, barley malt, and fructose. Nutritive sweeteners typically have about the same caloric impact as sugar. Saccharin was first developed in 1879—the result of an accidental spill during research on food preservatives. The sweetener saw huge jumps in popularity during World War I and World War II when sugar was being rationed. Some research starting in the 1960s suggested a link between saccharin and cancer. The U.S. Food and Drug Administration (FDA) considered banning it based on animal research that suggested the link to bladder cancer in rats. Indeed, it was banned in Canada in 1977, but it has never been banned in the United States. For 25 years, however, products that contain saccharin did carry a warning label that saccharin had caused cancer in lab animals. That label was a requirement of the 1977 Saccharin Study and Labeling Act. In December 2000, a bill passed that essentially gave saccharin a clean bill of health. Saccharin is between 200 and 700 times sweeter than sugar; Sweet and Low is a brand name.

Aspartame was discovered in 1965 and was first approved in 1981 as a tabletop sweetener. Aspartame breaks down as it heats up, so it is not an effective sugar substitute in most baked goods. As of 1996, it had been approved for use in foods and beverages, some snack foods, and products such as syrups and salad dressings. It is about 200 times sweeter than sugar. NutraSweet and Equal are well-known brands of aspartame sweetener.

According to an article in the *Journal of the American Dietetic Association*, "demand for aspartame in the United States rose from 8.4 million lb. in 1986 to 17.5 million lb. in 1992, a figure that represents more than 80% of the world demand. Although soft drinks account for more than 70% of aspartame consumption, this sweetener is added to more than 6,000 foods, personal care products, and pharmaceuticals." Overall, the United States consumes about 50 percent of the world's demand and leads the world in consumption of high-intensity sweeteners.

The third sweetener, acesulfame potassium, was approved in 1992 for gums and dry foods and its approval was expanded to liquid use in 1998. Pepsi immediately included it in its new Pepsi One drink. It is about 200 times sweeter than sugar, and according to its manufacturer, Nutrinova, it is used in more than 4,000 products.

The fourth sweetener is sucralose and its trade name is Splenda. It's 600 times sweeter than sugar and is the only artificial sweetener actually derived from table sugar. Sucralose cannot be digested; therefore, it adds no calories to food. Before approving sucralose in 1998, the FDA reviewed data from more than 110 studies in humans and animals.

Neotame, produced by the NutraSweet Company, was approved by the FDA in 2002. The manufacturer says it is 8,000 times sweeter than sugar.

Indeed, the FDA has determined that these five artificial sweeteners are safe for human consumption. However, computer users surfing the Internet can find many claims that artificial sweeteners are linked to the development of cancer, tumors, birth defects, brain damage, and other serious medical conditions. It is the role of the FDA to ensure that food products sold in the United States are safe. Indeed, the FDA banned the sweetener cyclamate in 1969 out of concerns that it could be carcinogenic to some people.

While the FDA and the medical establishment note that the approved sweeteners are generally recognized as safe, physicians and nutritionists recommend moderation in sweet foods. Whether the sugar is nutritive or artificial, sweetened foods with little or no nutritional value should be a small part of the U.S. FDA's ChooseMyPlate guidelines for daily eating.

See also: Calories; Food and Drug Administration.

FURTHER READING

FDA Talk Paper: "FDA Approves New High-Intensity Sweetener Sucralose." *FDA*, April 1, 1998.
Henkel, John. "Sugar Substitutes: Americans Opt for Sweetness and Lite." *FDA Consumer* (U.S. Food and Drug Administration) (November/December 1999).
"Use of Nutritive and Nonnutritive Sweeteners—Position of the ADA." *Journal of the American Dietetic Association* 98 (1998): 580–87.
www.aspartame.org.
www.caloriecontrol.org.
www.neotame.com.
www.saccharin.org.
www.sucralose.com.

Atkins, Robert C.

Dr. Robert C. Atkins (b. October 17, 1930, in Columbus, Ohio, d. April 18, 2003) was the founder and executive medical director of the Atkins Center for Complementary Medicine in New York City. The Center was founded in 1976 with the stated philosophy "that the best medicine integrates the safest and most effective therapies from all the healing arts, both traditional and alternative." Dr. Atkins was the author of several best-selling diet books, including *Dr. Atkins' Diet Revolution* (1972), as well as *Dr. Atkins' New Diet Revolution* (1992), and *Dr. Atkins' New Diet Revolution: Revised and Updated* (1999). His last book before his death was *Atkins for Life* (2003). He and his wife, Veronica, coauthored *Dr. Atkins' Quick and Easy New Diet Cookbook* (1997) and he wrote a guide to using vitamins, minerals, and other supplements, titled *Dr. Atkins' Vita-Nutrient Solution: Nature's Answer to Drugs* (1998).

Atkins began his study of medicine at the University of Michigan where he earned his bachelor of arts degree in 1951. He received his medical degree from Cornell University in 1955. Atkins practiced as an internist and cardiologist for

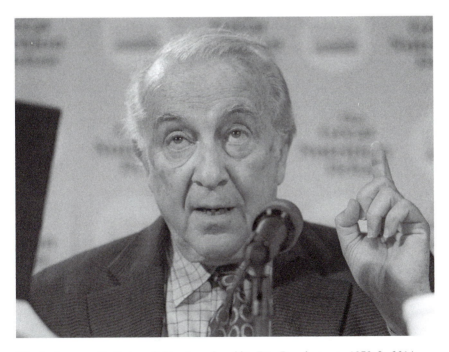

Weight-loss guru Dr. Robert Atkins introduced his Diet Revolution in 1972. In 2014, the company that uses his name sold prepackaged foods as well as books that explain the low-carbohydrate Atkins Diet. (AP Photo/Tyler Mallory)

some 20 years before he published his first book and best seller, *Dr. Atkins' Diet Revolution*. His diet was followed by another very popular high-protein, low-carbohydrate eating plan, *The Complete Scarsdale Medical Diet*, written in 1978 by physician and cardiologist Dr. Herman Tarnower.

Although he is better known for his work in weight control, Dr. Atkins also built a reputation as a supporter of what he called natural medicine and nutritional pharmacology, which he advocated as an alternative to pharmaceutical drugs and surgery for many debilitating illnesses. Criticism of Atkins's belief in alternative medicine reached its peak in 1993 when New York health commissioner Mark Chassin briefly suspended Atkins's medical license. Calling Atkins's medical practice "an imminent danger to the health of the people of this state," the commissioner's action was in response to how the doctor treated one of his patients who complained of headaches and weakness after injecting herself with ozone. Atkins at the time was a strong advocate of the use of ozone gas to treat cancer and AIDS. Atkins, in an August 1993 *Time* magazine article, called the commissioner's action harassment and said the suspension was a reaction to Atkins's belief in the use of alternative medicine. Atkins's medical license was restored less than a month later.

See also: Atkins Nutritional Approach; Ketones/Ketosis; Ornish, Dean; Scarsdale Diet.

FURTHER READING

"Atkins Diet." In *Gale Encyclopedia of Medicine*. Detroit: Gale Group, 2001.

Atkins, Robert C. *Atkins for Life*. New York: St. Martin's Press, 2003.

Atkins, Robert C. *Dr. Atkins' New Diet Revolution*. New York: Avon Books, 1992.

Brody, Jane E. "Senate Nutrition Panel to Focus on Perils of Being Overweight." *New York Times*, April 13, 1973, 18.

"Fad Diets: Don't Look for Magic Bullets." *Consumers' Research Magazine*, July 2000, 24–26.

"License Suspended, Dr. Robert Atkins." *Time*, August 23, 1993, 21.

Taubes, Gary. "The Soft Science of Dietary Fat." *Science* March 30, 2001, 2536–45.

"The Trendy Diet That Sizzles: A Counterintuitive Program Reaches Critical Mass." *Newsweek*, September 6, 1999, 60.

Underwood, Anne. "The Battle of Pork Rind Hill: When the Nation's Best-Selling Diet Gurus Squared Off in a Raucous Food Fight, One Thing Was Clear: There's No Easy Way to Shed That Ugly Flab. So Get Out the Jogging Shoes." *Newsweek*, March 6, 2000, 50–52.

Atkins Nutritional Approach

In the past several years, the Atkins diet has gone through some substantial changes, although the primary principle of a low-carbohydrate diet remains from the Atkins Nutritional Approach developed by the late Dr. Robert C. Atkins and published in his best-selling books, *Dr. Atkins' Diet Revolution* (1972) and *Dr. Atkins' New Diet Revolution* (1992).

In 2014, Atkins Nutritionals, a company that now includes the sales of frozen meals, nutrition bars, and shakes, released *The New Atkins Made Easy: A Faster, Simpler Way to Shed Weight and Feel Great—Starting Today*. This latest book includes recipes, detailed shopping lists to maintain a pantry full of Atkins-friendly foods and tips for dining out, which include downloading the latest Atkins smartphone or iPad application.

The 2014 volume follows the release of a more workable Atkins program in 2010, with the publication of *The New Atkins for a New You*. The 2010 changes included specific recommendations for eating vegetables daily and relented on its prohibition of caffeine drinks and alcohol, allowing those in small amounts.

The Atkins Center for Complementary Medicine calls its eating plan a controlled carbohydrate program for weight management and good health. Critics call the diet a high-protein, high-fat, and low-carbohydrate ketogenic diet. The Atkins theory is that excess carbohydrate intake prevents the body from burning fat efficiently. He maintained that drastically reducing the daily intake of carbohydrates will rebalance an individual's metabolism and force the body to burn reserves of stored fat for energy through a condition known as ketosis. Critics counter that a ketogenic diet lacks carbohydrates for fuel, which triggers the body's production of large amounts of ketone bodies, producing ketosis. Symptoms of ketosis include nausea, dehydration, constipation or diarrhea, and bad breath.

There are four phases to an Atkins diet plan: induction, ongoing weight loss, premaintenance, and maintenance. The first two weeks is called the induction, which severely limits carbohydrate intake to just 20 grams per day. Dietary intake recommendations from the U.S. Department of Agriculture (USDA) and the National Institutes of Health allow a daily intake of up to 300 grams of carbohydrates for a healthy adult male eating an average of 2,000 calories a day. During this induction, meals are planned around Atkins's acceptable foods, such as beef, pork, bacon, fish, chicken, eggs, and cheese. A typical breakfast might include a cheese omelet served with strips of bacon but no orange juice. In later phases, whole fruit, which is a healthy source of fiber, is introduced, but fruit juice is not recommended because it elevates blood sugar.

Depending upon food choices, a typical caloric intake during induction is between 1,800 and 2,400 calories. It is not necessary to count calories when following the Atkins program, since, according to Atkins representatives, there is ample food to allow dieters to feel satiated and to discourage cheating or overeating. According to the Atkins Center, the original edition of the diet did occasionally imply that individuals could eat unlimited portions of protein and fat. However, a spokesperson stressed that the newest edition of the book clears up this mixed message and anyone following the diet should eat these foods until satisfied but not stuffed.

Atkins in his book also encourages dieters on his plan to take vitamin supplements to correct any nutritional deficiencies they may encounter. The next phase is called the ongoing weight loss (OWL) phase, when weight loss is deliberately slowed in an effort to introduce more variety in foods. Now dieters can choose from more vegetables, as well as seeds and nuts, plus low-glycemic fruits such as strawberries and blueberries. According to the Atkins plan, as long as weight loss continues, individuals can gradually increase their carbohydrate intake. The first week they can eat 25 grams of carbohydrates per day; the second week, they move to 30 grams, and so forth until weight loss stalls. Premaintenance occurs when each dieter reaches his or her goal weight and begins to slowly consume increasing amounts of carbohydrates, but monitors that intake to prevent any weight gain. Finally at the maintenance stage dieters are allowed 60 to 90 grams of carbohydrates per day, which might include legumes and whole grains as well as other fruits.

By limiting carbohydrate intake, the Atkins diet eliminates many of the foods and food groups called for in the USDA MyPlate recommendations. Those include fruits, cereals, breads, grains, starches, dairy products, and starchy vegetables. However, in direct contrast to the Atkins plan, the USDA encourages people to eat sparingly foods high in fat like butter, oil, meat, poultry, fish, eggs, cheese, and cream and instead suggests that a healthy diet should include five servings of fruits and vegetables each day.

Critics of fad diets that eliminate several foods or food groups say studies show dieters following these plans have the worst failure rates over time. Nutritionists also criticize high-protein, high-fat, low-carbohydrate diets because they suggest the rapid initial weight loss is made primarily of water and lean muscle mass instead of fat. In response to critics, the Atkins Center says Dr. Atkins devoted a new chapter in the most recent edition of *Dr. Atkins' New Diet Revolution* to what they call repeated errors and misconceptions, such as the question of water-weight loss. Atkins explained that although early weight loss will be water, he identified research that shows water balance soon returns to normal and weight loss comes from burning body fat for energy.

On another front, the American Heart Association charges that high-protein diets are rich in saturated fat and can accelerate heart disease and dehydration. In rebuttal, the Atkins Center cites a growing body of scientific literature that demonstrates that a controlled carbohydrate eating plan, if followed correctly, promotes heart health. Atkins representatives point to the Harvard School of Public Health and its Nurses' Study. Those study results suggest that total fat consumed has no relation to heart disease risk; that monounsaturated fats like olive oil lower risk; and that saturated fats are little worse, if at all, than the pasta and other carbohydrates that the MyPlate suggests be eaten. According to the Atkins Center, the Nurses' Study research makes the case that consuming less fat and cholesterol actually resulted in more weight gain and higher blood cholesterol.

In his book, Atkins stated that people who follow his plan and then return to eating their prediet amount of carbohydrates would find the pounds returning.

The Atkins Lifetime Maintenance phase begins when dieters reach their goal weight. Then, depending upon age, gender, exercise level, and genetics a person can decide how much carbohydrate to consume, usually from 90 to 120 grams per day. For most people this means occasionally eating modest portions of foods like potatoes, other starchy vegetables, whole wheat pasta, and whole grain bread without regaining weight. The Atkins diet is not recommended for lacto-ovo vegetarians, since it would be difficult to find enough nonanimal sources of protein to eat. And vegans cannot follow this diet since a vegan diet is very high in carbohydrates, according to Atkins. Instead, the Atkins Center recommends that vegetarians with a serious weight problem give up vegetarianism, or at least include fish in their diet.

Atkins claimed that his eating plan causes no adverse side effects, yet many health care organizations disagree with his recommendations. Over the years, the American Medical Association (AMA), the American Dietetic Association, the American Society of Bariatric (controlled weight loss) Physicians, and the American Heart Association have criticized him. Critics also call attention to the fact that the Atkins diet has been in circulation for 30 years, but national obesity rates are continuing to rise at alarming rates. Atkins turned the tables on those critics by charging that Americans who follow the USDA-recommended daily allowances are becoming fatter and fatter. Plus, he called the rising incidence of Type 2 diabetes in this country part of the "twin epidemics of diabesity."

See also: Atkins, Robert C.; Food Guide Pyramid; Ketones/Ketosis; Ornish, Dean.

FURTHER READING

Atkins, Robert C. *Dr. Atkins' Health Revolution: How Complementary Medicine Can Extend Your Life.* New York: Houghton Mifflin Company, 1988.

Atkins, Robert C. *Dr. Atkins' New Diet Revolution.* New York: Avon Books, 1992.

Brody, Jane E. "Senate Nutrition Panel to Focus on Perils of Being Overweight." *New York Times*, April 13, 1973, 18.

Hellmich, Nanci. "Digesting the Facts on the 'New Atkins' Low-Carb Diet." *USA Today*, March 3, 2010. http://usatoday30.usatoday.com/news/health/weightloss/2010-03-03-atkins03_ST_N.htm.

Osterhout, Jacob. "New Atkins Diet Is Better than Ever: Flexibility in Veggies, Caffeine Revamps Popular Regimen." *New York Daily News*, March 23, 2010. http://www.nydailynews.com/life-style/health/new-atkins-diet-better-flexibilty-veggies-caffeine-revamps-popular-regimen-article-1.172516.

"Simplified Diet Book the New Atkins Made Easy Offers Easy Jumpstart Weight Loss for a New Year, New You," press release from Atkins Nutritionals, January 8, 2014. http://www.prnewswire.com/news-releases/simplified-diet-book-the-new-atkins-made-easy-offers-easy-jumpstart-weight-loss-for-a-new-year-new-you-239231071.html.

Taubes, Gary. "The Soft Science of Dietary Fat." *Science* 291, no. 5513 (March 30, 2001): 2536-45.

Underwood, Anne. "The Battle of Pork Rind Hill: When the Nation's Best-Selling Diet Gurus Squared Off in a Raucous Food Fight, One Thing Was Clear: There's No Easy Way to Shed That Ugly Flab. So Get Out the Jogging Shoes." *Newsweek*, March 6, 2000, 50.

Willett, Walter C. *Eat, Drink, and Be Healthy: The Harvard Medical School Guide to Healthy Eating.* New York: Simon and Schuster, 2001.

Baby Food Diet

The jars are filled with pureed meals like pears, bananas, carrots, peas, and sweet potatoes. They are designed to provide babies with the nutrition they need once they transition from milk to solid foods. For women intent on quickly losing weight, the idea is simple: substitute tiny jars of baby food for higher-calorie meals or snacks. Created by Tracy Anderson, often described as a health and fitness expert with clients including Madonna, Gwyneth Paltrow, Jennifer Aniston, Courtney Cox, and Reese Witherspoon, the idea is to prevent overeating and stay satisfied with the small servings in what amounts to a very low calorie diet.

There are lots of food choices for baby food dieters who can replace one meal each day with baby food or eat up to 14 jars each day and enjoy a meal of real, chewable food at dinner. In fact, the options are as endless as the varieties of baby food, but weight loss will depend on overall calories. That makes food choices extremely important since a jar of baby food can range anywhere from 20 to 100 calories. While the diet seems simple, there is still a need for dieters to carefully plan which jars of food they will eat throughout the day.

The advantages of eating baby food lies in the fact that infant food is free from most additives or preservatives. The jars are filled with pureed foods already low in fat, sugar, and salt, and baby food is considered nutritious, at least for babies. There are also organic brands and a great deal of variety. The drawbacks of this diet include lack of fiber, calcium, and many important vitamins at an adult level. Add that to lack of chewing and the absence of fiber, and dieters are left without a feeling of fullness and satisfaction.

Critics of the diet suggest that dieters who eat the pureed counterpart of an apple or carrot may feel hungrier by the end of the day and that feeling of hunger can easily lead to overeating or binging. Another problem pointed out by critics is that the baby food plan offers quick weight loss, which nutritionists predict will come back once the dieter stops, especially since poor eating habits are all but ignored.

While the specifics of the diet have never been published in a book, word of mouth and rumors have spread the details. Several celebrities have been linked to it in the tabloids but they have publicly denied eating baby food for weight loss. Even its reported founder Anderson has both advocated the diet as a way to eliminate toxicity and break bad habits and at other times has denied any connection to it. Anderson has also partnered with Paltrow and opened workout studios in California and New York that feature muscle strengthening and cardio dancing classes with her signature system of resistance bands that hang from the ceilings.

See also: Bulimia Nervosa; Vitamins.

FURTHER READING

Hartmann, Margaret. "Tracy Anderson's Singular Focus on Being Teeny Tiny." Jezebel. com. http://jezebel.com/5646226/tracy-andersons-singular-focus-on-being-teeny-tiny.

Pogrebin, Robin. "Building on the Abs of Madonna and Gwyneth." *The New York Times*, February 8, 2009, ST10.

Rubin, Courtney. "High Energy Is Part of the Package." *The New York Times*, December 20, 2012, ST8.

Zelman, Kathleen. "The Baby Food Diet: Review." *WebMD*. http://www.webmd.com/fiet/features/baby-food-diet-review.

Banana Diet

Successful weight loss comes from eating fewer calories than are burned and from eating in a way that can be maintained long term. Diets that follow arbitrary rules may seem like they work at first but people rarely keep the weight off and often gain back more than they lost when they return to their old eating habits.

The banana diet, which gained international notice in 2006, is a classic example of a "successful" diet that is more likely to hurt in the long term even though it may seem wildly successful in the short term. The diet gained international recognition when a Japanese celebrity reported losing some 37 pounds. Hitoshi Watanabe, a former printing company worker, had tried many diets in his efforts to lose weight. When his girlfriend, a pharmacist in training, suggested he eat as many bananas as he wanted for breakfast along with tepid water, then eat whatever he liked for the rest of the day. But she admonished him to stop eating by 8 P.M.

The story goes that for the next half year. Watanabe continued to lose weight, and then he married Sumiko and posted his success story online to instant acclaim. The idea behind the banana diet is that the starch found in the bananas is said to speed up fat burning as it boosts the body's metabolism. The Watanabes have become celebrities since they published their diet book and the diet became even more popular after a popular Japanese singer reported she lost 26 pounds in just six weeks. Following the release of the diet book, the banana craze swept Japan. During the height of its popularity, grocery stores and shops could not keep bananas on the shelves. Bananas are not the first diet fad to cause shortages in Japan. Other fads have included chili pepper, oolong tea, and boiled eggs.

Directions are simple; for breakfast eat bananas and drink room-temperature water. The bananas should not be cooked or frozen and only one other type of fruit can be substituted each meal. The dieter should eat a regular lunch and dinner and the diet recommends Japanese food, which includes lots of vegetables and plain rice. There is only one snack allowed each day and it should be eaten in the afternoon. Sweets are allowed only during the afternoon and dairy should be avoided. The diet also calls for reducing stress whenever possible, recording food in a diet journal and going to bed by midnight with no eating after 8 P.M.

Critics of the diet say any weight loss may come from the fiber in the bananas, which provides a feeling of fullness and from the other diet rule to stop eating by 8 P.M. Weight loss may also come simply from eating fewer calories. While bananas are a good source of carbohydrates and potassium, the sugars in bananas can adhere to teeth more than other fruits and can increase the risk of cavities. Plus, eating one food, no matter how healthy, can be a prelude to a binge and sooner or later dieters may overeat in response to the feeling of deprivation.

Bananas are not the only fruit to launch a diet fad. The grapefruit diet has been popular for many years because people want to believe the citrus fruit has special fat-burning properties. The dieting properties of citrus may also have added to the popularity of the lemonade diet, also known as the Master Cleanse, which calls for dieters to drink "lemonade" made from lemon juice, maple syrup, and cayenne pepper. The coconut diet is based on the idea that coconut oil metabolizes more efficiently than other fats but like any fat, eating too much of it will cause weight gain rather than weight loss.

See also: Coconut Diet; Grapefruit Diet; Master Cleanse Diet.

FURTHER READING

Chen, Joanne. "The New Japanese Fad Diet: Going Bananas." *Marie Claire,* January 15, 2009. http://www.marieclaire.com/health-fitness/news/japanese-banana-diet-fad.

Parker, Eloise. "Morning Banana Diet May Be the Cheapest, Easiest Ever. But Does It Work?" *New York Daily News,* October 22, 2008. http://www.nydailynews.com/lifestyle/health/morning-banana-diet-cheapest-easiest-work-article-1.304041.

Shaw, Daisy. "Top Banana." *Allure* 19, no. 11 (November 2009): 151.

Toyama, Michiko. "Japan Goes Bananas for a New Diet." *Time.com.* October 17, 2008. http://content.time.com/time/world/article/0,8599,1850454,00.html.

Barnard, Neal

Dr. Neal Barnard, a psychiatrist by training, has made a name for himself as a champion of the critical role diet plays in maintaining good health. He is a strong supporter of vegan and vegetarian diets. He is also known for his work advocating animal-rights issues, including the end of reliance on animals as experimental models for humans. Barnard founded the Physicians Committee for Responsible Medicine (PCRM) in 1985 with the stated mission of promoting preventive medicine through exercise and diet. He has written several books about nutrition and its impact on health. His latest title, *Power Foods for the Brain* (2013), looks at the impact that diet can have on conditions such as memory loss, stroke, and Alzheimer's. His 2011 book, *21-Day Weight Loss Kickstart: Boost Metabolism, Lower Cholesterol, and Dramatically Improve Your Health* provides a game plan for a three-week immersion into a plant-based diet.

As part of his dietary tips, Barnard divides different foods into those that release sugars slowly and those that release them quickly. He blames the American tendency to overeat on the rapid rise and fall of blood sugar and the signal to eat again that it produces. According to Barnard, the best choices for a slow, steady energy release are beans, vegetables, fruits, and certain grains and grain products like pasta, barley, bulgur, and whole grain breads. However, refined sugars found in food like white bread, white potatoes, and some sweeteners release their natural sugars more rapidly. He added that weight loss is often seen in people who consume large amounts of raw foods like melons, carrots, and apples, since these foods contain natural sugars but release them only gradually.

Barnard has been recommending a low-fat, high-fiber, vegetarian diet for many years. This opposition to eating meat and dairy is apparent in all of his books, including the earlier titles *The Get Healthy, Go Vegan Cookbook* (2010); *Dr. Neal Barnard's Program for Reversing Diabetes* (2007); *Turn Off the Fat Genes* (2001); *Foods That Fight Pain: Revolutionary New Strategies for Maximum Pain Relief* (1998); *Food for Life* (1994); and *Eat Right, Live Longer* (1997). Physical activity is another important part of Barnard's message. He recommends brisk walking for a half-hour three times per week as a way to burn calories and to counteract the fat-storage effect of lipoprotein lipase or LPL, which he believes plays a role in whether calories are stored as fat or lost as body heat. Barnard also suggests that exercise can help raise a naturally low metabolism and it can help control eating binges by taking the dieter away from temptation and replacing eating with activity.

Barnard's interest in healthy eating evolved over many years, according to a biography released by the PCRM. Before going to medical school he worked as an autopsy assistant, where he observed heart disease and other deadly effects of an unhealthy diet. Barnard received his medical degree in 1980 from the George Washington University School of Medicine and Health Sciences in Washington, D.C. As president of the PCRM, he currently works to promote preventive medicine and to address controversies in modern medicine as well as ethical issues in research.

See also: Atkins, Robert C.; McDougall Program; Ornish, Dean; Sears, Barry; The Zone.

FURTHER READING

Barnard, Neal. *Dr. Neal Barnard's Program for Reversing Diabetes*. Emmaus, PA: Rodale, 2007.

Barnard, Neal. *Eat Right, Live Longer*. New York: Harmony Books, 1995.

Barnard, Neal. *Power Foods for the Brain*. New York: Grand Central Life & Style, 2013.

Barnard, Neal. *Turn Off the Fat Genes: The Revolutionary Guide to Taking Charge of the Genes That Control Your Weight*. New York: Harmony Books, 2001.

Brandt, Peter. "Dr. Neal Barnard." *Salon.com*. March 12, 2001.

"Eat Right, Live Longer: Using the Natural Power of Foods to Age-Proof Your Body." *Publishers Weekly* 242, no. 33 (August 14, 1995): 80.

Kennedy, Barbara Ferguson. "Turn Off the Fat Genes and Control Your Weight." *Health Science* 24, no. 3 (Summer 2001): 16.

Belviq

Belviq (lorcaserin HCl) is one of two prescription weight-loss medications that was approved by the U.S. Food and Drug Administration (FDA) in 2012. Prior to that, the FDA had not approved a prescription weight-loss medication in 13 years. The other drug approved in 2013 is called Qsymia.

In order to get a prescription for Belviq, a patient must have an official designation as being obese, with a body mass index (BMI) of at least 30, or overweight, with a BMI of 27 or higher and have at least one weight-related medical condition, such as high cholesterol, high blood pressure, or Type 2 diabetes. According to the Belviq Web site, the results of two FDA clinical trials for patients who added Belviq to their diet and exercise showed that 47.1 percent of the people taking Belviq lost 5 percent or more of their body weight after one year of treatment, compared with 22.6 percent of those using diet and exercise along. Just more than 22 percent of those taking Belviq lost as much as 10 percent of their body weight after one year of treatment, compared to 8.7 percent who did so with just diet and exercise.

According to the FDA press release announcing its approval, "Belviq works by activating the serotonin 2C receptor in the brain. Activation of this receptor may help a person eat less and feel full after eating smaller amounts of food." The drug's maker, Arena Pharmaceuticals, is being required to conduct six post-approval studies, including a long-term study to look at any health risks to the cardiovascular system. This is the precaution required because other weight-loss drugs, fenfluramine and dexfenfluramine, had to be withdrawn from the market in 1997, after it was found they caused heart valve damage. The FDA wrote, "This effect is assumed to be related to activation of the serotonin 2B receptor on heart tissue. When used at the approved dose of 10 milligrams twice a day, Belviq does not appear to activate the serotonin 2B receptor."

See also: Body Mass Index; Qsymia.

FURTHER READING

"FDA Approves Belviq to Treat Some Overweight or Obese Adults." U.S. Food and
    Drug Administration press release. June 27, 2012. http://www.fda.gov/NewsEvents/
    Newsroom/PressAnnouncements/ucm309993.htm.
Grohol, J. "Qsymia and Belviq Drugs for Obesity, Weight Loss." *Psych Central* (2012). http://
    psychcentral.com/lib/qsymia-and-belviq-drugs-for-obesity-weight-loss/00013443.
Park, Alice. "Belviq: 5 Things You Need to Know about the New Weight-Loss Pill." *Time*,
    June 28, 2012. http://healthland.time.com/2012/06/28/belviq-5-things-you-need-to-
    know-about-the-new-diet-pill/.
"Weight-Loss Pill Belviq Is Now Available, but We Say Skip It." *Consumer Reports*, June 13,
    2013. http://www.consumerreports.org/cro/news/2013/06/weight-loss-pill-belviq-is-
    now-available-but-we-say-skip-it/index.htm.
www.belviq.com.

Beverly Hills Diet

The Beverly Hills Diet by Judy Mazel has been labeled among the most nutritionally outrageous of the fad diets. The original six-week plan, published in 1981, began with 10 days of eating only fruit in unlimited amounts. Pineapples, bananas, papayas, mangoes, watermelon, blueberries, strawberries, apples, prunes, raisins, and grapes were all to be eaten in a certain order on specific days. In *The New Beverly Hills Diet* (1996), Mazel said she fine-tuned the plan following 15 years of research and experimentation. The book calls this newest diet "a lifestyle eating plan" and says the changes help the plan "meet all standards set by the Senate Committee on Nutrition and Human Needs as recommended for a balanced weekly diet." A key change: the original diet did not include any animal protein until day 19, but the new diet allows foods from all food groups, including protein, in the first week.

Mazel tells readers they will see how successfully "the right combination of foods can trigger astonishing weight loss and weight maintenance." Those combinations start with day 1 when dieters can eat only pineapple, corn on the cob, and the author's favorite LTO Salad—iceberg lettuce, tomatoes, onion, cucumbers, and the Mazel dressing. Minor substitutions can be made, for example, when fruits like watermelon are not in season or readily available. Day 2 allows limitless strawberries, a half-pound of prunes, and baked potatoes. Mazel reminds dieters of the "Waiting Rule"; when going from one fruit to another, dieters must wait one hour, when moving from food group to food group, wait two hours.

Fruit portions are generous, from the half a pound of prunes on day 2 to five pounds of grapes on day 3. Nutritionists say five pounds of grapes would equal only 1,350 calories. But nearly all those calories come from sugar; only a small portion would provide any protein or dietary fat. Critics say that eating so little protein means dieters quickly become protein deficient and are likely to lose lean muscle tissue rather than fat. That happens because the human body has no storage organ for protein and when there isn't enough to meet daily needs, the protein in body tissues is broken down to fill in. However, when normal eating patterns return, so do the pounds in the form of increased body fat.

The theory behind the Beverly Hills Diet is simple, according to Mazel. She writes that when food isn't digested properly due to enzyme confusion, unused food turns to fat. Mazel says this confusion develops when proteins, carbohydrates, and fats are mixed together during meals. Calling this Conscious Combining, Mazel explains that the enzymes in each specific fruit along with the combination of foods eaten are critical to the success of her diet. "It isn't what you eat or how much you eat that makes you fat; it is when you eat and what you eat together!" Critics argue that all foods except for plain sugar or fat are a mixture of carbohydrates, protein, and fat and the body produces all the enzymes needed to digest them without complicated food-combining plans. According to Mazel, the principles of Conscious Combining go back thousands of years to China and ancient Persia. This theory has had its supporters more recently, too, such as the Somersizing diet promoted by actress Suzanne Somers.

Weight loss comes easily on the Beverly Hills Diet, since fruits are very low in calories, but the generous portions of fruit can also cause diarrhea and gastric problems. Even though the diet quickly became a best seller, critics were also quick to point out concerns with its basic lack of standard nutrition. In a report released in 1981 in the *Journal of the American Medical Association*, doctors called the Beverly Hills Diet "full of medical inaccuracies" and criticized Mazel's claim that undigested food causes weight gain. Doctors disagreed, saying the undigested food is not absorbed as fat but instead passes through the digestive tract to the large intestine where it is broken down by bacteria, forming gases, or eliminated as body waste. In an August 1981 *New York Times* interview, Dr. Philip White, director of the AMA's department of foods and nutrition, said, "There is very little in the book in the way of explanation of nutrition, biology or digestion that is in fact the truth." Health organizations say the real solution to being overweight is solved by eating a nutritionally balanced diet and combining that with increased exercise.

See also: Somers, Suzanne.

FURTHER READING

Brody, Jane E. "Another Entry in the Annals of Fad Diets." *New York Times*, June 3, 1981, C17.

Hevesi, Dennis. "Judy Mazel, Creator of Best-Selling 'Beverly Hills Diet,' Is Dead at 63." *New York Times*, October 27, 2007. http://www.nytimes.com/2007/10/27/health/nutrition/27mazel.html?_r=0.

Mazel, Judy. *The New Beverly Hills Diet*. Deer-field Beach, FL: Health Communications, Inc., 1996.

McDowell, Edwin. "Behind the Best Sellers." *New York Times*, August 23, 1981, 26.

Rhodes, Maura. "America's Top 6 Fad Diets." *Good Housekeeping*, July 1996, 100–103.

The Biggest Loser

The reality in the United States when it comes to obesity statistics is staggering. According to figures from the Centers from Disease Control and Prevention (CDC), more than 35 percent or 78 million adults and over 17 percent or more than 12 million children and teens are obese or overweight. The estimated medical costs of obesity in the United States is more than $147 billion each year and has driven incidence of diabetes, high blood pressure, and heart disease to record levels.

Reality television programming has paid attention to these facts and figures and in 2004 aired *The Biggest Loser*, a show that chronicles the attempts of severely obese individuals as they struggle to lose weight through a combination of intensive fitness training, nutritional instruction, and behavior modification that is supervised by a team of trainers, doctors, and dietitians. The cameras have been rolling ever since even though this reality show, like all the others, is not reality

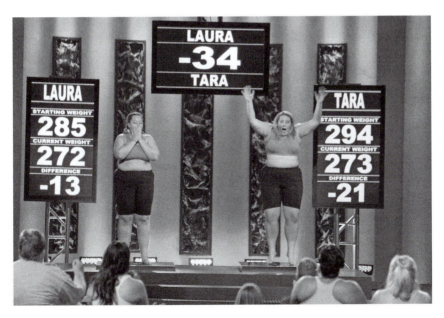

The *Biggest Loser* on NBC became a reality TV hit chronicling the attempts of severely obese individuals as they work to lose weight. (Trae Patton/NBC/Photofest)

and does not represent an acceptable weight-loss program that would be safe for overweight or obese people to follow.

Considered a ratings giant for NBC, the show sequesters the contestants at a private ranch in Southern California, and the winner, the one who loses the biggest percentage of weight, walks away with $250,000 and the potential for a new, thinner lease on life. Those players who drop the least weight each week are eliminated until a live finale where the final three contestants are pitted against each other. The payoff for the network is also measured in dollars with a reported $50 million in related consumer spending for tools and products inspired by the show and approved by their team of professionals.

Researchers studying the phenomenon of reality television report that viewers enjoy the show and may even find it inspirational, but it does little to create healthy behavior changes in those watching. Those same viewers also registered disapproval of how the contestants are presented in unflattering and sometimes humiliating ways. Still, people watch because the self-help movement is a big part of the U.S. culture. In a weight-loss reality show, the societal belief that all people should seek to achieve and maintain a specific body size and should continue to work on their failures is as American as apple pie. When surveyed, viewers suggested the show is ultimately about positive change in an individual's life and about being able to overcome any obstacles to achieve a goal.

Where *The Biggest Loser* may fail both audience members and participants is in the follow-up. Statistics show that maintaining weight loss can be more difficult than losing it in the first place. The American Council on Exercise (ACE) released a statement warning against setting unrealistic expectations for weight loss and recommended clients not to exceed a loss of more than one to two pounds per week. The organization also reinforced the fact that weight-loss maintenance is more difficult than weight loss and the key to success is the ability to make slow, permanent lifestyle changes. The ACE is a nonprofit fitness certification organization that provides continuing education to professionals and conducts science-based research on weight-loss and fitness products.

See also: Obesity.

FURTHER READING

"Adult Obesity Facts." The Centers for Disease Control and Prevention. http://www.cdc .gov/obesity/data/adult.html.

"American Council on Exercise Tackles the Reality of Reality TV Weight Loss." *Obesity, Fitness & Wellness Week*, April 6, 2013, 238.

"Biggest Loser Study Finds Modest Diet and Exercise Can Sustain Weight Loss." National Institutes of Health: News and Events. October 15, 2012. http://www.nih.gov/news/ health/oct2012/niddk-15.htm.

Odgen, Cynthia L., Margaret D. Carroll, Brian K. Kit, and Katherine M. Flegal. "Prevalence of Obesity in the United States, 2009–2010." U.S. Department of Health and

Human Services, NCHS Data Brief, No. 82 January 2012. http://www.cdc.gov/nchs/data/databriefs/db82.pdf.

Readdy, Tucker, and Vicki Ebbeck. "Weighing in on NBC's the Biggest Loser, Governmentality and Self-Concept on the Scale." *Research Quarterly for Exercise and Sport* 83, no. 4 (December 2012): 579(8).

Ross, Brooke. "Losing to Win: The Biggest Loser Tackles Teen Obesity." *Junior Scholastic/Current Events* 115, no. 13 (February 4, 2013): 5.

Body for Life

Body for Life: 12 Weeks to Mental and Physical Strength by Bill Phillips and Michael D'Orso, published in 1999 by HarperCollins, tells dieters they can change the shape and the fitness of their body in 12 weeks with reasonably hard work. Pound for pound, this is a very specific diet with precise exercise requirements and limited food choices, although the program has one "free" day per week where the dieter can eat anything he or she wants.

It is now also an Internet-based challenge program that includes online resources at the user's fingertips, as well as a chance to post "before" and "after" photos and compete for reimbursement of the supplement costs.

The eating plan warns users away from a majority of carbohydrates. Phillips and D'Orso say eating too many carbohydrates over a long period of time can create "insulin resistance." Instead they encourage a diet that features protein, which they suggest can provide stable energy levels and help control appetite. With its focus on protein foods, the *Body for Life* eating plan shares characteristics with several other diets like *The Zone* and Dr. *Atkins's New Diet Revolution*.

Critics of Atkins, the Zone, and other high-protein, low-carbohydrate diets contend that there is no reliable scientific evidence that insulin resistance develops from eating a reasonable amount of carbohydrates such as the serving recommendations in the MyPlate guide.

The diet instructs users to count "portions" of food rather than calories and includes a chart of some 18 authorized food choices that dieters can mix and match. Another important component in the *Body for Life* eating plan is the Myoplex drink mix, designed and distributed by Phillips's company, Experimental and Applied Sciences (EAS). The powdered formula contained a "precise blend of nutrients" that Phillips designed to help dieters maintain proper health and recover quickly from strenuous workouts. He writes, "Without the advantage it offers, I don't believe I would have been able to stick with this nutrition method," something critics say is a problem with diets that rely heavily on special foods or shakes. Statistics show that a large percentage of dieters who use prepackaged foods or shakes fail to learn to make healthy food selections or to eat sensible meals and are often at the greatest risk of regaining weight after the program ends. Phillips has since sold his interest in EAS and *Body for Life*. And the

Body for Life offerings have expanded to include ready-to-drink Myoplex products, nutrition bars, protein powders, and other supplements, with formulas based on the goals of managing weight, building performance and strength, and general fitness.

For each meal, dieters choose 1 of the 18 protein options along with something from the carbohydrate column. A vegetable serving is recommended for two of the daily meals. Dieters eat a grand total of six small meals per day, spread out to reduce feelings of hunger and fatigue. The book includes suggestions for six weeks' worth of meals, which dieters can then repeat again during the 12-week period. Nutritionists agree that more frequent, small meals and snacks can help dieters maintain a steady energy level and avoid intense feelings of hunger that can trigger unhealthy eating.

The book lists sample menus such as the Wednesday meals that start with a breakfast of one vanilla Myoplex shake made with half a fresh orange and three ice cubes. Midmorning, the meal is a portion of cottage cheese along with a portion of fat-free, sugar-free yogurt and two cups of water. Lunch is a skinless chicken breast with freshly squeezed lemon and lime juice plus a plain potato served with fresh carrots and a tall glass of iced tea. Midafternoon calls for another Myoplex shake. Dinner includes a serving each of steak and brown rice. And the final meal that day is a chocolate Myoplex shake blended together with one serving of fat-free, sugar-free hot cocoa mix and three ice cubes.

Phillips and D'Orso then add a strenuous exercise program, something critics consider to be a plus, since many other diets fail to emphasize the importance of physical exercise. *Body for Life* offers a number of success stories along with before and after pictures on the dust jacket in an effort to prove that the program works. What is lacking, critics say, is any mention of long-term weight-loss success or any nutritional studies that support the diet.

Phillips defends his 20-minute aerobics solution and high-point technique as a way to create a more metabolically efficient body. He charts a six-day exercise program, with aerobics three times a week and intense weight-training workouts three days a week, on alternate days. What sets this plan apart is the intensity of the sets at the end of each exercise designed to compound the training effect on each muscle group. The same is true for the cardiovascular exercise, which follows a schedule of increasing and decreasing intensity. This up and down, according to Phillips, allows dieters to burn more calories in less time.

He also suggests that dieters can keep metabolism levels from slowing by setting aside one free day each week—free of exercise and diet restrictions. The free day stems from Phillips's theory that eating regularly one day every week tricks the body into holding metabolism levels steady rather than letting them slow down in response to perceived starvation. The weightlifting program is simple; anyone who has spent time in a gym will immediately be comfortable following Phillips's directions. As founder and executive editor of *Muscle Media*, a strength-training magazine, Phillips knows his way around exercise equipment.

With a detailed 12-week training schedule and daily progress reports, users can easily follow the exercise script and chart their progress in the back of the book. Phillips predicts people can lose up to 25 pounds of body fat in the 12-week program but cautions that losing more than 2 pounds per week could signal the loss of muscle tissue as well. Critics say that in the short term any diet will cause a weight loss but because of its many restrictions, this diet and other low-carbohydrate, high-protein eating plans are difficult to follow for long periods. The fact remains that carbohydrates help store fluid in the body, so when a dieter restricts carbohydrates the body releases some of those fluids. And when dieters resume eating carbohydrates they can expect a quick weight gain of from 5 to 10 pounds as the lost fluid returns.

See also: Atkins Nutritional Approach; Food Guide Pyramid; MyPlate; The Zone.

FURTHER READING

Phillips, Bill, and Michael D'Orso. *Body for Life: 12 Weeks to Mental and Physical Strength.* New York: HarperCollins, 1999.
www.bodyforlife.com.
www.eas.com.

Body Mass Index

Researchers developed the body mass index (BMI) to help people gauge a healthy weight range for their age. Originally, there was only a BMI calculator for adults, but in recent years, a calculator for children and teens has been added. The child and teen calculator accounts for variables such as age, height, and gender and measures weight in 1/4 pound increments, so it would be easiest for a user to use an online calculator, such as this one offered by the Centers for Disease Control and Prevention (CDC) at http://apps.nccd.cdc.gov/dnpabmi/.

While there are also numerous BMI calculators for adults online, the formula to calculate it is this:

#1. Multiply your weight in pounds by 703.
#2. Multiply your height in inches by your height in inches.*

Divide answer #1 by answer #2.
* If you're 5'5", your height in inches would be 65 inches so the 65 × 65 would equal 4,225.

People who have a BMI of 30 or higher, or those who are considered overweight and have two or more other health risk factors, should know that even a small weight loss could help lower their risk of developing diseases associated with obesity.

Table B.1   BMI Weight Indicator

If Your BMI Is	Your Weight Status Is
Below 18.5	Underweight
18.5–24.9	Normal
25–29.9	Overweight
30 and above	Obese

See also: Belviq; Obesity.

FURTHER READING

"Healthy Weight—It's Not a Diet, It's a Lifestyle." Centers for Disease Control and Prevention. http://www.cdc.gov/healthyweight/assessing/bmi/index.html.

Bulimia Nervosa

Bulimia nervosa is an eating disorder characterized by a binge-and-purge eating pattern. Either by forcing herself to vomit, taking laxatives or diuretics, or giving herself enemas, the bulimic is purging to rid herself of the food she ate. There is also a nonpurging form of bulimia, characterized by some other method of keeping the weight off, such as compulsive exercising or fasting.

Binges and purges can range from once or twice a week to several times a day. What is visible to family and friends, however, may only be strident dieting. Symptomatic of the disorder is the excessive amount of food being eaten. Someone with bulimia will eat more food and more frequently than most people. Often, while eating, the person seems to lack control or feels as if he or she can't stop eating. For example, normal food intake for women and teens is between 2,000 and 3,000 calories per day. But bulimic binges often consume more than that in a span of less than two hours. Some people with the disorder have reported consuming up to 20,000 calories in binges lasting up to eight hours.

Rapidly purging food, either through abuse of laxatives, enemas, and diuretics, or induced vomiting, upsets the body's balance of chemicals, including sodium and potassium. The result is often fatigue, irregular heartbeat, thinner bones, and seizures. Repeated vomiting can also damage the stomach and esophagus and can erode tooth enamel. It can also result in skin rashes and broken blood vessels in the face.

Bulimia typically begins during adolescence and can continue for years undetected by others. The longer someone with an eating disorder waits to seek help, the more ingrained his or her eating habits become and the more difficult the recovery.

See also: Anorexia Nervosa; Eating Disorders.

FURTHER READING

Firth, Shannon. "Study: Bulimics 4 Times Likely to Get Diabetes." *U.S. News & World Report,* January 30, 2014. http://www.usnews.com/news/articles/2014/01/30/study-bulimics-4-times-more-likely-to-get-diabetes.

Mills, Tara. "Eating Disorders: Sufferers Unaware Condition Can Be 'Fatal.'" *BBC.com,* February 18, 2014. http://www.bbc.com/news/uk-northern-ireland-26227243.

Cabbage Soup Diet

The cabbage soup diet is a quick weight-loss plan that has circulated like a chain letter across the United States for decades via photocopiers, fax machines, and word of mouth. The diet promises a 17-pound weight loss in one week and requires followers to adhere to a rigid eating schedule to achieve that goal. Many versions of this anonymously created diet have surfaced over the years. The basic soup recipe has also been attributed to many sources, including Raymond Dietz, a doctor who proposed it to his patients in the 1930s. J. T. Cooper published the soup recipe in the 1960s as *Dr. Cooper's Super Soup* in *The Doctors' Clinic 30 Program.* In 1975, another version of the soup and eating plan appeared in the *Oriental Seven Day Quick Weight-Off Diet,* by the one-name author Norvell. Both titles were re-released by the publishers in 1996. The diet has also been called "the Skinny," and the "Basic Fat Burning Soup Diet."

The recipe is simple and consists of one head of cabbage, six large onions, two green peppers, one 28-ounce can of tomatoes, one bunch of celery, one packet of onion soup mix, and water. The cook is instructed to chop the vegetables, boil all the ingredients rapidly for 10 minutes, and then simmer. For one week, dieters eat all the soup they want plus a specified food, mostly in unlimited amounts. Meals for Day 1 include soup and any fruit except bananas; Day 2 is soup and vegetables, including a baked potato with butter for dinner. Potatoes are off-limits on the other six days. Day 3 is soup, fruits, and vegetables; Day 4 allows up to eight bananas and skim milk plus soup; Day 5 is soup and six tomatoes plus 20 ounces of beef, chicken, or fish; Day 6 is the same and vegetables are not limited to tomatoes; and Day 7 is soup, brown rice, unsweetened fruit juice, and vegetables.

Nutrition experts call the diet an unbalanced, unrealistic plan, and say pounds shed are mostly water weight. Critics acknowledge that the soup is filling, but add that eating two bowls of any low-carbohydrate soup will act as an appetite suppressant. Cabbage soup dieters complain of gas, nausea, and fatigue after a few days on this diet, but nutritionists say the one-week duration isn't long enough for most people to suffer any serious health problems. But people on this plan can expect to suffer from extreme boredom and a return of lost pounds once they resume their normal eating patterns.

See also: Carbohydrates; Dietary Fat; Yo-Yo Dieting.

FURTHER READING

Cooper, Sharon, and J. T. Cooper. *The Doctor's Clinic 30 Program*. Erie, PA: Green Tree Press, 1996.

Norvell. *The Oriental Seven Day Quick Weight-Off Diet*. West Nyack, NY: Parker Publishing Co., 1996.

Rubin, Rita, and Leonard Wiener. "A Bad Diet with Phony Credentials." *U.S. News & World Report*, June 24, 1996, 69.

Weinraub, Judith. "A Closer Look into the Cabbage Soup Diet." *Washington Post*, March 6, 1996, E5.

Yazigi, Monique P. "The Cabbage-Soup Diet That Came from Nowhere." *New York Times*, March 20, 1996, C3.

Caffeine

Caffeine is a natural substance found in the leaves, seeds, or fruits of over 63 plant species worldwide and is part of a group of compounds known as methylxanthines. The most commonly known sources of caffeine are coffee and cocoa beans, kola nuts, and tea leaves. Diets high in sodium and caffeine negatively affect calcium levels because calcium is lost through urine.

See also: Calcium; Osteoporosis.

Calcium

Calcium is a mineral that contributes to strong bones and teeth. It's found naturally in dairy products, green leafy vegetables, and soy products, including tofu. Calcium requirements are highest for adolescents, whose bones are growing rapidly, and pregnant and lactating women. In the winter of 2011, the National Institutes of Health included the updated calcium requirement for various life stages. Young people, aged 14 to 18, should consume 1,300 mg/day of calcium. After age 19, all the way to age 51 when women become at risk for osteoporosis—a weakening of the bones—the Recommended Dietary Allowance is 1,000 mg/day for men and women. Even for women over the age of 19, who are pregnant or lactating, 1,000 mg/day remains the recommended amount.

The NIH also recommends exercise as an important component in achieving maximal peak bone mass and stresses that fat-reduced dairy products such as skim milk are just as nutritious for older children.

So how do you get enough calcium? Consuming four to five glasses of low-fat milk per day is one way. Other milk products are also good sources of calcium. Green leafy vegetables, such as kale, collards, beets, and turnip tops, are also natural sources of calcium, so are tofu, dried peas and beans, the soft bones of canned fish, and calcium-fortified orange juice. Many people find they can get enough calcium through a healthy diet, but calcium supplements do exist for those who cannot or who are at particularly high risk for osteoporosis. Read the label of a calcium supplement carefully to find the amount of "elemental" calcium. There are different kinds of calcium supplements—including calcium citrate (which is generally the most easily absorbed), calcium carbonate, and calcium phosphate—that include other elements such as vitamin D, which help with absorption.

Overdoses of calcium can interfere with the absorption of other nutrients such as zinc and iron.

Bone mass is also affected by how you use your body. Weight-bearing exercise, such as dancing and running, can increase bone mass and strength. Unhealthy activities, such as smoking, alcohol use, and a poor diet, contribute to losing bone mass. Diets high in sodium and caffeine negatively affect calcium levels because calcium is lost through urine.

See also: Caffeine; Exercise; Osteoporosis.

FURTHER READING

"New Recommended Daily Amounts of Calcium and Vitamin D." *NIH MedLine Plus,* Winter 2011. http://www.nlm.nih.gov/medlineplus/magazine/issues/winter11/articles/winter11pg12.html.

Calorad

Calorad is a weight-loss product, advertised as a collagen protein supplement. According to the manufacturer, Essentially Yours Industries, dieters who take one tablespoon of Calorad with eight ounces of water just before bed and don't eat or drink anything but water for three hours before taking the supplement will lose excess fat and toxins naturally and will see an increase in lean body mass.

Collagen hydrolysat, the main ingredient listed on the label, is the scientific name for gelatin. Other ingredients in Calorad include aloe vera, which has a laxative effect when taken orally; glycerin, a sugar alcohol traditionally used as a mild sweetener; and potassium sorbate and methyl paraben, preservatives to keep the collagen from spoiling. Critics like the National Council against Health Fraud say that the manufacturer's claims that Calorad helps build lean muscle mass and burn more calories during sleep are inaccurate. They suggest that weight loss associated with Calorad may stem from the fact that users do not eat for three hours before bed. In many adults, this would amount to a reduced intake of daily calories, resulting in weight loss.

Critics say studies show human muscle tissue does not spontaneously generate with increased protein consumption; instead, muscle mass is increased through various types of resistance training. Calorad packaging and advertising claims that users can increase muscle mass without exercise. Critics also cite the lack of peer-reviewed research published to support the scientific claims of the product. The manufacturer points to anecdotal testimonials as proof of Calorad's effectiveness.

See also: Body Mass Index; Calories.

FURTHER READING

Czarnecki, Joanne, and Shelley Drozd. "Rating the Fat-Fighters." *Men's Health,* January 1999, 60.

Calories

A calorie is a measure of heat needed to raise the temperature of 1 kilogram of water by 1 degree Celsius. Since food "stokes the furnace" of our bodies, foods have assigned calorie values. The number of calories in a food can be found on the Nutrition Facts label on any packaged food. Realize, however, that these are calories per serving. If the nutrition label claims the package has two servings—and you've eaten it all—you've eaten double the calories that the label says.

Fat and alcohol are high in calories. Foods high in both sugars and fat contain many calories but often are low in vitamins, minerals, or fiber. There are numerous calorie counters readily available—online and often in cookbooks. If you reduce your caloric intake, you'll lose weight. If you increase the amount of calories you consume, you'll gain weight. A pound equals 3,500 calories. So to lose a pound in, say, a week, you'll either have to eat 3,500 calories less or burn off 3,500 calories in exercise, or some combination of the two.

It is possible to estimate about how many calories per day you need to eat to maintain your body weight. Once you use the following formula to calculate that number, you can tweak it. If you want to lose weight, cut the calories or increase your level of activity.

Moderately active males should multiply their weight in pounds by 15. For example, if you weigh 170 pounds, you need about 2,500 calories per day. Moderately active females should multiply their weight by 12. A 130-pound female needs about 1,560 calories per day.

However, if you are not regularly active, you'll need to use a different formula because the number of calories needed per day decreases as the level of activity decreases. In other words, if you burn fewer calories a day, you'll need

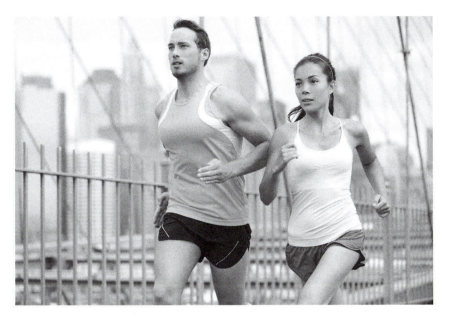

Running burns calories and builds muscles. Plus, it's easy to do just about anywhere. (Martinmark/Dreamstime)

fewer of them to maintain your weight. Relatively inactive men should multiply their weight in pounds by 13 and women in that category should multiply their weight by 10. So that a 170-pound inactive man needs only 2,210 calories and a 130-pound inactive woman needs only 1,300 calories to maintain body weight.

CALORIES FROM FAT

Numerous health and government authorities, including the U.S. Surgeon General, the National Academy of Sciences, the American Heart Association, and the American Dietetic Association, recommend reducing dietary fat to 30 percent or less of total calories. However, that doesn't mean you have to give up all high-fat food products. For example, peanut butter with sugar added has 200 calories in a two-tablespoon serving. Of those, 140 calories are from fat— 70 percent. Add that peanut butter to two slices of whole wheat bread, which have 120 calories and 20 calories from fat, and the equation is different: now the fat is down to about 48 percent. It's still higher than the recommendation, but by adding a glass of skim milk and an apple, you start to bring it down to a healthy level.

Keep in mind that the information on nutrition labels is based on a 2,000-calorie-per-day diet. So if your average caloric intake is lower, realize that the overall percentage of fat is higher than what's listed on the label. For example, back to the peanut butter with its 16 grams of total fat and 3 grams of saturated fat. The total fat is 25 percent of the daily value and the saturated fat is 15 percent of the daily value—based on a 2,000-calorie diet, which calls for less than 65 grams of total fat and less than 20 grams of saturated fat per day. Now let's say you're inactive and need only 1,300 calories per day to maintain your body weight. You'd need to cut your overall dietary fat intake accordingly.

In general, restoring physical activity to our daily routines is critical. According to surveys conducted in 1999–2000 and 2009–2010, reported daily caloric intakes remained high from 2,239 kcal (calories) to 2,455 kcal in men and from 1,534 kcal to 1,646 kcal in women.

Eating more frequently is encouraged by numerous environmental changes: a greater variety of foods, some with higher caloric content; the growth of the fast-food industry; the increased numbers and marketing of snack foods; and a growing tendency to socialize with food and drink. At the same time, there are fewer opportunities in daily life to burn calories: children watch more television daily; many schools have done away with or cut back on physical education; many neighborhoods lack sidewalks for safe walking; the workplace has become increasingly automated; household chores are assisted by labor-saving machinery; and walking and cycling have been replaced by automobile travel for all but the shortest distances.

Consider this: the American Institute for Cancer Research says Americans' snack-food intake has tripled since the 1980s. An average American now consumes 16 to 20 pounds of snack food, or 40,000 snack calories, a year.

CALORIES BURNED DURING EXERCISE

Exercise burns calories. For example, walking briskly can burn off about 100 calories per mile. Bicycling for half an hour at nearly 10 mph will burn about 195 calories. The specific number is dependent on the person's weight and the intensity of the activity. A variety of interactive exercise counters, available on the Internet, allow you to plug in your weight and age, and change variables such as the length of time and intensity of the activity. For someone working to lose weight, the combination of exercise and a healthy diet works more effectively than either method by itself. Eat less and you'll lose weight; exercise more and you'll lose weight and tone muscles and build aerobic endurance. Do both and they'll complement each other.

The more you weigh, the more calories you'll burn. The reason is that your heart has to pump harder to get the blood to the different parts of your body. So a 130-pound person doing medium-intensity aerobic dancing for 30 minutes will burn about 174 calories in that time. A 150-pound person will burn about 201 calories in the same amount of time.

Today, there are smartphone apps and Web-based calculators that help determine how many calories you can burn doing different activities.

Let's say you eat 2,000 calories worth of food. But your physical activity uses only 1,500 of these. The extra calories are stored in your body—as fat. When you exercise, your body uses fuel, which comes from one of two forms: stored carbohydrates called glycogen or stored body fat. Stored body fat is found in fat cells and is also stored as small droplets in the muscles.

Most activities use both carbohydrates and fat for fuel. Lower-intensity workouts, such as walking, use fat as the primary fuel. As the workout intensifies, the fuel reserves come increasingly from carbohydrates. But that doesn't mean that walking burns more fat than running. When the carbohydrate or glycogen source runs low, the body releases fats for fuels. Also, a higher-intensity workout, such as running, continues to burn fat even after the physical activity is over. As the body works to restore glycogen, it continues to use fat to do so. And because higher-intensity workouts burn more calories overall, even though the mix of carbohydrates and fats may be different, you're still burning more fat in the workout.

See also: Aerobic Activity; Anaerobic Activity.

FURTHER READING

Choi, Candice. "Dieters Move Past Calories, Food Makers Follow." *The Washington Post,* April 10, 2014. http://www.washingtonpost.com/business/dieters-move-past-calories-food-makers-follow/2014/04/10/cc064404-c0bc-11e3-9ee7-02c1e10a03f0_story.html.
Kaplan, Karen. "Bright Light—Early and Often—Linked to Lower BMI." *Los Angeles Times,* April 2, 2014. http://www.latimes.com/science/sciencenow/la-sci-sn-early-morning-light-exposure-weight-gain-20140402,0,5265290.story.

Carbohydrate Addict's Diet

The husband and wife team of Rachael F. Heller and Richard F. Heller, who hold PhD in psychology and biology, respectively, developed the Carbohydrate Addict's Diet. It is a low-carbohydrate diet based on the theory that as many as 75 percent of people who are overweight have a carbohydrate addiction. On their Web site, such an addiction is defined as having "a compelling hunger, craving, or desire for carbohydrate-rich foods; an escalating, recurring need or drive for starches, snack foods, junk food, or sweets."

The body counteracts carbohydrate consumption by releasing the hormone insulin. The Hellers say that people with carbohydrate addictions have a hormonal imbalance. The body releases too much insulin when they eat carbohydrates. As a result, they feel hungry again sooner as the excess insulin signals their body to take in more food. Insulin also signals the body to store food energy as fat.

That's why carbohydrate addicts, who may be eating low-fat meals, still gain weight. The diet plan outlined in the *Carbohydrate Addict's Diet* consists of two carbohydrate-restricted meals and one "reward meal" in which anything can be eaten up to one hour following a high-protein meal.

The Web site offers a quiz to help determine if you're a "carbohydrate addict." It asks questions about eating habits: do you eat even though you're not really hungry or if you finish a meal and don't feel satisfied? If so, you may be a carbohydrate addict. Is it hard for you to resist snacking at night and is it difficult to stop snacking once you've started? If so, you may also be a carb addict.

The Hellers, who are carbohydrate addicts themselves, say this diet plan has done much to both help them lose weight and maintain weight loss. They followed up on the *Carbohydrate Addict's Diet* with other books, among them, *The Carbohydrate Addict's Program for Success* and *The Carbohydrate Addict's Gram Counter.*

Are Americans eating too many carbohydrates? Carbohydrate consumption has increased by 50 pounds per person per year over the past decade. As people have turned away from high-fat foods, carbohydrates may have become a greater share of most Americans' diets.

An article in the *Journal of the American Dietetic Association* suggested that carbohydrates became the dieter's taboo "because the low-fat diets of the 1980s and 1990s failed consumers who mistakenly believed that consumption of low-fat products was license to eat voraciously while paying no mind to the amount of sugar and energy being consumed. Many people find irresistible the basis of low-carbohydrate diets: eating as much protein as desired—including steaks, eggs, and other fatty foods that they had previously been told by media reports and medical practitioners to shun—and still losing weight, so long as intake of carbohydrates is strictly limited."

Yet many critics of these restrictive carbohydrate plans say severely limiting carbohydrates is not good either. All high-protein, low-carbohydrate plans put the dieter at risk of loss of vitamin B, calcium, and potassium, resulting from lack of carbohydrates in the diet, and risk of coronary heart disease from eating more high-protein foods that are also high in fat.

While a low-carbohydrate diet will help a dieter lose weight initially, critics say the dieter will feel lethargic. Because there are so few carbohydrates to burn as energy, the body begins to burn lean muscle mass for energy. The Physicians Committee for Responsible Medicine rated the *Carbohydrate Addict's Program* as unsafe.

See also: Carbohydrates; Insulin.

FURTHER READING

Davis, Caroline, and Carter, Jacqueline. "Compulsive Overeating as an Addiction Disorder. A Review of Theory and Evidence." *Appetite* 53, no.1 (August 2009): 1–8.

Gotthardt, Melissa Meyers. "The New Low-Carb Diet Craze." *Cosmopolitan*, February 2000, 148.

Heller, Rachael F., and Richard F. Heller. *Carbohydrate Addicted Kids: Help Your Child or Teen Break Free of Junk Food or Sugar Cravings for Life*. New York: HarperCollins, 1998.

Heller, Rachael F., and Richard F. Heller. *The Carbohydrate Addict's Cookbook*. Hoboken, NJ: John Wiley & Sons, 2000.

Heller, Rachael F., and Richard F. Heller. *The Carbohydrate Addict's Diet: The Lifelong Solution to Yo-Yo Dieting*. New York: New American Library, 1999.

Heller, Rachael F., and Richard F. Heller. *The Carbohydrate Addict's Program for Success*. New York: Plume, 1993.

Physicians Committee for Responsible Medicine press release: "Doctors Rate Popular Diet Books." January 9, 2001.

Stein, Joel. "The Low-Carb Diet Craze." *Time*, November 1, 1999, 71–79.

Stein, Karen. "High Protein, Low-Carbohydrate Diets: Do They Work?" *Journal of the American Dietetic Association* 100, no. 7 (July 2000): 760.

Turner, Richard, and Joan Raymond. "The Trendy Diet That Sizzles: A Counterintuitive Program Reaches Critical Mass." *Newsweek International*, September 13, 1999, 62.

Wilgoren, Jodi. "Low-Carb Diet: Lose the Bun, Not the Burger." *New York Times*, January 11, 2000, D7. www.carbohydrateaddict.com.

Carbohydrates

Carbohydrates provide energy for the brain, central nervous system, and muscle cells. They are found largely in sugars, fruits, vegetables, and cereals and grains. Meats generally have no carbohydrates. Carbohydrates can be classified as simple, such as sugars, or complex, such as breads and pastas, which are broken down into sugars in the body. Someone with a 2,000-calorie-per-day diet should limit carbohydrates to 300 grams. Someone with a 2,500-calorie-per-day diet can consume up to 375 grams of carbohydrates. A medium-baked potato with skin has 51 grams of carbohydrates. An apple has about 21 grams of carbohydrates, a tablespoon of sugar has 12 grams, and a slice of pie can pack 60 or more grams of carbohydrates.

All carbohydrates eventually break down into sugars in your body. The difference is that complex carbohydrates do so more gradually, providing energy over a longer period of time. And complex carbohydrates also contain other nutrients, whereas simple sugars generally do not. That's particularly true of "empty" calories, such as soft drinks and candy.

Consuming carbohydrates raises insulin, which then lowers blood sugar levels. That, in turn, can leave the dieter feeling hungry or even jittery. The need for carbohydrates is one of the key differentiating points in diet plans. Many diet plans seem to fall either under the low-fat, high-carb category or the low-carb, high-protein diets, such as Atkins.

See also: Calories; Nutrition Facts Label.

FURTHER READING

"Carbohydrates: How Carbs Fit into a Healthy Diet." Mayo Clinic. http://www.mayoclinic
    .org/healthy-living/nutrition-and-healthy-eating/in-depth/carbohydrates/art-
    20045705.
Jameson, Marni. "A Reversal on Carbs." *Los Angeles Times*, December 20, 2010. http://
    articles.latimes.com/2010/dec/20/health/la-he-carbs-20101220.
Taubes, Gary. "What Really Makes Us Fat." *The New York Times*, June 30, 2012. http://
    www.nytimes.com/2012/07/01/opinion/sunday/what-really-makes-us-fat.html?_r=0.

Celebrity Doctors

Need advice on nutrition? Not sure about which vitamins to take? Want to know which is the best diet to lose those last 10 pounds? Ask the doctor, the one that makes house calls via the Internet, television, on Facebook or Twitter, the celebrity doctor. American society has revered the family physician for decades, and now this growing medical group with their fame and name recognition is even more trusted to help with diet, health, and medical concerns.

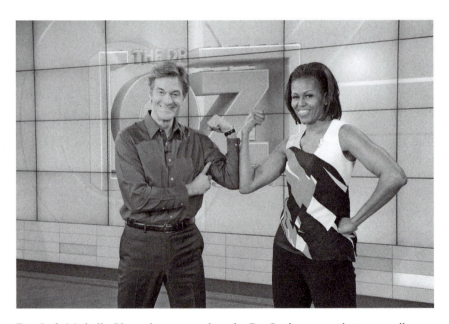

First Lady Michelle Obama has appeared on the *Dr. Oz* show several times to talk about her efforts to encourage physical activity and healthy eating. (PRNewsFoto/ The Dr. Oz Show/AP Images)

In fact, according to research, the impact of social media on bringing these medical professionals into American homes is the reason for the difference between celebrity doctors of the past and those of today. Today's celebrity docs are on TV every day, they have Facebook fan pages, they write best-selling books, and they promote their own products on their Web sites while they tweet or blog about their latest discovery. No more than 20 years ago celebrity doctors reached consumers through their books and the occasional television interview. It's no wonder they are stars, appearing everywhere and fueling the growing appetite in the United States for immediate diet and health information.

Another factor for their success can be attributed to the rising cost of medicine, which makes a trip to the doctor a luxury for some Americans. When that cost is combined with less access to specialists, it stands to reason more consumers would start looking for advice and a medical diagnosis on the computer or from a television show. With movie star–good looks, impressive credentials, and larger-than-life personalities, these medical stars use the exposure to reach more people, which can perpetuate the cycle.

Unfortunately, getting medical advice from a celebrity is a prescription for problems. So who are these medical stars? Turn on the television for a session with Dr. Mehmet Oz or Dr. Phil McGraw. Browse through magazines and books to find Dr. Andrew Weil, Dr. Arthur, Agatston of South Beach Diet fame, or the late Robert Atkins of the Atkins Diet, Deepak Chopra called the "poet prophet of alternative medicine," or Dr. Joel Fuhrman and his Nutrient Density program.

Consumers looking for answers should check the credibility of any celebrity who has a "doctor" in his or her title. If there is a discussion of something on a show or on the Internet that looks interesting or of value, the best advice is to check with a credible source. Most importantly, seek the advice of a trusted personal physician before taking any supplement or over-the-counter medication. A second opinion in this situation can be the difference between good or bad decisions.

See also: Atkins Nutritional Approach; South Beach Diet.

FURTHER READING

Jameson, Marni. "The Cult of Celebrity Doctors." *The Los Angeles Times,* June 14, 2010. http://articles.latimes.com/2010/jun/14/health/la-he-celeb-docs-20100614.

LaPook, Jon. "VIPs and Lousy Healthcare: Poor Celebrity Care May Provide Lessons for Everyone." *Huffington Post Healthy Living,* July 9, 2009. http://www.huffingtonpost.com.

McEvoy, Victoria. "Celebrity Doctors, Beware." *CNN Opinion,* November 8, 2011. http://www.cnn.com/2011/11/08/opinion/mcevoy-murray-verdict/.

Celebrity Endorsements

What do the actress Lynn Redgrave, former NBA basketball star Charles Barkley, actress and writer Carrie Fisher, and 1994 Playmate of the Year Jenny McCarthy have in common? At one time or another, they have all been a spokesperson for a weight-loss company.

Redgrave, the noted English actress, was the first celebrity spokesperson for Weight Watchers beginning in 1984. The commercials featured Redgrave and the signature line for the ads, "This Is Living." She later wrote a book with the same title that featured some Weight Watcher recipes. Other prominent people who promoted Weight Watchers included Sarah Ferguson, the Duchess of York, Playmate Jenny McCarthy, NBA great Charles Barkley, Grammy-winning singer Jennifer Hudson, and singer and actress Jessica Simpson.

Many celebrities have endorsed other well-known weight-loss plans, such as Jenny Craig and Nutrisystem. Jenny Craig has featured Fisher as well as actress Kirstie Alley, actor Jason Alexander of Seinfeld fame, actress Valerie Bertinelli, and singer Mariah Carey. Nutrisystem continues to use spokesperson Marie Osmond and actress Melissa Joan Hart, and has also worked with football quarterback Dan Marino and singer Janet Jackson.

Hiring a celebrity is a risk for the companies since celebrities are people, too. Sometimes they succeed at losing weight, and other times they fail or regain the weight, as in the case of Kirstie Alley. However, many companies think it is worth the risk since celebrities can also create a greater awareness of their brand. They can reach their already-developed fan base, especially in this age of social media. The use of stars to endorse any kind of product is nothing new and dates back to stage actress Lillie Langtry who allowed her name and likeness to appear on packages of Pears Soap beginning in the late 1800s.

Marketers know that a recognizable person lends "star quality" to any brand, and if that person uses the brand there is a bigger wow factor. While the number of dieters has started to drop—currently 25 percent of American women are dieting compared to some 36 percent in 1991—there is still a great deal of money to be made in the weight-loss business. Figures released by a research company, NPD Group, suggest dieters continue to pay billions of dollars each year for diet-related products.

See also: Hudson, Jennifer; Nutrisystem; Weight Watchers.

FURTHER READING

Brodesser-Akner, Taffy. "When Dieting Becomes a Role to Play." *The New York Times,* August 4, 2011, E1.
Olson, Elizabeth. "For Weight Watchers, Jennifer Hudson Wins a Losing Battle." *The New York Times,* April 6, 2010, B3.

Celiac Disease

Celiac disease is an immune response to eating gluten that causes inflammation and eventual damage to the lining of the small intestine. This damage then prevents absorption of needed nutrients and can also cause diarrhea, bloating, and other physical symptoms. If left untreated, over time complications such as autoimmune diseases, osteoporosis, thyroid disease, and cancer can also develop.

About 1 percent of the U.S. population, or just more than 3 million people, are affected with celiac disease. However, research shows that some 18 million Americans may be suffering from non-celiac gluten sensitivity. According to the National Association for Celiac Awareness Foundation, this figure is six times the number of people who have been diagnosed with celiac disease.

See also: Gluten-Free.

FURTHER READING

Beck, Melinda. "Clues to Gluten Sensitivity." *Wall Street Journal*, March 15, 2011. http://online.wsj.com/news/articles/SB10001424052748704893604576200393522456636.
Velasquez-Manoff, Moises. "Who Has the Guts for Gluten?" *The New York Times*, February 23, 2013. http://www.nytimes.com/2013/02/24/opinion/sunday/what-really-causes-celiac-disease.html?_r=0.
www.americanceliac.org.
www.celiaccentral.org.
www.digestive.niddk.nih.gov/ddiseases/pubs/celiac/.

Childhood Obesity

The combination of diets filled with high-fat foods, sugary drinks, and too little exercise continues to keep obesity rates for American children and teens at about 17 percent. The good news, according to the Centers for Disease Control and Prevention (CDC), is that the prevalence of obesity among children aged two to five years decreased significantly from 13.9 percent in 2003–2004 to 8.4 percent in 2011–2012. The CDC also noted that in 2011–2012, obesity prevalence was higher among Hispanics (22.4%) and non-Hispanic black youth (20.2%) than non-Hispanic white youth (14.1%). Non-Hispanic Asian youth had the lowest prevalence of obesity, at 8.6 percent.

The Children's Defense Fund notes that children's lifestyles and diets are a potent combination for poor nutrition and weight gain. The group says, "Only one in five high school children eats the five recommended servings of fruits and vegetables a day and fast food consumption has increased fivefold among children since 1970. Nearly one-third of American children ages 4 to 19 eat fast food every day, resulting in about six extra pounds per year for each child."

Sugar-sweetened beverages—a key contributor to weight gain and obesity—constitute nearly 11 percent of children's total calorie consumption.

An April 2014 article in the magazine *Pediatrics* examined six studies to determine the incremental lifetime direct medical cost from the perspective of a 10-year-old obese child compared to a 10-year-old child of normal weight. The studies found a range of $12,660 to $19, 630, when weight gain through adulthood among normal weight children is accounted for and from $16,310 to $39,080 when this adjustment is not made. In other words, an obese child who remains obese for most of his or her life could require nearly $40,000 in additional costs for medical care and treatment. The authors concluded that $19,000 was a reasonable estimate for the added medical costs for an obese child. *USA Today* and other media outlets pointed out that the amount is higher than an average year of college costs at a four-year public institution.

The study, also conducted by the CDC, showed that childhood diabetes doubled during the last two decades, gall bladder disease tripled, and sleep apnea increased fivefold, a substantial increase. Sleep apnea, a disorder in which a sleeping person repeatedly stops breathing for long enough to lower the amount of oxygen in the blood and brain, is more common among overweight children because fat gathers at the back of the neck and can block the airway.

The researchers also found that obesity, in addition to directly contributing to childhood diseases, is turning up more often as a secondary factor in illnesses such as asthma and mental health disorders. A statement issued by Dr. Jeffrey P. Koplan, director of the CDC, said the figures show a growing epidemic of obesity, which must be addressed so that American children can lead healthier lives. Koplan added that overweight children, like their adult counterparts, would continue to be at increasing risk for cardiovascular diseases, diabetes, and other serious health problems as long as childhood obesity remained a major health problem in the United States.

Parents can exacerbate the problems of overweight children. A press release from the Bassett Healthcare Research Institute in Cooperstown, New York, noted that research found that most parents of overweight children do not think of their children as overweight. Physician and researcher Barbara A. Dennison said, "For example, 68 percent of parents of obese children, those with a BMI above the 95th percentile, reported that their child's weight was 'OK, just right,' and 8 percent even reported their child was 'underweight.'"

The press release also cited research that showed parents could do more harm than good by using dessert as a reward for finishing dinner. "Using foods like desserts as rewards tends to increase the child's preference for those foods, while rewarding a child for finishing dinner may actually encourage overeating," Dennison said.

See also: Obesity; Television.

FURTHER READING

Finkelstein, Eric, et al. "Lifetime Medical Direct Costs of Childhood Obesity." *Pediatrics*, April 2014.

Healy, Michelle. "Price Tag for Childhood Obesity: $19,000 per Kid." *USA Today*, April 7, 2014.

Ogden, Cynthia, et al. "Prevalence of Childhood and Adult Obesity in the United States, 2011–2012." *The Journal of the American Medical Association*, February 26, 2014: 806–14.

www.cdc.gov/obesity/data/adult.html.

www.childrensdefense.org.

www.healthypeople.gov.

Cholesterol (Blood Types)

Blood cholesterol is divided into three separate classes of lipoproteins: very-low density lipoprotein (VLDL); low-density lipoprotein (LDL), which contains most of the cholesterol found in the blood; and high-density lipoprotein (HDL).

LDL seems to be the culprit in coronary heart disease and is popularly known as bad cholesterol. Too much LDL in the bloodstream can build up within the walls of the arteries and contribute to the formation of plaque, which can ultimately clog the arteries. A blood test can measure cholesterol levels. Ideally, LDL levels should be below 130.

By contrast, HDL is increasingly considered desirable and known as good cholesterol. HDL levels typically range from 40 to 50 mg/dL for men and 50 to 60 mg/dL for women. Levels below 35 mg/dL are abnormally low and pose a risk factor for cardiac problems. Cigarette smoking, obesity, and lack of physical activity can cause low HDL levels.

See also: Exercise; Obesity.

Cholesterol (Dietary)

Dietary cholesterol is found only in animal foods. Abundant in organ meats and egg yolks, cholesterol is also contained in meats and poultry. Vegetable oils and shortenings are cholesterol free.

Foods high in saturated fat raise blood cholesterol more than other forms of fat. Limiting saturated fats to less than 10 percent of calories should help lower blood cholesterol levels. While polyunsaturated and monounsaturated fats could help lower blood cholesterol levels, the recommendation still holds that total fat should account for no more than 30 percent of daily calorie intake.

See also: Dietary Fat; Fat.

Christian Diets

With the 1957 publication of Charlie Shedd's book, *Pray Your Weight Away,* Christian-oriented weight-loss programs set their sights on an audience beyond church walls. Today faith-based dieting programs, books, and workouts continue to grow in popularity. Dieting programs such as Gwen Shamblin's Weigh Down workshop are held in thousands of churches across the United States. Book titles such as *Slim for Him, More of Jesus, Less of Me,* and *What Would Jesus Eat?* preach the gospel of eating right for God. And Christian exercise videos like Sheri Chamber's *Praise Aerobics* link exercise and spirituality.

Shamblin is one among a growing list of Christian diet creators. Her approach, grounded in a conservative form of Protestant Christianity, requires no calorie counting or measuring. Instead, she suggests that a person with unhealthy food cravings may be suffering from a real spiritual hunger. Shamblin advocates eating only when truly hungry and she believes that eating when the body doesn't need food is a sign that an individual needs to get right with God. If overeating is a problem of the soul, she suggests that putting your spiritual life in order will bring weight loss without cutting out foods you love. To illustrate that point, she teaches people to stop midway through a candy bar, or eat M&M's one by one, to let their taste buds savor the flavor without feeling guilty. Shamblin organized her first support group in 1986 and now counts over 10,000 Weigh Down workshops with a quarter of a million participants. Shamblin and others find willing followers among the estimated 39 percent of born-again Christians in the United States.

Conservative estimates place the total worth of the American dieting industry at over $30 billion a year and economists say a healthy 5 percent of that is Christian money.

Christian dieting programs, like their secular counterparts, are not created equal. First come the programs that avoid strict rules and focus instead on the spiritual side of eating rather than the calorie counting. At the top of the list in popularity is Shamblin's Weigh Down Workshop. But newer titles, like Dr. Don Colbert's *What Would Jesus Eat?: The Ultimate Program for Eating Well, Feeling Great, and Living Longer,* go beyond Shamblin's comfort food choices. Colbert, a family physician, tells dieters to examine and emulate the simple diet of Jesus. Basically he advocates the Mediterranean diet favored by many nutritionists—a diet low in saturated fat, sugar, and red meat and high in whole grains, fruits, and vegetables. Plus he encourages the consumption of fish, the use of olive oil, and a daily exercise regimen.

Colbert received his medical degree from Oral Roberts School of Medicine in Tulsa, Oklahoma. After developing chronic fatigue syndrome as a young doctor, he began looking more closely at the links between physical, spiritual, and mental health. He detailed his experiences in his first book, *What You Don't Know May Be Killing You*, which he wrote after he quit eating processed and fatty foods and took up exercise. He describes his newest plan in *What Would Jesus Eat?* as an "all-natural diet from biblical times," and says those who follow his suggestions can expect good health, fitness, longevity, and spiritual health. In his book, Colbert acknowledges the similarities between his diet and other nutrition plans, but writes that his program has a healthy difference. "The low-fat diets, such as the Pritikin and Ornish Diets, also work. People lose weight. However, the low-fat diet doesn't taste as good, and after eating a meal, a person often leaves the table without feeling satisfied. This can lead to binge eating. For all of these diets, an equal and opposite 'binge response' seems to be waiting around the corner." He goes on to suggest that binge eating can be avoided by choosing simpler foods. He writes that foods cooked in olive oil and seasoned with herbs and spices and meals of fresh fruits, vegetables, and whole grains leave a person feeling full and nourished. Even less traditional than Colbert's plan is the Hallelujah Diet, founded by George Malkmus. He preaches the benefits of vegetarianism and a raw food diet based on foods found in the Garden of Eden.

Still other Christian dieting programs more closely resemble their secular counterparts and advocate food exchanges, measuring amounts, and counting calories. Carol Showalter's *3D: Diet, Discipline, and Discipleship* is a faith-based 12-week plan that relies on the American Diabetes Association food exchange lists in a style similar to the Weight Watchers program, but unlike Weight Watchers it draws inspiration from the Bible. Founded in 1973 by Showalter, a Presbyterian pastor's wife, this program teaches that Christians can lose weight successfully by meeting in small groups and by leading disciplined lives with disciplined eating and disciplined prayer. The book also emphasizes good nutrition, proper eating habits, sensible weight loss, and a long-term exercise program.

First Place is yet another Christian-based diet program, founded in 1981 in Houston's First Baptist Church. Carole Lewis, national director of the group, said in an article in the September 2000 issue of *Christianity Today* that the group supports a recognized food plan, using food exchanges and the Food Guide Pyramid developed by the U.S. Department of Agriculture with the added goal of drawing dieters closer to Christ.

While no formal studies have looked at faith-based weight-loss programs, experts say that adding a spiritual component can be a positive step, since the most successful programs do incorporate a lot of social support. In response to suggestions that there is a link between spiritual hunger and physiological hunger, Shape Up America! even added a "soul food" section to its Web site, featuring a series of tutorials that explore the actual concept of spiritual hunger. Ultimately, nutritionists say any faith-based diet must still be based on healthy eating and regular exercise, not just on the notion that God wants us to be thin.

See also: Ornish, Dean; Pritikin, Nathan; Shamblin, Gwen; Weigh Down Diet; Weight Watchers.

FURTHER READING

Barrett, Stephen. "Rev. George Malkmus and His Hallelujah Diet." http://www.quackwatch .org/11Ind/malkmus.html.
Brown, Deneen. "Dieting Faithfully; Proponents of the Weigh Down Diet Turn to God for the Will to Resist Overeating." *Washington Post,* April 11, 2000, Z14.
Colbert, Don. *What Would Jesus Eat?: The Ultimate Program for Eating Well, Feeling Great, and Living Longer.* Nashville, TN: Thomas Nelson Publishers, 2002.
Ellin, Abby. "Seeing Overeating as a Sin, and God as the Diet Coach." *The New York Times,* May 29, 2004, A13.
Hancock, Rita. *The Eden Diet.* Oklahoma City: Personalized Fitness Products, 2008.
Showalter, Carol. *3D: Diet, Discipline & Discipleship.* Brewster, MA: Paraclete Press, 1973; new, rev. ed. 2002.
Turner, Susie. "New Weight Loss Devotional via YouVersion Bible App." *Christian Today,* September 11, 2013. http://www.christiantoday.com/article/new.weight.loss .devotional.via.youversion.bible.app/33929.htm.
Winner, Lauren F. "The Weigh & the Truth." *Christianity Today,* September 4, 2000, 50.
www.danielsdiet.com.
www.takebackyourtemple.com.

Coconut Diet

Americans are notorious for embracing unusual diets, even when it is clear that a diet is a poor nutritional choice. In fact, though some diets are unhealthy they have redeemed themselves years after being introduced. A classic example of diet redemption is the re-emergence of coconut oil. Decades ago saturated fats like coconut oil, butter, and lard were commonplace. However, in the 1990s, they disappeared, driven underground by all the information about the danger of saturated fats. It appeared they were gone for good when movie theaters stopped cooking popcorn in coconut oil, thanks to a study released by the Center for Science in the Public Interest which showed that the saturated fat in theater popcorn matched the unhealthy saturated fat in fast food.

Now, annual sales of coconut oil in places like Whole Foods have doubled in the last several years, thanks to some backtracking by scientists along with the growing number of vegans and individuals following paleo and gluten-free diets. Scientists even recanted the earlier studies that warned consumers away from coconut oil, suggesting the research was done using partially hydrogenated coconut oil rather than the virgin coconut oil now available in health food and regular grocery stories.

While the current Dietary Guidelines for Americans recommends a limit on daily calories from saturated fat, groups like the American Dietetic Association are suggesting not all saturated fats are created equal. Coconut oil differs from other saturated fats because it contains medium-chain triglycerides (MCTs), which enter the bloodstream when eaten and quickly raise triglyceride levels. The body responds by rapidly releasing fat-burning enzymes, a big difference from how most dietary fats digest slowly and take hours to become available as energy.

Another difference in coconut oil is that it raises LDL (low-density lipoprotein) while at the same time raises HDL (high-density lipoprotein) cholesterol. The LDL cholesterol has been labeled the "bad" cholesterol as it collects in the blood vessel walls and can lead to blockages and to an increased risk of heart disease and heart attack. The HDL cholesterol is the "good" guy and it removes the bad cholesterol when it collects in the bloodstream and reduces the risk of heart disease.

While researchers have not gone as far as to call coconut oil healthy, there is a shift in opinion and it appears that coconut oil is considered healthier than other saturated animal fats. It stacks up even better when compared to trans fats. This change in thinking has led to the creation of a variety of coconut and coconut oil diets. The diets share the central theme that to lose weight the body needs a specific balance between fats, carbohydrates, and protein. Like the Atkins diet, any basic coconut diet severely limits carbohydrates and replaces them with protein-rich foods. The coconut diet also includes the addition of daily coconut oil.

Divided into four phases, a coconut dieter begins with the strictest phase when food choices are severely limited to lean proteins, nonstarchy vegetables, and water. The second phase calls for a cleanse that resembles the Master Cleanse and uses lemon juice, cayenne, and little else. The third phase slowly adds back a few carbohydrates and the final phase is the maintenance phase that allows healthy carbs in moderation along with lean meats and, of course, coconut oil. Similar to other elimination diets, health professionals caution that the lack of variety and the severe limitations on healthy fruits and vegetables can create health problems. When coupled with the lack of scientific evidence that coconut oil, a saturated fat, is healthy, there is little to recommend this plan to dieters. Finally, like any change in eating habits, nutritionists caution that moderation is the key to staying healthy, and suggest individuals can occasionally eat coconut oil and remain healthy but they caution that too much of any fat is still a recipe for weight gain.

See also: Atkins Nutritional Approach; Cholesterol (Dietary); Dietary Guidelines for Americans; Gluten-Free; Master Cleanse Diet; Paleo Diet.

FURTHER READING

"Coconut Oil." *Shape*, January 2012, 68.

Cullum-Dugan, Diana. "Get the Facts on Coconut Oil: Coconut Oil is One of the Hottest Foods on the Market with Exuberant Claims Made for Its Health Potential." *Environmental Nutrition* 37, no. 1 (January 2014): 6.

Lillien, Lisa. "Diet-Food Fakers: In Honor of April Fools' Day, Hungry Girl Lisa Lillien Warns You Off 4 Foods That Seem Low-Cal but Aren't." *Redbook* 218, no. 4 (April 2012): 170.

"Two Thumbs Down for Movie Theater Popcorn. New Lab Tests of Movie Theater Popcorn Show It's Still the Godzilla of Snacks." *Center for Science in the Public Interest.* November 18, 2009. https://www.cspinet.org/new/200911182.html.

D'Adamo, Peter J.

Peter J. D'Adamo (b. 1956, New York) is a naturopathic physician and researcher who developed the blood type diet, Eat Right 4 Your Type. The diet suggests that one's blood type is the key to healthy eating and living. For example, people with type O blood are descended from earliest man; a high-protein diet and strenuous physical activities are best suited to them. Type As are descended from a gentler agrarian culture, and therefore type As do best with a vegetarian diet and noncompetitive physical activity.

In D'Adamo's 1996 book, he explained that he is a second-generation naturopathic physician and credited the genesis of blood type diets to his father, James D'Adamo. The Eat Right diet plan has its share of critics who say that categorizing people by their blood type is a flawed basis on which to build a successful diet.

In 1990, D'Adamo was selected Physician of the Year by the American Association of Naturopathic Physicians. He founded *The Journal of Naturopathic Medicine* and works in a private practice in Stamford, Connecticut.

See also: Eat Right 4 Your Type.

FURTHER READING

D'Adamo, Peter J. *Change Your Genetic Destiny*. New York: Harmony, 2007.
D'Adamo, Peter J. *Eat Right 4 Your Type*. New York: Putnam Adult, 1997.
www.dadamo.com.

DASH Diet

The sale of weight-loss products and services is now a billion-dollar business as millions of Americans look for an easy way to lose weight. Yet, the answer to weight loss is the simple rule that calories in must be less than calories out. The Dietary Approaches to Stop Hypertension (DASH) diet is a commonsense, healthy, effective, and sustainable approach to lose weight and keep it off. The diet is based on the work of researchers who were actually looking for a way to lower blood pressure. What they discovered with the DASH plan was the added benefit of weight loss, as well as protection from heart disease and diabetes.

What is the DASH diet? It is a blueprint for healthy eating that is low in saturated fat; low in sodium; high in fiber, vitamins, and minerals; and centers on eating a large variety of fresh fruits, vegetables, whole grains, and lean proteins. Developed by the National Heart, Lung, and Blood Institute, the diet limits sodium consumption to 2,300 milligrams or less per day, a substantial difference from the 3,500 milligrams of sodium or more commonly eaten by most Americans. Studies that examined the DASH diet have shown consuming 2,300 milligrams or the lower sodium DASH version of 1,500 milligrams can lower systolic blood pressure by up to 16 points in less than half a year for people with high blood pressure.

Hypertension or high blood pressure is an important health concern because it causes the heart to work too hard while it also hardens arteries and can even cause poor kidney function or brain hemorrhage in its most extreme cases. High blood pressure is classified as blood pressure measured at above 140/90 mm Hg. It is believed that over 59 million Americans are at risk for high blood pressure or have been diagnosed with it.

The DASH diet is a far cry from the typical American diet filled with high-sodium processed foods like canned soups, lunch meats, cold cereals, salad dressings, cheese, potato chips, hot dogs, frozen pizza, or frozen dinners. In fact, studies show only 5 percent of sodium in the standard American diet is added during cooking as table salt.

The *U.S. News & World Report* ranked the DASH diet number one overall in healthy diets for several years as part of their analysis of weight-loss programs. The DASH diet has also been incorporated into MinuteClinic, a division of CVS Caremark, the largest provider of walk-in medical clinics in the United States as part of their weight-loss program. The MinuteClinic plan includes nutrition and weight-loss advice provided through the online DASH Web site where dieters can find meal plans, exercise tips, recipes, and other weight-loss tools. The DASH diet is also an eating model that supports the objectives of the Dietary Guidelines for Americans, and the 2010 guidelines recommend the DASH eating plan for all Americans. The U.S. Departments of Agriculture and Health and Human Services update the guidelines every five years.

HISTORY

The study that leads to the development of the DASH diet was published in 1997 in the *New England Journal of Medicine*. The study, conducted by the National Institutes of Health along with hundreds of doctors, nurses, nutritionists, and other health care professionals from Harvard, Duke, and Johns Hopkins medical schools, showed promising results of how diet was able to control blood pressure in study participants. Reports showed that some study participants were even able to stop using their prescribed blood pressure medications after they followed the DASH diet. Follow-up research, including the 2005 OmniHeart Study, once again showed positive results with participants demonstrating improvements that matched the effects of some antihypertensive drugs. The Omni-Heart Study was undertaken to examine the diet's effects on both hypertension and cholesterol.

NUTRITIONAL FACTORS

Nutrition on the DASH diet includes lots of whole grains, fruits, vegetables, low-fat dairy, and lean proteins such as fish, chicken, and legumes. While red meat, sweets, and fats are included they are only added in small amounts. DASH guidelines also suggest limiting alcohol to two or fewer drinks a day for men and just one or less per day for women since alcohol can increase blood pressure. Caffeine is the one item the DASH diet doesn't address since there is no consensus on how caffeine does or does not affect blood pressure. For those who think caffeine may influence their health, it is important to discuss the issue with their primary health care provider.

A DASH daily eating plan would include six to eight servings of whole grains each day such as bread, cereal, rice, or pasta. Vegetables should include four to five servings per day of everything from tomatoes, carrots, and broccoli to sweet potatoes or other greens in order to take advantage of the fiber, vitamins, and minerals they provide. Studies have shown that too little potassium can raise blood pressure, which increases the risk of stroke. Current guidelines for potassium recommend 4,700 milligrams per day for adults and dietary potassium can come from dark leafy greens, squash, baked potatoes, beans such as kidney or garbanzo beans, avocados, and bananas. Studies have shown that increased dietary potassium can even allow patients to reduce blood pressure medications. However, it is important to check with a primary care doctor, as potassium and salt can create problems for people with kidney disease and some medications can be influenced by potassium.

The diet suggests eating four to five servings of fruits per day since they are loaded with fiber, potassium, and magnesium while at the same time when fresh they are typically low in fat. Dairy servings should be limited to two or three each day and should include low-fat milk, yogurt, cheese, and other dairy products, especially since they are major sources of calcium. Researchers have determined that low calcium intake can be a contributing factor to high blood pressure. Good sources of dietary calcium include greens like collards, kale, bok choy, and broccoli rabe, along with salmon or other fish, cheeses like ricotta, and fortified orange juice or beverages like almond milk. To make sure calcium is absorbed, it is important to maintain an adequate level of vitamin D as well. While health care professionals do not recommend calcium supplements to lower blood pressure it is recognized that many Americans do not get enough calcium in their diets and overall health of many Americans would benefit from a boost in calcium intake.

Current guidelines recommend 1,000 milligrams daily for adults and 1,200 milligrams per day for adults over age 50.

Protein is an important component of a healthy diet and the DASH plan calls for six or fewer servings each day of lean meats, poultry, or fish, with a recommendation to be especially careful to avoid proteins that contain fat and cholesterol. Healthy proteins include heart-healthy fish like salmon and tuna, as well as skinless poultry. Nuts, seeds, and legumes are another important aspect of the diet, which recommend four to five servings per week. At the lower end of the diet are fats and oils, which should be restricted to two to three servings each day of monounsaturated fats rather than the saturated fats or trans fats known to raise blood cholesterol and increase the risk of heart disease. Sweets should also be consumed less frequently, no more than five or fewer servings each week. When eating sweets, use moderation and cut back on the ones especially high in sugar and fat.

The DASH plan also calls for regular activity such as walking or swimming that adds up to 30 minutes of moderate activity on most days. This will help avoid weight gain and can also prevent and control high blood pressure.

See also: Dietary Guidelines for Americans.

FURTHER READING

Appel, L. J., et al. "A Clinical Trial of the Effects of Dietary Patterns on Blood Pressure." *New England Journal of Medicine* 336, no. 11 (April 1997): 1117.

"DASH Diet: Healthy Eating to Lower Your Blood Pressure." *Mayo Clinic*, May 15, 2013. http://www.mayoclinic.com/health/dash-diet/HI00047.

"MinuteClinic Partners with DASH for Health to Create Personalized Weight Loss Program." *Diabetes Week*, July 29, 2013, 81.

Moore, Thomas. *The DASH Diet for Hypertension.* Pocket Books, 2003.

Palmer, Sharon. "The Top-Rated Diet of the Year: DASH Diet." *Environmental Nutrition* 36, no. 4 (April 2013): 2.

Sacks, F. M., L. P. Svetkey, W. M., Vollmer, L. J. Appel, G. A. Bray, D., Harsha, E. Obarzanek, P. R., Conlin, E. R., Miller, D. G. Simons-Morton, N. Karanja, P. H. Lin. "The DASH-Sodium Trial: The Effects on Blood Pressure of Reduced Sodium and the DASH Dietary Program." *New England Journal of Medicine* 344, no. 1 (2001): 3–10.

Dehydration

Dehydration occurs when the body loses too much water or the intake of water is too low. Severe diarrhea or vomiting can cause dehydration. Fitness experts suggest drinking a cup of water about half an hour before exercising and immediately after a 20- to 30-minute workout to keep the body adequately hydrated.

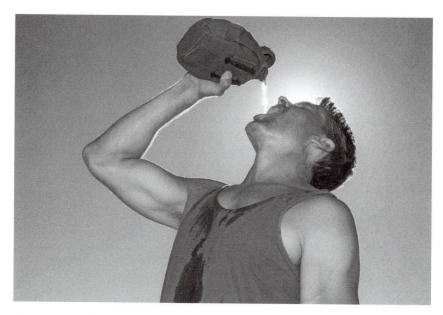

For most physical activities, water is the perfect drink to stay hydrated. (Czuber/
Dreamstime)

Don't drink beverages containing alcohol or caffeine, since both promote dehydration. Whether it is necessary to drink electrolyte-type sports drinks depends
on the intensity and duration of the exercise. Water may well be sufficient, and
it contains no calories.

Some symptoms of dehydration include a dry or sticky mouth, a low output of
urine, and dizziness or weakness.

Dehydration as an area of study, especially in connection with sports performance, is relatively new. More research is underway, too. As an article in the
Canadian Journal of Applied Physiology states, "Although the negative effects of
exercise-induced dehydration on exercise performance were clearly demonstrated in the 1940s, athletes continued to believe for years thereafter that fluid
intake was not beneficial. More recently, negative effects on performance have
been demonstrated with modest (<2%) dehydration, and these effects are exac-
erbated when the exercise is performed in a hot environment."

See also: Caffeine; Exercise.

FURTHER READING

Barr, S.I. "Effects of Dehydration on Exercise Performance." *Canadian Journal of Applied
Physiology* 24, no. 2 (April 1999): 164–72.

Wall, Bradley, Greig Watson, Jeremiah J. Peiffer, Chris R. Abbiss, Rodney Siegel, Paul B. Laursen. "Current Hydration Guidelines Are Erroneous: Dehydration Does Not Impair Exercise Performance in the Heat." *British Journal of Sports Medicine*, September 2013. http://bjsm.bmj.com/content/early/2013/09/20/bjsports-2013-092417.

Dehydroepiandrosterone (DHEA)

Dehydroepiandrosterone (DHEA) is a hormone produced by the body, now being used as a supplement in weight-loss and other health-boosting formulas. DHEA supplements are typically made from wild yams or soy. Manufacturers of these products say that DHEA helps the body fight aging, provides energy, and builds muscle strength.

Natural DHEA levels, produced in the adrenal gland, begin to decline around age 30. Because DHEA produces the male and female sex hormones, low levels of DHEA have been considered possible factors in depression, hormonal disorders, and more. Although DHEA is being studied to gauge its impact on depression, obesity, and treatment for schizophrenia, medical researchers say there's still much research to be done.

According to the Mayo Clinic, there does seem to be a building body of evidence that DHEA supplements can help with weight loss because of a boost in metabolism. However, the long-term impact of hormonal therapies is often not known for years. There are concerns that DHEA can trigger aggressiveness, trouble sleeping, and even increase the risk for certain diseases, such as breast cancer.

The U.S. Food and Drug Administration banned DHEA in 1985, but that ban was removed in 1994. However, the National Football League, for example, still bans its use among players because of the concern that DHEA works similarly to muscle-building steroids.

See also: Dexatrim.

FURTHER READING

DHEA Fact Sheet. American Cancer Society. http://www.cancer.org/treatment/treat mentsandsideeffects/complementaryandalternativemedicine/pharmacologicaland biologicaltreatment/dhea.

Haiken, Melanie. "3 New Weight Loss Supplements Getting Buzz." *Forbes*, June 22, 2013. http://www.forbes.com/sites/melaniehaiken/2013/06/22/3-new-fat-busting-supplements-for-speedy-weight-loss/2/.

http://www.mayoclinic.org/drugs-supplements/dhea/background/hrb-20059173.

Kornblut, Anne, and Wilson, Duff. "How One Pill Escaped the List of Controlled Steroids." *The New York Times*, April 17, 2005. http://www.nytimes.com/2005/04/17/national/17steroid.html?_r=0.

Skerret, P.J. "DHEA: Ignore the Hype." QuackWatch. http://www.quackwatch.com/
    01QuackeryRelatedTopics/dhea.html.

Dexatrim

Dexatrim is a once-a-day diet pill originally formulated with the controversial appetite suppressant phenylpropanolamine, or PPA. It became a best seller among over-the-counter weight-loss pills following its introduction in 1976. In 2000, company officials pulled Dexatrim from drugstore shelves following a November 2000 public health warning to consumers by the U.S. Food and Drug Administration (FDA), saying PPA was no longer safe for consumption and had been shown to increase the risk of stroke in young women.

The FDA also asked manufacturers of products containing PPA—diet drugs as well as over-the-counter allergy and cold medications—to use another active ingredient in their formulas. Dexatrim, with sales of $200 million in 1999, responded.

> Chattem, Inc. withdrew the original formula and released an herbal alternative, Dexatrim Natural. The replacement uses the herb ephedra in place of PPA; an ingredient critics say may be just as dangerous as PPA. Derived from a Chinese herb called mahuang, ephedra/ephedrine is a stimulant used for short-term energy boosts and to increase metabolism and suppress the appetite. Researchers are studying the possibility that the human body may convert ephedra to PPA. Information on the Dexatrim Web site informs consumers that Dexatrim Natural follows the FDA's recommended daily dosage limit of 24 milligrams of ephedrine. In 1997 the FDA called for ephedra labeling to recommend a daily dosage limit after serious complications, including heart attacks, strokes, and several deaths, were linked to the ephedra in some dietary supplements.

In the meantime, Chattem launched another new diet drug, Dexatrim Natural Ephedrine-Free. According to its packaging, it contains bitter orange peel, caffeine, and ginger root, plus green tea leaf and guarana, both herbal forms of caffeine. Critics argue that these new formulas share the same side effects as products containing ephedrine, including insomnia, restlessness, nausea, dizziness, irritability, anxiety, high blood pressure, and strokes. Diet pills, both prescription and over the counter, when used with increased exercise and behavior modification do play a role in short-term weight loss. There are a variety of Dexatrim products on the market in 2014; the key ingredients in those products are caffeine, green tea extract, ginseng root extract, and dehydroepiandrosterone, known as DHEA.

However, health professionals continue to question the long-term effects of these medications and they raise concerns that repeated unsuccessful attempts to diet using pills may lead to eating disorders such as anorexia and bulimia in some teenage users. Even though suppliers of weight-control products like Dexatrim Natural do not target teens and have warning labels on their products, younger teens are turning to over-the-counter weight-control products in growing numbers in response to rising teen obesity levels. According to the FDA, a national survey of high school students conducted by the National CDC found that the most common dieting methods used were skipping meals, taking diet pills, and inducing vomiting after eating.

Diet pills at best offer a temporary solution and at worst may jeopardize health. The safest way for anyone to control his or her weight, according to health professionals, is to eat a healthy diet, using the USDA MyPlate guide as a blueprint, and get enough exercise.

See also: Ephedra/Ephedrine; Phenylpropanolamine (PPA).

FURTHER READING

Berman, Phyllis, and Amy Feldman. "An Extraordinary Peddler." *Forbes*, December 9, 1991, 136–39.
Brink, Susan. *U.S. News & World Report*, November 20, 2000, 74.
"Marketing to Teens a Complex Issue." *Chain Drug Review* 23, no. 7 (April 9, 2001): 29.
www.dexatrim.com.

Diabetes

Diabetes is a disease in which the body can no longer produce or properly use insulin, a hormone required to convert sugars and starches from the food we eat into the energy we need. It is one of the most common chronic illnesses today, affecting an estimated 25.8 million people in the United States. It is affecting an increasing number of people. Another 79 million adults aged 20 and older have prediabetes, a condition where blood glucose levels are higher than normal but not high enough to be called diabetes.

There are two major types of diabetes, In Type 1, sometimes called juvenile diabetes or insulin-dependent diabetes, the pancreas no longer produces insulin. Approximately 5 percent of people diagnosed with diabetes have Type 1 diabetes. It usually strikes children or young adults, though it can develop at any age. It occurs when the body's immune system mistakenly attacks the insulin-producing cells in the pancreas. People with Type 1 diabetes must take daily insulin injections to stay alive. While the cause of Type 1 diabetes is unknown, it is likely that heredity plays a role. However, in susceptible individuals, a virus can trigger the disease.

In Type 2 diabetes, the body does produce insulin, but either makes too little or has become resistant to it. More than 90 percent of people with diabetes have Type 2, and it most often strikes older people and those with a history of obesity and inactivity, though increasingly it is appearing in younger people—even children—who are overweight and inactive. Type 2 diabetics can often control their blood-sugar levels through weight loss, exercise, and better nutrition, but many also need oral medications and/or insulin. A third type of diabetes, gestational diabetes, is a temporary condition that occurs during pregnancy, when the body fails to produce the extra insulin needed during some pregnancies. Gestational diabetes requires that the pregnant woman monitor her food and blood-sugar levels carefully. It usually goes away after the pregnancy, but women who have had it are at an increased risk of later developing Type 2 diabetes.

Heredity plays a role in the development of Type 1 diabetes. Siblings of people with Type 1 as well as children of parents with Type 1 are at a higher risk of developing the disease. Type 1 most often strikes in puberty, according to researchers, though it can occur at any age. Type 2 diabetes has a hereditary factor as well—people with a family history of Type 2 are more likely to develop the disease themselves. And some racial and ethnic groups have higher rates of diabetes. African Americans and Latinos are nearly twice as likely to develop Type 2 diabetes as the general population.

The warning signs for Type 1 diabetes include frequent urination, excessive thirst, unusual hunger, extreme fatigue, and unexplained weight loss. Victims of Type 2 diabetes can experience the same symptoms, as well as blurred vision, tingling or numbness in the hands or feet, and cuts, bruises, and infections that are slow to heal. Often, though, people with Type 2 diabetes will have no symptoms at all, and the disease won't be discovered until they have developed complications.

Diabetes is the seventh leading cause of death in the United States, and the sixth leading cause of death by disease. Each year, nearly 200,000 people die as a result of diabetes and its long-term complications, which include blindness, kidney disease, heart disease, stroke, nerve disease, and amputations. It is often described as a "silent killer" because in its Type 2 form, it can go undetected for years. It is only when serious and sometimes life-threatening complications develop that many people learn they have the disease. Complications of diabetes—which often take years to develop—stem in many instances from the damage that high blood-sugar levels do to the tiny blood vessels in the body. In instances of kidney failure, for example, damage has been done to the blood vessels inside the kidney that act as filters to remove wastes, chemicals, and excess water from the blood. Poorly controlled diabetes can cause blindness by damaging the tiny blood vessels in the retina.

The most serious short-term complication of Type 1 diabetes is called ketoacidosis. When the body doesn't have enough insulin, it begins to burn fat for energy. Burning fat produces ketones, an acid that can poison the body, leading to coma and even death. Ketoacidosis usually develops slowly—early warning signs include thirst, a dry mouth, frequent urination, and high levels of ketones in the urine. Later, the person may feel nausea, have a fruity odor on the breath, or have difficulty breathing. Ketoacidosis is a serious condition that requires immediate medical attention.

People with diabetes must take a lot of responsibility to make sure their treatment plan works. People with diabetes must balance a variety of factors every day—deciding what to eat and when, or determining how much medication to take and when to take it. Physical activity or illness can also mean adjusting the treatment regimen. The best way to learn that responsibility is to seek advice from a team of health care professionals. A primary care physician is a good place to start, but treating diabetes almost always involves specialists in other areas as well. A diabetes care team usually involves an eye doctor, a dietitian, and a certified diabetes educator. If complications arise, a patient might be sent to other specialists.

For people with Type 1 diabetes, insulin is the only option. But there are a wide variety of approaches to insulin therapy. There are more than 20 kinds of insulin available—some act very quickly or peak at different times, and some last all day long. There are also different ways to deliver insulin—syringes, insulin pens, and insulin pumps.

Most people with Type 1 begin by taking injections of two types of insulin per day, a fast-acting insulin immediately before meals and a slower-acting insulin that helps keep blood glucose levels steady over a longer term. Depending on what they're eating or their level of activity, diabetics monitor their own blood glucose levels and inject themselves or program an insulin-delivery pump as needed. A person with Type 1 diabetes often calculates the amount of carbohydrates she will consume and then injects herself with a number of units of insulin. This formula depends on the individual's reaction to insulin as well as expected activity level.

Injecting insulin before every meal or snack is the most targeted approach to diabetes treatment and allows the greatest flexibility, but some diabetics find it cumbersome. Another approach is to inject a specific amount of insulin in the morning and then eat only those foods that will be covered by that amount of insulin. The second approach is more regimented and doesn't allow for spontaneous snacking.

Another recent innovation in insulin delivery is the insulin pump, a device that looks like a beeper and provides a steady, incremental dose of fast-acting insulin through a tiny tube inserted in the person's abdomen. Insulin pumps are the most expensive approach to diabetes care, but the device is the closest thing to the normal delivery of insulin that a person with diabetes can achieve. Pumps can be programmed to deliver different amounts of insulin at different times of the day or night, giving the person the ability to fine-tune their treatment regimen.

If you have an insulin-dependent diabetic friend, or if you are insulin-dependent yourself, make sure you discuss this openly with your friends. There's the possibility that insulin-dependent diabetics may need help at some point.

They may experience an episode of hypoglycemia (low blood sugar) and need help getting a snack or sugared drink. Hypoglycemia occurs when the person has either taken more insulin than needed for the carbohydrates consumed, or is particularly active. The other risk is developing hyperglycemia, or high blood sugar. That happens when the person hasn't taken enough insulin or has eaten more carbohydrates than the insulin can cover. A fast-acting insulin can help counteract these spikes. It's much less intimidating to help a diabetic prepare an insulin injection or provide a sweet snack if you've discussed the symptoms and what to do in advance.

People with Type 2 diabetes have a different set of treatment options. Sometimes, Type 2 diabetes can be controlled through diet and exercise alone. In many cases, though, the body needs help. In people with Type 2, the body doesn't make enough insulin or doesn't use the insulin it does make properly.

Oral medications can help the body reduce blood-sugar levels. There are three classes of drugs for Type 2. The first kind stimulates the body to produce more insulin. The second makes the body more sensitive to the insulin it does have. The third blocks the breakdown of starches and certain sugars, which slows the rise of blood-sugar levels. Sometimes people with Type 2 will take a combination of oral medications, or take pills in combination with insulin. For every person with Type 2, medication combined with improved nutrition and regular exercise is the best treatment.

A key part of self-treatment of diabetes is frequent blood-sugar testing. Pharmacies sell a variety of small blood glucose monitors and test strips that diabetics can (and should) carry with them. The diabetic places a drop of blood on the test strip and within a minute or so has a reading of the blood-sugar levels. The general goal is to achieve blood-sugar levels as close to normal as possible. People without diabetes generally maintain blood-sugar levels between 70 and 120 mg/dL before eating and less than 180 mg/dL after eating.

People with diabetes can also gauge how well they're controlling their blood sugar by taking a glycated hemoglobin test every three months. The test, done through a doctor's office, measures the presence of excess glucose in the blood over a three- or four-month period and gives a better picture of the effectiveness of the person's diabetes care than a single test on a glucose monitor.

Research has shown that the best way to avoid complications is to keep blood-sugar levels as close to normal as possible. A 10-year study that was completed in 1993 showed the benefits of tight control. The Diabetes Control and Complications Trial (DCCT) followed 1,441 people with Type 1 diabetes for several years. Half of the participants followed a standard diabetes treatment, while the other half followed an intensive-control regimen of multiple injections and frequent blood-sugar testing.

Those who followed the intensive-control regimen had significantly fewer complications. Only half as many developed signs of kidney disease, nerve disease was reduced by two-thirds, and only one-quarter as many developed diabetic eye disease.

Achieving tight control means taking several injections of insulin every day, or using an insulin pump to mimic the release of insulin that occurs in people without diabetes. It also means doing several blood tests a day to gauge how much insulin is needed.

Though the DCCT only followed people with Type 1, researchers believe tight control can have the same effect on people with Type 2. Since most people with Type 2 diabetes do not take insulin, they must take a different approach to tight control. Losing weight is one of the best ways to bring down glucose levels. Regular exercise helps, too, not only in bringing down weight but in helping to reduce glucose levels. A recent study of 1,263 men with Type 2 diabetes showed that, over 12 years, the men who did not exercise and stay active were more than twice as likely to die as those who exercised.

Tight control has obvious benefits, but it's not necessarily the right choice for everyone. The DCCT found that people who followed tight control had three times the number of low blood glucose episodes as those using conventional treatment. Plus, people using the tight control approach gained more weight than those on conventional treatment—an average of 10 pounds, according to the DCCT.

Those who should avoid tight control include people who already have complications; young children, whose developing brains need glucose; and the elderly, who can suffer strokes or heart attacks from episodes of hypoglycemia.

See also: Insulin; Obesity.

FURTHER READING

American Diabetes Association. www.diabetes.org.
National Diabetes Education Program. www.ndep.nih.gov/diabetes-facts/#howmany.
2011 National Diabetes Fact Sheet. Centers for Disease Control and Prevention. http://www.cdc.gov/diabetes/pubs/factsheet11.htm.

Dietary Fat

Dietary fat is the amount of fat consumed in the foods we eat. Numerous health and government authorities, including the U.S. Surgeon General, the National Academy of Sciences, the American Heart Association, and the American Dietetic Association, recommend reducing dietary fat to 30 percent or less of total calories.

See also: Calories; Fat.

FURTHER READING

"Dietary Fats Explained." National Institutes of Health. July 26, 2014. http://www.nlm.nih.gov/medlineplus/ency/patientinstructions/000104.htm

Dietary Guidelines for Americans

In 2015, the U.S. Department of Agriculture will release its revised Dietary Guidelines for Americans. These guidelines are revised every five years, based on new evidence and findings. However, the fundamentals don't change drastically. It's considered more of a refinement. For example, in 1995, the following were the seven dietary guidelines: eat a variety of foods; balance the foods you eat with physical activity—to maintain or improve your weight; choose a diet with plenty of grain products, vegetables, and fruits; choose a diet low in fat, saturated fat, and cholesterol; choose a diet moderate in sugars; choose a diet moderate in salt and sodium; and if you drink alcoholic beverages, do so in moderation.

The 2010 guidelines emphasized the following three major goals:

- Balance calories with physical activity to manage weight.
- Consume more of certain foods and nutrients such as fruits, vegetables, whole grains, fat-free and low-fat dairy products, and seafood.
- Consume fewer foods with sodium (salt), saturated fats, trans fats, cholesterol, added sugars, and refined grains.

A total of 23 key recommendations for the general population, and 6 additional guidelines for specific population groups (such as pregnant women) were part of the 2010 report.

The 2010 guidelines also recommend the following three healthy eating patterns:

- Select an eating pattern that meets nutrient needs over time at an appropriate calorie level.
- Account for all foods and beverages consumed and assess how they fit within a total healthy eating pattern.
- Follow food safety recommendations when preparing and eating foods to reduce the risk of foodborne illnesses.

The 2010 revision of the guidelines also addressed eating habits of children, noting that there is a "growing body of evidence documenting the vital role that optimal nutrition plays throughout the lifespan. Today, too many children are consuming diets with too many calories and not enough nutrients and are not getting enough physical activity. Approximately 32 percent of children and adolescents ages 2 to 19 years are overweight or obese, with 17 percent of children being obese.11 In addition, risk factors for adult chronic diseases are increasingly found in younger ages. Eating patterns established in child- hood often track into later life, making intervention on adopting healthy nutrition and physical activity behaviors a priority."

See also: Calories; Exercise; Obesity.

FURTHER READING

Dietary Guidelines for Americans 2010. www.dietaryguidelines.gov.

Dietary Supplement Health and Education Act (DSHEA)

President Bill Clinton signed the Dietary Supplement Health and Education Act (DSHEA) of 1994 into law on October 25, 1994. Congress included several provisions applying strictly to dietary supplements and their ingredients in the DSHEA, hoping to improve the earlier 1958 Food Additive Amendments to the federal Food, Drug, and Cosmetic Act (FD&C Act). In findings associated with

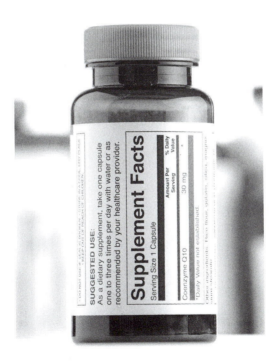

Research the ingredients in dietary supplements. Even natural ingredients can be harmful in large doses. In 2004, the government banned the sale of supplements containing ephedra. (Monticelllo/ Dreamstime)

the DSHEA, Congress stated that there may be a positive link between good dietary practice and good health, and there may also be a connection between dietary supplement use, reduced health care expenses, and disease prevention. The provisions of DSHEA are designed to ensure that safe and appropriately labeled products remain available to consumers by defining dietary supplements and dietary ingredients; establishing a new framework for assuring their safety; outlining literature guidelines to be displayed where supplements are sold; requiring ingredient and nutrition labeling; providing for use of claims and nutritional support statements; and granting the Food and Drug Administration (FDA) the authority to establish good manufacturing practice (GMP) regulations.

A dietary supplement is now formally defined as a product other than tobacco intended to supplement the diet that bears or contains one or more of the following ingredients: a vitamin; a mineral; an herb or other botanical; an amino acid; a dietary substance used to supplement the diet by increasing the total daily intake; or a concentrate, metabolite, constitute, extract, or combination of these ingredients. A dietary supplement, under the DSHEA, is intended for ingestion in pill, capsule, tablet, or liquid form; is not represented for use as a conventional food or as the sole item of a meal or diet; is labeled as a dietary supplement; includes products such as approved drugs, certified antibiotics, or licensed biologics that were marketed as a dietary supplement or food before approval, certification, or license.

The DSHEA also allows the secretary of Health and Human Services (HHS) to declare that a dietary supplement or dietary ingredient poses an imminent hazard to public health or safety. And the DSHEA restricts manufacturers from statements about the use of a dietary supplement to diagnose, prevent, mitigate, treat, or cure a specific disease.

Under the provisions of the DSHEA, the HHS Secretary may establish an office within the National Institutes of Health to explore the potential role of supplements to improve health care in the United States, to promote scientific study of supplements and their value in preventing chronic diseases, to collect scientific research, and to serve as a scientific adviser to the HHS and the FDA.

See also: Nutrition Facts Label.

FURTHER READING

Nestle, Marion. *Food Politics: How the Food Industry Influences Nutrition and Health.* Berkeley: University of California Press, 2007.

Dimethylamylamine HCl (DMAA)

Dimethylamylamine (DMAA) HCl is an amphetamine-like additive in some dietary supplements. DMAA can elevate blood pressure and could lead to cardiovascular problems, including heart attack, shortness of breath, and tightening of the chest, and it can be particularly dangerous when used with caffeine. In November 2013, the U.S. Food and Drug Administration (FDA) said the product is referred to on dietary supplements using 11 possible names: 1,3-DMAA; 1,3-dimethylamylamine; 1,3-dimethylpentylamine; 2-amino-4-methylhexane; 2-hexanamine, 4-methyl-2-hexanamine; 4-methyl-2-hexylamin; 4-methyl- (9CI); dimethylamylamine; geranamine; methylhexanamine; and methylhexaneamine. Products listing *Pelargonium graveolens* extract or Geranium extract might also contain DMAA.

The health nutrition chain GNC destroyed its supplements that contained DMAA, OxyElite Pro, and Jack3D, in July 2013.

In November 2013, scientists were trying to determine whether supplements with the ingredient *Acacia rigidula* contained DMAA. Extracts of *Acacia rigidula* leaves are used in weight-loss products sold in vitamin shops and over the Internet. In late 2013, press reports stated that the FDA scientists found an amphetamine-like compound in selected dietary supplements that included *Acacia rigidula* as an ingredient. The stimulant apparently is not found to be naturally occurring in the plant. However, press reports questioned whether these supplements contained DMAA, which has been flagged by the FDA as dangerous.

The FDA has a webpage exclusively devoted to DMAA that includes the variety of names of ingredients that might indicate DMAA.

http://www.fda.gov/Food/DietarySupplements/QADietarySupplements/ucm 346576.htm.

See also: Caffeine.

FURTHER READING

Press release. U.S. Marshals Seize More than $2 million in Adulterated Dietary Supplements from Georgia Company? In *FDA Acts to Prevent Distribution of Products Containing Unapproved Food Additive*. U.S. FDA, November 18, 2013. http://www.fda.gov/ NewsEvents/Newsroom/PressAnnouncements/ucm375458.htm.
Young, Alison. Nine Diet Supplements Contain Amphetamine-Like Compound. *USA Today*, November 18, 2013.

Dukan Diet

French nutritionist Pierre Dukan considers overweight and obesity to be a major health concern and he is doing everything he can to fight against it. He published his solution in 2000 and is now considered a weight-loss guru to the international audience. And if you ask millions of fans, his system is working. *The Dukan Diet* has been translated from French into English and 14 other languages, and sold millions of copies around the world as well as topping the *New York Times* best-seller list. Those rumored to have followed the diet include Catherine, the Duchess of Cambridge, her mother Carole Middleton, model Gisele Bundchen, and singer Jennifer Lopez.

Similar to the Atkins diet made popular by American Dr. Robert Atkins in the 1970s and 1980s and the South Beach created by Dr. Arthur Agatston in the 2000s, the Dukan diet kick-starts dieters with an intense protein-only phase. And like other high-protein diets, followers should expect to find themselves in a state of ketosis, thanks to the complete lack of carbohydrates.

Ketosis is a condition that occurs when the body does not have enough carbohydrates to burn for fuel. Without adequate carbohydrate sources, the body instead uses stored fat for energy. When the fat stores break down they create ketones, the small carbon fragments used as fuel. Ketosis can become serious if ketone levels get too high, something Atkins's followers used to monitor in the early stages of the diet.

The Dukan eating plan has four phases or stages that could be defined as mini-diets, the first known as the attack phase lasts for about five days and has dieters fill up on lots of high-protein foods along with plenty of water and oat bran to avoid constipation. Dukan provides a list of more than 60 acceptable high-protein foods including seafood and game meats. The second phase, for three days, is called the cruise phase, which allows mostly protein foods along with a small list of approved vegetables. The third stage, known as consolidation, should go on for three days for every pound the dieter wants to lose and reintroduces dairy and grain foods like cheese and bread. The last phase is the stabilization stage, when dieters are expected to resume normal eating, with the addition of oat bran every day as well as one day a week eating only protein foods.

Dukan, in discussing the success of his diet, suggests that other diet fail while his succeeds because it provides a structured plan, gives immediate results, and offers long-term support. However, Dukan's critics say his diet fails to teach healthy food habits and puts an emphasis on quick weight loss, often as much as seven pounds each week. The British Dietetic Association (BDA) named the Dukan diet the worst celebrity weight-loss plan of 2013. The BDA criticized how the diet cut out whole groups of foods, suggesting it was unhealthy for most people and dangerous for others. They also found fault with the amount of saturated fat in the form of protein foods, calling it a sure way to increase cholesterol levels. The association called on dieters to look for more long-term solutions that include a variety of healthy foods along with exercise.

The doctor has been harshly criticized by his French peers who accuse him of practicing medicine like a business with more interest in his personal fame than the health of his patients. Critics of Dukan's diet include members of the French National Order of Doctors, the British Medical Association, as well as members of its Paris branch. In a poll of former Dukan dieters, numbers indicate that as many as 80 percent regained the weight they lost in just three years.

See also: Atkins Nutritional Approach; South Beach Diet.

FURTHER READING

"The Dukan Diet: A Fad with a French Accent." *Prevention*, July 2011, 70.
"Dukan Diet Tops BDA List of 2013s Worst Celebrity Diets." *International Business Times*, November 22, 2012.
"The Middleton Diet." *Marie Claire* 18, no. 11 (November 2011): 228.
"Weighing in on the Dukan Diet: Don't Believe the Hype." *Food & Fitness Advisor* 14, no. 6 (June 2011): 5.
Willsher, Kim. "French Doctors Put Squeeze on Diet Guru." *The Guardian (London, England)*, March 27, 2012, News, 19. http://www.theguardian.com/world/2012/mar/26/dukan-diet-inventor-faces-censure.

Eat Right 4 Your Type

The Eat Right 4 Your Type diet plan suggests that there are four different ideal diets. One for blood type O people, one for blood type A, one for blood type B, and one for blood type AB. Peter J. D'Adamo wrote in the introduction to the 1996 book by the same name, stating that your blood type is the key to understanding much of what your body wants and needs. He breaks down foods into three categories—highly beneficial, neutral, or avoid—for each blood type. His suggestion is that people stop eating the avoid category foods for their blood type. However, people are encouraged to balance their diets by including selections from the neutral categories. "Eating only 'highly beneficial' foods and eliminating all others will result in too rapid a weight loss and an unhealthy diet," he writes.

He also suggests that some forms of exercise are more beneficial to certain blood types than others. As he writes in the book, "Your blood type plan lets you zero in on the health and nutrition that corresponds to your exact biological profile."

The type O diet, for example, should mimic the ancestral high-protein, hunter-gatherer diet, as type O blood was the earliest in the evolution. Type Os who adopt the Eat Right 4 Your Type diet plan will lose weight because they restrict the amount of grains, breads, legumes, and beans they consume. These foods encourage weight gain in type Os. Foods that encourage weight loss are seafood, red meat, liver, and some of the leafy green vegetables and kelp. Most meat and fish are either highly beneficial or neutral to type Os, although bacon, ham, pork, catfish, caviar, and some others should be avoided. Wheat products overall aren't recommended for this blood type; cereals and breads are generally considered neutral at best and the list of grains to avoid is long.

Type Os should exercise vigorously to relieve stress and to lose weight, if needed. Type Os "have the immediate and physical response of our hunter ancestors: stress goes directly to your muscles."

Type A people, however, are the descendants of the "more settled and less warlike farmer ancestors" and therefore, a vegetarian diet suits them best. Type As who cut meat out of their diets will lose weight rapidly "as you eliminate the toxic foods from your diet." That's because type As store their meat as fat. Most meat should be avoided; seafood can be substituted for red meats. Beans, grains, cereals, breads, vegetables, and fruit are staples of this diet. Stress relief for type As comes through "quieting techniques" such as yoga and meditation. Competitive sports "will only exhaust your nervous energy, make you tense all over again, and leave your immune system open to illness or disease."

The other two blood types are more difficult to peg. Type Bs, for example, display many of the characteristics of type Os, but show "a sophisticated refinement in the evolutionary journey, an effort to join together divergent peoples and cultures." Wheats and grains encourage weight gain; green vegetables, meats, eggs, and low-fat dairy products encourage weight loss. In terms of stress reduction and physical activity, type Bs again show their hybrid past, represented by "both barbarians and agrarians. . . . You're less confrontational than Type Os, but more physically charged than Type As." So physical activities should be a balance between the competitive and the psychic—group hiking, biking, tennis, and aerobics classes are suggested.

Type ABs, which make up only between 2 and 5 percent of the population, should take their cues from types A and B. Red meats and poultry should be limited; seafood is typically recommended. Tai chi, golf, walking, swimming, hiking, and low-impact aerobics are good for this group, according to the plan.

Eat Right 4 Your Type provides detailed suggestions for beneficial foods and those to avoid. It further specifies how often certain foods should be eaten, based on the individual's ethnic background. The chapters include menus, beneficial beverages, condiments, and listings of supplements that are best suited for each blood type.

In 2001, D'Adamo followed up with another book, *Live Right 4 Your Type*, suggesting that blood types are not just the key to diet, but the key to each individual's lifestyle. In this volume, D'Adamo lists the characteristics of certain blood types and develops "lifestyle strategies." For example, type Os are typically impulsive. Therefore, they shouldn't make big decisions when feeling stressed. Methodical eating is recommended—type Os should sit at the table for each meal and put down the fork and knife between bites. Physical activity is a good outlet for them.

Type As crave consistency in all aspects of their lives. Smaller more frequent meals suit them better. Type Bs also benefit from smaller, more frequent meals. They should seek out ways to connect to their community and find methods to express their nonconformity. Type ABs take their cues from a combination of other blood types—small, frequent meals; a combination of aerobic activity and relaxing techniques; and time alone and time spent with others are all recommended as lifestyle strategies for these people.

The eat right endeavor has expanded to an organization called D'Adamo Personalized Nutrition, where consumers can purchase books and supplements formulated for each blood type and also according to the GenoType (hunter-gatherer, teacher, explorer, warrior, or nomad). D'Adamo calls the GenoType the refinement of his work on blood types. The six genetic types given evolved differently and have different predispositions for weight loss/gain, immune function, disease propensity, and a comprehensive diet, exercise and life style profile tailored to fit their type.

The diet has its share of critics. *The Tufts University Health & Nutrition Letter* gave the diet plan an F. Even its fundamental philosophy of tracing blood types back to ancestors is flawed, the review said. "It is a fallacy even to speak of 'original' type Os or 'original' type As because blood types did not originate with humans," explains Stephen Bailey, PhD, a nutritional anthropologist at Tufts. "They came on the biologic scene long before humans did. Furthermore, there is no anthropologic evidence whatsoever that all prehistoric people with a particular blood type ate the same diet."

See also: Exercise; Paleo Diet.

FURTHER READING

D'Adamo, Peter J. *Change Your Genetic Destiny*. New York: Harmony, 2007.

D'Adamo, Peter J. *Live Right 4 Your Type*. New York: G. P. Putnam's Sons, 2001.

D'Adamo, Peter J., with Catherine Whitney. *Eat Right 4 Your Type*. New York: G. P. Putnam's Sons, 1996.

"Eat Right 4 Your Type." Book Review. *Tufts University Health & Nutrition Letter* 15, no. 6 (August 1997): 6.

Williams, Deirdre B., and John J. McMahon. "The Blood Type Diet: Latest Diet Scam." http://www.vegsource.com/articles/blood_hype.htm. Accessed June 12, 2003.

Eating Disorders

Anorexia nervosa and bulimia nervosa are eating disorders. Food and weight control are the avenues through which the eating disorders are expressed, but eating disorders aren't just about food. People with eating disorders often have issues with self-esteem, stress, fear of becoming overweight, and a feeling of helplessness. What they eat or don't eat becomes a tool of control, either as self-control or even control over others.

Researchers are not precisely sure of what causes eating disorders. They suspect these disorders may stem from a combination of factors—behavioral, genetic, and biochemical. People who develop anorexia often share some similar characteristics: they tend to be obedient, perfectionists, good students, and often excellent athletes. People who develop bulimia and binge eating often eat large amounts of junk food and then feel guilty about it. They eat to relieve stress, but the subsequent guilt increases stress. And the cycle continues.

See also: Anorexia Nervosa; Bulimia Nervosa.

FURTHER READING

Chang, Samantha. "More Men and Teens Suffer from the Eating Disorders Anorexia and Bulimia." *Examiner.com,* February 23, 2014. http://www.examiner.com/article/increase-eating-disorders-among-men-women-and-teens-a-cause-for-alarm.

Hartung, L. "Disordered Eating Patterns in Relation to Gender in the College Environment." *Journal of the American Dietetic Association* 97, no. 9 (1997): A-60.

Eicosanoids

Eicosanoids are powerful, hormone-like substances that help control many body processes, including the transfer of oxygen into muscles and the use of fat and carbohydrate as energy sources. Eicosanoids have very diverse effects and are extremely short lived and hard to study.

In the current culture and its obsession with thinness and weight loss, fats have almost been eliminated from our diet. However, the human body needs small amounts of two types of essential fatty acids that it cannot manufacture. The omega-3s include EPA and DHA. Top sources of omega-3 fats are fish high in oil, like salmon and mackerel. The average American consumes a minuscule one-quarter of a teaspoon of EPA and DHA daily. The second variety of omega-3 fatty acid is alpha-linolenic acid, which comes from plant foods and is then converted to EPA and DHA. Top sources of this fat are flaxseed oil and canola oil. Most average Americans consume less than a third of a teaspoon of alpha-linolenic acid per day.

The second variety of essential fatty acid the body needs is linolenic acid and it is plentiful in modern diets. In fact, today's foods are saturated with it in the form of vegetable oils like corn, soybean, and safflower oils, and it can be found in margarine, mayonnaise, and other processed foods; our current ratio of linolenic acid to the omega-3s is now 10 to 1. Scientists say early diets had a ratio of 1 or 2 to 1, which amounted to a more equal balance between the two essential fats.

What scientists now suspect is that when the linolenic acid predominates, as it does today, and when omega-3s are in short supply, this affects the kind of eicosanoids our bodies produce as well as the overall health of our cardiovascular and immune systems. Eicosanoids that lack omega-3s tend to provoke inflammation, blood clots, and so forth. This has led to the label of "good" or "bad" eicosanoids.

Researchers are now examining the role of omega-3 fatty acids in our diet and their effects on cell functions. In November 2000, based on the strength of current omega-3 research, the FDA determined that manufacturers could promote evidence that omega-3 supplements may reduce the risk of coronary heart disease.

While research continues, some diet promoters have taken that need for essential fatty acids and turned it to their own advantage by calling for diets higher in protein and lower in carbohydrates than what nutritionists and health experts suggest. For example, in his book *The Zone*, Dr. Barry Sears supports a daily intake of 30 percent fat, 30 percent protein, and 40 percent carbohydrates. He says that ratio will cause weight loss while at the same time it will keep eicosanoids in balance. By eating this way, dieters are in what he calls "the Zone." His theory also claims that the traditional carbohydrate-rich American diet dramatically raises the level of insulin in the bloodstream, which in turn influences the production of too many "bad" and not enough "good" eicosanoids.

Even though critics call this an oversimplification of the problem, there is agreement that it is just as unhealthy to eliminate all fat from the diet as it is to eat those fats to excess. So even though not everyone agrees on the numbers, they all agree that a balanced ratio of fats in the diet is essential for normal growth and development and good health.

See also: Sears, Barry; The Zone.

FURTHER READING

Lawrence, Ronald M. "Fat in the Diet: How to Retain the 'Good' Fats and Avoid the 'Bad.'" *Total Health*, March 1, 2001, 50.
McCord, Holly, R.D., and Teresa Yeykal. "The Fat You Need: Can This Forgotten Nutrient Ward Off Illness from Head to Toe?" *Prevention*, January 1, 1997, 100–104.

Ephedra/Ephedrine

Ephedrine is a drug from the plants of the genus *Ephedra*, and is promoted in many herbal diet remedies as a "natural" weight-loss product. Derived from a Chinese herb called ma huang, ephedra is a stimulant, used for short-term energy boosts to enhance athletic performance and endurance, to help people exercise longer and feel more alert, to increase metabolism, and to dampen or suppress appetite. Ephedra has been an ingredient in several popular diet supplements, including Metabolife, Diet Pet, and Dexatrim, all part of the multibillion-dollar weight-loss industry.

In February 2004, the U.S. FDA prohibited the sale of dietary supplements containing ephedrine alkaloids (ephedra), saying the supplements present an unreasonable risk of illness and injury.

Research published in the December 2000 issue of the *New England Journal of Medicine* outlined serious complications from dietary supplements containing ephedra, including 10 deaths, 32 heart attacks, 62 cases of cardiac arrhythmia, 91 reports of hypertension, 69 strokes, and 70 seizures. Those figures were compiled between 1993 and 2000. Another possible problem with ephedrine, according to researchers, is that the human body may convert ephedra to PPA, short for phenylpropanolamine, an ingredient the FDA banned after it was shown to increase the risk of a kind of stroke in young women. Although the FDA has taken no formal action, in 1997 the agency called for ephedra labeling recommending that daily consumption be held to 24 milligrams. The agency also suggested that users take the supplements no more than seven days in response to studies showing that users who take ephedrine-containing supplements may develop a tolerance to it and must take more of the supplement to achieve the same effect.

The alarm over ephedra use rose after the drug was considered a factor in the death of several high-profile athletes such as Steve Bechler, a 23-year-old minor-league baseball player who collapsed and died while training with the Baltimore Orioles in February 2003. Bechler had been taking a weight-loss supplement containing ephedra at the time of his death. Illinois governor Rod Blagojevich signed the first statewide ban on ephedra use into law in May 2003 after the death of a 16-year-old high school football player. The governor has urged other states and the federal government to adopt similar bans.

Health organizations, businesses, and professional athletes have all started to distance themselves from the use of ephedra. Nutritional supplement retailer General Nutrition Centers announced in May 2003 that it would stop selling products containing ephedra. Following Bechler's death, minor-league baseball officials took steps to stop their players from using supplements with ephedra, a restriction already in place for professional and college football players as well as for NCAA and Olympic athletes. Ephedra was considered a factor in the deaths of college football players Rashidi Wheeler and Devaughn Darling and Minnesota Viking Korey Stringer. One baseball agent quoted in the March 2003 *Sporting News* estimated that 75 percent of ball players use ephedrine.

The American Medical Association continues its efforts to remove ephedra from the market. Following Bechler's death, Health and Human Services secretary Tommy G. Thompson called for warnings on ephedra labels and for a ban on its use. The American Heart Association has also been vocal in its opposition to supplements containing ephedra.

Researchers also caution that supplements containing ephedrine and caffeine, when used in combination, can produce dangerous side effects similar to those of the banned drug methamphetamine. Those side effects include insomnia, restlessness, euphoria, palpitations or cardiac arrhythmia, high blood pressure, strokes, and seizures. The information, featured in the December 2000 issue of the *New England Journal of Medicine,* prompted critics to call for a halt in the production and sale of dietary supplements containing ephedrine alkaloids, charging they increase the already apparent risk for heart attacks, strokes, seizures, and hypertension. Industry officials, quoted in a 2001 article in *Drug Topics*, maintain that the 200 products containing ephedra aimed at U.S. dieters and bodybuilders are not a health risk. However, in response to the continuing controversy, some of those manufacturers are now marketing an ephedra-free version of their product, such as Metabolife and Dexatrim. Nutritionists say the safest way to increase metabolism is to increase physical activity.

See also: Dexatrim; Metabolife.

FURTHER READING

Brink, Susan. "Diet Drugs: What a Pill." *U.S. News & World Report*, November 20, 2000, 74.

The Columbia Encyclopedia. 6th ed. New York: Columbia University Press, 2000.

Conlan, Michael F. "Consumer Groups Want FDA to Ban Dietary Supplements with Ephedra." *Drug Topics* 145, no. 18 (September 17, 2001): 18.

Haller, C.A., and N.L. Benowitz. "Adverse Cardiovascular and Central Nervous System Events Associated with Dietary Supplements Containing Ephedra Alkaloids." *New England Journal of Medicine* 343, no. 25 (December 21, 2000): 1833–38.

http://www.fda.gov/NewsEvents/Newsroom/PressAnnouncements/2004/ucm108242.htm.

Rosenthal, Ken. "No More Delays on Drug Testing." *The Sporting News* 227, no. 9 (March 3, 2003): 50–52.

Smith, Ian K. "The Trouble with Fat-Burner Pills: Be Suspicious of the Dramatic Weight-Loss Claims of These Supplements." *Time*, August 27, 2001, 66.

U.S. Food and Drug Administration. "Final Rule Declaring Dietary Supplements Containing Ephedrine Alkaloids Adulterated Because They Present an Unreasonable Risk." *Federal Register* 69, no. 28 (2004): 6788–6854.

Exercise

Trying to lose weight without increasing your level of physical activity is like driving a car with no gas in the tank. You may roll forward a little, but you're not really going to get anywhere. Remember that a pound equals 3,500 calories. So to lose a pound in, say, a week, you'll either have to eat 3,500 calories less or burn off 3,500 calories in exercise, or some combination of the two. Some combination of the two is easier and healthier in the long run.

Exercise burns calories. While the specific rate at which you burn calories depends on your weight and the intensity with which you perform the activity, here are some examples of calorie-burning activities. Walking briskly can burn off about 100 calories per mile. Bicycling for a half-hour at nearly 10 mph will burn about 195 calories. Experts recommend at least 30 minutes of vigorous activity five days a week. If you can't find 30 minutes, try two 15-minute intervals, or even three 10-minute intervals. And realize that what's vigorous for a sedentary person is different from a vigorous workout for an athlete. Work at your own pace.

In 2008, the U.S. Department of Health and Human Services issued its *Physical Activity Guidelines for Americans*. The guidelines describe the major research findings on exercise and physical activity. According to the guidelines:

- Regular physical activity reduces the risk of many adverse health outcomes.
- Some physical activity is better than none.
- For most health outcomes, additional benefits occur as the amount of physical activity increases through higher intensity, greater frequency, and/or longer duration.
- Most health benefits occur with at least 150 minutes (2 hours and 30 minutes) a week of moderate-intensity physical activity, such as brisk walking. Additional benefits occur with more physical activity.
- Both aerobic (endurance) and muscle-strengthening (resistance) physical activities are beneficial.
- Health benefits occur for children and adolescents, young and middle-aged adults, older adults, and those in every studied racial and ethnic group.
- The health benefits of physical activity occur for people with disabilities.
- The benefits of physical activity far outweigh the possibility of adverse outcomes.

Specifically, the guidelines emphasize four guidelines for adults: avoid inactivity; engage in a minimum of 150 minutes of moderate-intensity activity or 75 minutes of vigorous-intensity activity every week; recognize that more activity results in greater benefits; and include muscle-strengthening exercises.

In 1998, the American College of Sports Medicine (ACSM) created a new Physical Activity Pyramid. It's similar in design to the nutritional pyramid, with the bottom or base, showing the activities that should be performed the most. The pyramid narrows, with less vigorous activity being required less often.

The base of the pyramid, or the bottom level, is "everyday activities," which could include walking, house or yard work, outdoor play, and walking the dog. These bottom-level activities should total 30 minutes done most days of the week. While that satisfies the basic requirement, there's much more people can do to become fit.

The second level of the pyramid is divided between active aerobics and sports and recreation, which should be done at least three times a week. These are more vigorous activities, which involve speeding up the heart rate. These activities could involve aerobic exercises, basketball, tennis, bicycling, soccer, jump roping, and hiking. Because these activities elevate the heart rate, three 20-minute intervals per week have about the same health benefits as the activities done every day.

The third level of the pyramid is divided into flexibility and muscle fitness exercises, which should be done two or three times a week. These activities improve motion and flexibility and include golf, bowling, softball, and yard work. Muscle strength activities include stretching, light weight-lifting, push-ups, curl ups, and gymnastics. The ACSM recommends that people exercise each major muscle group three to seven days a week and stretch to the point of mild discomfort, but not pain. For strength, the ACSM recommends doing muscle fitness exercises for each major muscle group two or three days a week with a day of rest in between.

The top level of the pyramid is inactivity. Remember that in the nutritional pyramid, fats and sugars are at this level. Some are required, but they shouldn't be the mainstay of one's diet. Likewise in the activity pyramid, inactivity should be the exception, not the rule. Inactivity should be a small portion of your day—and no more than 30 minutes at a time.

See also: Aerobic Activity; Anaerobic Activity.

FURTHER READING

Physical Activity Guidelines for Americans. www.health.gov/PAGuidelines/guidelines/.

Fat

The reason many people start an exercise program or diet is to lose weight—particularly fat. It's an excellent strategy, and combined with proper nutrition and diet, it should begin to show results fairly soon. Every human body has some fat in

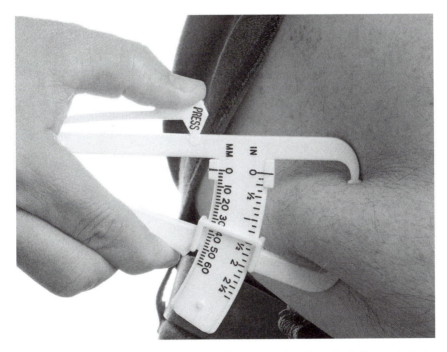

Fat calipers are one device used to measure body fat. A simple scale and calculations for body mass index are other easy-to-use ways to measure weight loss. (jimd_stock/iStockphoto.com)

it. A healthy adult male's body should have about 12 to 18 percent fat. Healthy adult females have a slightly higher body fat composition—about 15 to 22 percent fat. Fitness centers often offer body composition tests using calipers or pinchers. People can buy these in fitness and sports stores, too. It's a painless test measuring a fold of skin in several places on your body. Fat lies just below skin level. By measuring a small fold of skin, these calipers can measure how much fat is accumulated. It's a more precise measure of body composition than a simple weigh-in.

However, the bathroom or exercise-room scale is still a good indicator, too. Remember, though, that muscle weighs more than fat. So a person beginning to exercise, turning fat into muscle, may not see as dramatic a weight loss. Don't let that deter you, though. What you'll see and feel is a transformation of your body that will be longer lasting and easier to maintain.

Here's how exercise helps burn fat. Let's say you eat 2,000 calories worth of food. But your physical activity only uses 1,500 of these. The extra calories are stored in your body—as fat. When you exercise, your body uses fuel that comes from one of two forms: stored carbohydrates called glycogen and stored body fat. Stored body fat is found in fat cells and is also stored in small droplets in the muscles.

Most activities use both carbohydrates and fat for fuel. Lower intensity workouts, such as walking, use fat as the primary fuel. As the workout intensifies, the fuel reserves come increasingly from carbohydrates. But that doesn't mean that walking burns more fat than running. When the carbohydrate or glycogen source runs low, the body releases fats for fuels. Also, a higher intensity workout, such as running, continues to burn fat even after the physical activity itself is over. As the body works to restore glycogen, it continues to use fat to do so. And because higher intensity workouts burn more calories overall, even though the mix of carbohydrates and fats may be different, you're still burning more fat in the workout.

It's not necessary to create a workout regimen that burns the most fat when you're starting out. Create an exercise program that you like and can stick with. As long as you keep using more calories than you consume and start getting those muscle groups active, you will burn fat, strengthen your muscles and your heart, feel better, and lose weight.

See also: Calories; Dietary Fat; Exercise.

FURTHER READING

"Dietary Fats: Know Which Types to Choose." Mayo Clinic. www.mayoclinic.org/healthy-living/nutrition-and-healthy-eating/in-depth/fat/art-20045550.

Fat Blockers

Imagine a product that lets dieters eat exactly what they want, including cake, pie, candy, and cookies, and still lose weight. Fat blockers, another weapon in the war against obesity, promise "miracles" but deliver health problems.

During the early 1990s, Cal-Ban 3000, a fat blocker, was advertised as an automatic weight-loss solution. Made of guar gum, a soluble fiber used in small amounts as a thickener in sauces, desserts, syrups, and other processed foods, the pills were supposed to decrease appetite and block absorption of fat. Instead, the fiber in Cal-Ban 3000 swelled four or five times its original size and created havoc for users. The Food and Drug Administration (FDA) received reports of at least 17 cases of esophageal obstruction among users. According to the FDA, at least 10 of those people with obstructions were hospitalized; one reportedly died. Other side effects included stomach obstruction and intestinal blockages, along with nausea and vomiting.

Guar gum is a complex sugar that swells when wet, forms a gel in the stomach, and can create a feeling of fullness. But, unfortunately, in the case of Cal-Ban 3000, the guar gum stuck in the wrong places, in the throat and intestines, forming dangerous obstructions. And critics say that along with the obvious health risks, taking fat blockers does not help those overweight people who eat even when they feel full.

According to the FDA Consumer, the FDA had been moving to ban guar gum and some 100 other diet products, whose ingredients had not been proven when reports of serious problems with Cal-Ban 3000 prompted them to halt its distribution. Guar gum is still considered safe for use in small amounts in foods like salad dressings, cheese, and ice cream where it acts as a stabilizer, thickener, or binder.

Chitosan is another fat blocker used in weight-loss supplements. Made from the chitin, the outer skeleton of shellfish such as shrimp, lobster, and crabs, chitosan allegedly works as a "fat magnet," according to manufacturers, by binding fats in the stomach and preventing them from being digested and absorbed. The fat is then theoretically excreted via the body's feces.

A study by Judith Stern, a nutrition researcher at the University of California at Davis, showed that chitosan products have no weight-loss value. The results of her study, reported in the May 2001 issue of the American Journal of Clinical Nutrition, evaluated subjects taking daily doses of chitosan. Stern measured no change in fecal fat content, debunking the claim that chitosan blocked and then excreted large amounts of dietary fat.

Stern is cofounder of the American Obesity Association and a member of the obesity task force of the National Institute for Diabetes and Digestive and Kidney Diseases. The Napa County, California, district attorney's office partially funded Stern's study and later used the results to bring charges against Enforma, the manufacturer of Fat Trapper Plus, a fat blocker containing chitosan. The company was accused of making false advertising claims and they eventually settled with the government, paying $10 million to the Federal Trade Commission, to be returned to consumers who purchased the product or to the U.S. treasury if that repayment was impractical.

Interest in chitosan as a weight-loss aid grew dramatically in 1997 with the publication of The Fat Blocker Diet. Written by Dr. Arnold Fox, the best seller instructs dieters to eat a healthful diet, exercise, practice positive thinking, and take "something extra, a little lift" of chitosan to help start their weight loss and to keep them going through difficult periods. Fox maintains that chitosan helps dieters avoid any slowing of metabolism, which routinely occurs during low-calorie diets. Instead, Fox suggests that because users do not cut down on calories there is no corresponding message to the body to slow its metabolism. Instead, calorie levels are cut simply because fat is not being digested or absorbed as it was before the dieter took chitosan. Fox tells dieters to follow the U.S. Department of Agriculture Food Guide Pyramid (now MyPlate) and to eat the recommended daily servings of grains, vegetables, and fruits, and drink at least eight glasses of water per day. He recommends a daily intake of no more than 20 percent of calories from fat, 10 percent from protein, and 70 percent from carbohydrates. In other words, he calls for a basic high-fiber, low-fat eating plan with the addition of daily chitosan supplements. He also goes on to warn against fad diets and provides an eating disorder questionnaire for readers who may show early signs of eating disorders such as anorexia nervosa or bulimia. He recommends they see a physician or registered dietitian before using his diet or taking chitosan.

See also: Anorexia Nervosa; Food Guide Pyramid; MyPlate, Starch Blockers; Xenical.

FURTHER READING

Barrett, Stephen. "Be Wary of Calorie-Blockers." www.quackwatch.com.

"Better Not Swallow This: Accident Potential of Guar Gum." *Tufts University Diet & Nutrition Letter* 8, no. 9 (November 1990): 7.

Fox, Arnold. *The Fat Blocker Diet*. New York: St. Martin's Press, 1997.

"Guar Gum Diet Products under Investigation." *FDA Consumer* 24, no. 8 (October 1990): 3–5.

Healy, Melissa. "Next Miracle Fat Blocker? Grapefruit Derivative Promotes Weight Loss, Stabilizes Blood Sugar in Mice." *Los Angeles Times,* July 13, 2009. www.latimesblogs .latimes.com/booster_shots/2009/07/next-miracle-fatblocker-grapefruitderivative-promotes-weight-loss-stabilizes-blood-sugar-.html.

Wallace, Phil. "Study Finds Chitosan Doesn't Block or Trap Fat." *Food Chemical News* 43, no. 5 (March 19, 2001): 11.

Feingold Diet

While most people think of diet plans as a way to lose weight, some diets have different purposes. For example, the Feingold diet program is based on the concept that certain foods can affect behavior—particularly attention deficit hyperactivity disorder (ADHD), which affects either 3 to 5 percent of school-aged children or as many as 17 percent of school-aged children, depending on the source. ADHD is commonly treated with stimulants such as Ritalin. In 1974, Dr. Benjamin Feingold wrote the book *Why Your Child Is Hyperactive*, espousing what was then called "KP" or the "Kaiser-Permanente" diet—named after the medical center where he practiced and taught. In 1979, Dr. Feingold and his wife wrote *The Feingold Cookbook,* at which time the name Feingold diet began to stick.

The diet program is based on the idea that some people have difficulty tolerating salicylates, natural chemicals made by many plants and chemically related to aspirin. The program also states that other common additives and preservatives can also be difficult to tolerate. This intolerance can show itself in many ways, according to Dr. Feingold and his supporters—including symptoms of ADHD, and other behavioral or physical problems sometimes associated with ADHD, such as bedwetting, asthma, sleep disorders, and frequent ear infections.

Salicylates occur naturally in some fruits such as apples and oranges, and they are synthetic additives to other foods or products. Some people are intolerant of only a few different salicylates; others are intolerant of many different kinds. Therefore, the diet program starts by eliminating most salicylate foods and products at the beginning and reintroducing some slowly as behavior or other symptoms improve. The program also calls for eliminating artificial food dyes and flavors, which are petroleum-based additives, and petroleum-based preservatives, such as BHA, BHT, and TBHQ. Eliminating foods and products with these additives will generally show results in one to four weeks, according to the Web site. Younger children typically respond more quickly.

The Feingold program offers participants a food list, a shopping guide with acceptable name brand products. On the Feingold Association Web site it explains that the level of salicylates in foods cannot simply be determined by looking at the Nutrition Facts label or the product contents. For example, Eggo Homestyle Waffles are not acceptable, but Eggo Buttermilk Waffles are, the site says. Sugar isn't restricted, but corn syrup, which is more processed and chemical-laden, is. In fact, the Web site notes that some children who overdo their consumption of candy and seem pumped up on sugar may instead be reacting to the corn syrup, a common ingredient in some candy.

While the Web site offers information about the program and many research links, it doesn't provide someone with the details he or she needs to get started on the program. For that, U.S. members pay $77 for a Foodlist and Shopping Guide and regular updates about new product tests and research. There's also a 393-page companion book, *Why Can't My Child Behave?*

While the Feingold Web site is filled with testimonials from harried parents who say they've been able to take their children off other medication, or have seen marked improvement in behavior and demeanor since starting the diet, there are critics who say the underlying premise that food additives are the root cause of these problems has not been adequately determined.

On the "pro-Feingold" side are the nonprofit Center for Science in the Public Interest, which issued a 32-page report in 1999 titled, "Diet, ADHD, and Behavior." The report cites 17 controlled studies that found that diet can adversely affect behavior. It also cites six studies that did not detect any change in behavior when a child's diet was changed. In the report, Dr. Marvin Boris, a pediatrician and author of a 1994 study, found that diet affected the behavior of two-thirds of his subjects. "It makes a lot more sense to try modifying a child's diet before treating him or her with a stimulant drug. Health organizations and professionals should recognize that avoiding certain foods and additives could greatly benefit some troubled children."

Among criticism of the program are those studies that show no behavioral changes based on diet. The opposition is summarized in an article by Stephen Barrett, MD, "The Feingold Diet: Dubious Benefits, Subtle Risks." Dr. Barrett writes that, "Because the Feingold diet does no physical harm, it might appear to be helpful in some instances. However, the potential benefits should be weighed against the potential harm of (1) teaching children that their behavior and school performance are related to what they eat rather than what they feel, (2) undermining their self esteem by implanting notions that they are unhealthy and fragile, (3) creating situations in which their eating behavior or fear of chemicals are regarded as peculiar by other children, and (4) depriving them of the opportunity to receive appropriate professional help."

A fact sheet from the Web site of Children and Adults with Attention-Deficit/Hyperactivity Disorder lists the Feingold diet as a controversial treatment for ADHD. It says, "Over the years, proponents of the Feingold Diet have made many dramatic claims. They state that the diet—which promotes the elimination of most additives from food—will improve most (if not all) children's learning and attention problems. In the past 15 years, dozens of well-controlled studies published in peer-reviewed journals have consistently failed to find support for the Feingold diet. While a few studies have reported some limited success with this approach, at best this suggests that there may be a very small group of children who are responsive to additive-free diets. At this time, it has not been shown that dietary intervention offers significant help to children with learning and attention problems."

The good news for parents of children or young adults diagnosed with ADHD is that research into this condition is continuing and seems to be taking a more holistic approach than purely pharmaceutical approach.

See also: Nutrition Facts Label.

FURTHER READING

Jaslow, Ryan. "ADHD Diet Study Suggests Healthy Eating Might Help Kids." *CBS News,* January 9, 2012. http://www.cbsnews.com/news/adhd-diet-study-suggests-healthy-eating-might-help-kids/.

Rowe, K. S., and K. J. Rowe. "Diagnosis and Treatment of Attention Deficit Hyperactivity Disorder." *NIH Consensus Statement Online* 16, no. 2 (November 16–18, 1998): 1–37.

Rowe, K. S., and K. J. Rowe. "Synthetic Food Coloring and Behavior: A Dose Response Effect in a Double-Blind, Placebo-Controlled, Repeated-Measures Study." *Journal of Pediatrics* 125 (1994): 691–98.

Williams, J. I., D. M. Cram, F. T. Tausig, and E. Webster. "Relative Effects of Drugs and Diet on Hyperactive Behaviors: An Experimental Study." *Pediatrics* 61, no. 6 (1978): 811.

Fen-Phen

Fen-phen, a popular combination of the diet drugs fenfluramine and phentermine, sounded almost too good to be true when dieters first discovered the powerful duo. And the pills were a huge success right up until their dangerous side effects prompted the U.S. Food and Drug Administration (FDA) to call for their removal in 1997. While the drugs were supposed to be prescribed for seriously obese patients, doctors wrote millions of prescriptions for women who only wanted to lose a few pounds. Unfortunately, many of those women lost more than weight, some suffered permanent heart damage while others died from a rare lung disease.

In fact, from 1995 until September 1997, before fenfluramine and dexfenfluramine were taken off the market, an estimated 14 million prescriptions were written for them. FDA statistics also show that up to a total of 4.7 million people were eventually exposed to these deadly diet drugs. Finally, on September 15, 1997, the FDA announced that some 30 percent of patients taking the weight-loss pills had developed a fatal form of heart-valve disease. Manufacturers immediately pulled the drugs from the shelves.

Although fenfluramine was regularly combined with phentermine, another diet drug, to produce the popular fen-phen combination, it was the "fen" that was eventually singled out as the problem. No one taking phentermine alone developed any signs of the disease. Dexfenfluramine, sold under the brand name Redux, was the other deadly diet pill identified by the FDA. It had entered the market in 1996 when manufacturers refined fenfluramine into just its serotonin-stimulating portion, and removed the part that caused extreme drowsiness in users. The diet pills were developed to increase the amount of serotonin, a neurotransmitter released by the brain. This would then suppress a dieter's appetite.

Phentermine was first introduced to dieters in 1959 but was not immediately popular because of its side effects, which included inability to sleep, jitteriness, and constipation. Fenfluramine appeared on the market, approved for short-term obesity treatment, in 1973. Although fenfluramine helped some dieters, its side effects of extreme drowsiness and diarrhea held its popularity in check. But their use rose dramatically in 1992 when the results of a government-funded study published in the journal *Clinical Pharmacology & Therapeutics* showed that the two diet drugs given in combination canceled each other's unappealing side effects. Best of all the fen-phen combination doubled the weight loss of study participants when added to a diet and exercise program.

Meanwhile, in 1996, dexfenfluramine received FDA approval for use in obese patients for one year or less. The pills had already been taken by European dieters for about a year with no unmanageable side effects. Redux, like the earlier fen-phen combination, was hailed as a revolutionary breakthrough in weight management and doctors wrote tens of thousands of prescriptions for the medications every week.

Until the reports of heart-valve disease surfaced, the only serious side effect of fenfluramine or Redux had been a rare but fatal type of primary pulmonary hypertension or lung condition known as PPH, which occurred in those taking the drugs for more than three months. In PPH the arteries taking blood from the heart to the lungs thicken, creating high blood pressure in the lungs. Diseases like emphysema or chronic bronchitis typically cause this. But now PPH was showing up in dieters who had no previous history of lung disease but who were taking Redux or fenfluramine. Still, at the time any risk involved with taking the drugs seemed small compared with the serious health problems caused by obesity. And even after the risks of taking fen-phen and Redux were known, patients were willing to continue using the drugs because of the success they experienced. At the time there were few comparable diet drugs on the market. Since then manufacturers developed other obesity drugs like Meridia, which was removed from the market in October 2010, and Xenical. Xenical, and its non-prescription, lower-dosage related medication Alli, works by preventing the body from absorbing up to 30 percent of ingested fat but side effects include loose, fatty stools and an urgency to urinate.

Initial concerns about fen-phen's safety came from doctors who detected new heart-valve damage in patients with previously diagnosed heart disease who were also taking the diet drugs. Soon, researchers started finding fen-phen users with no previous heart disease were developing leaky heart valves. As evidence about the severity of the problem grew, the FDA issued new warnings. More and more cases of the rare valve disease were being reported. These reports and a Mayo Clinic study about the valvular disease were described in the August 28, 1997, *New England Journal of Medicine*. A few of the patients with newly diagnosed heart-valve abnormalities were so ill they required valve-replacement surgery. Two weeks before the Mayo Clinic study results were released, Jenny Craig Weight Loss Centres stopped staff doctors from prescribing dexfenfluramine (Redux) over concerns about the drug's side effects.

In calling for voluntary withdrawal of the diet drugs, Michael A. Friedman, the FDA's Lead Deputy Commissioner, said the data indicated that "fenfluramine and the chemically closely related dexfenfluramine, present an unacceptable risk to patients who take them." The FDA recommended that patients stop taking the pills and contact their doctors to be tested for heart and lung disease and to discuss treatment. The Department of Health and Human Services also announced its own list of recommendations for patients who had taken the drugs.

In 2000, the largest wrongful death award in the history of Massachusetts was given to the family of a woman whose death was linked to fen-phen. Although the settlement figure was not disclosed, until this time the highest award in the state was $7 million. The settlement also asked for a substantial portion of the damages to fund a foundation, set up by the patient's family, to study and treat primary pulmonary hypertension (PPH). Although the woman only took fen-phen for 11 days, she developed the incurable and fatal PPH, a side effect strongly linked to fenfluramine.

More recent studies show that some 30 percent of those who took dexfenfluramine alone or took fenfluramine in the fen-phen combination developed heart-valve disease, and the longer dieters used the drugs, the more likely they were to become sick. Sadly, researchers have also found that the majority of those who lost weight with Redux or fen-phen gained it back once the drugs were no longer available.

See also: Jenny Craig; Xenical.

FURTHER READING

Cowley, Geoffrey, and Karen Springen. "After Fen-Phen." *Newsweek,* September 29, 1997, 46–49.

"Fen-Phen Maker AHP Settles Lawsuits." *Claims,* March 2000, 18.

Levine, Hallie. "Fen-Phen Killed My Wife." *Cosmopolitan,* December 1997, 196–200.

Rover, Elena. "Rethinking Diet Pills." *Ladies Home Journal,* March 1997, 60.

Stapleton, Stephanie. "Diet Drugs: Problems and Prospects." *American Medical News,* November 9, 1998, 31.

Ukens, Carol. "Fat's in the Fire: Obesity Drugs Pose Weighty Problems for Pharmacists." *Drug Topics* 141, no. 7 (April 7, 1997): 54–56.

Welch, Christine B. "The Miracle that Wasn't: Fen-Phen and Redux." *Diabetes Forecast* 51, no. 4 (April 1998): 40–46.

Five a Day

Five a Day for Better Health is the healthy eating program spearheaded by the National Cancer Institute (NCI). The goal is to encourage Americans to eat at least five servings of fruits and vegetables per day. The effort includes government and private industry sources, including the U.S. Department of Agriculture and the Centers for Disease Control and Prevention. The actual recommendation is that women should eat at least seven and men should eat at least nine servings of fruits and vegetables each day. They add, however, that it's relatively easy to do. For example, the sliced onion on a sandwich counts or a healthy salad with a variety of greens and sliced vegetables would count as several servings in one.

In 2002, the NCI added the concept that these fruits and vegetables should cover the range of color with its "Savor the Spectrum" campaign.

By selecting fruits and vegetables from different color groups, people can get a wider range of phytochemicals—disease-fighting substances found in foods. Specifically, here are the benefits available in different colors of the spectrum.

Blue and purple fruits and vegetables have either anthocyanins or phenolics. Anthocyanins are antioxidants that help control high blood pressure and protect against diabetes-related circulatory problems. Anthocyanins and phenolics help reduce the risk of cancer, heart disease, and Alzheimer's disease, and they may even slow down the aging process. The best sources of anthocyanins are blackberries, blueberries, elderberries, purple grapes, and black currants. The best sources of phenolics are prunes, plums, raisins, and eggplant.

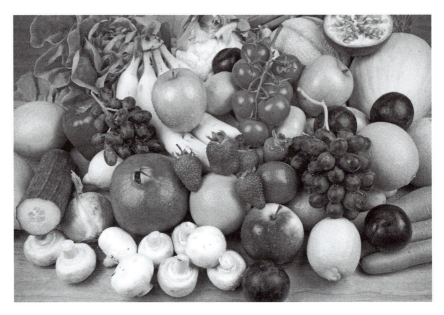

Aim for five servings of fruits and vegetables each day. Select from different color groups to get the widest variety of nutrients. (Dreamstime.com)

Green fruits and vegetables provide two more important phytochemicals—lutein and indoles. Lutein is an antioxidant that has been connected with better eye health. Lutein helps reduce the risk of forming cataracts and macular degeneration, both of which can cause vision loss in older people. The best sources of lutein can be found in green leafy vegetables such as turnip, collard, and mustard greens; kale; romaine lettuce; green peas; kiwi fruit; spinach; broccoli; and honeydew melon. Cruciferous vegetables—broccoli, cauliflower, cabbage, and brussels sprouts—are excellent sources of indoles, phytochemicals that are linked to a lower risk of breast cancer and prostate cancer. One study showed a 42-percent reduction in the risk of prostate cancer for men who ate cruciferous vegetables at least three times a week. Other sources of indoles are rutabaga, watercress, kale, arugula, turnips, cabbage, bok choy, and Swiss chard.

Deep orange and bright yellow fruits and vegetables contain two other phytochemicals: beta-carotene and bioflavonoids. Beta-carotene, the antioxidant that has been linked to a reduction in cancer risk and heart disease, also boosts the body's immune system and helps maintain eye health. Excellent sources of beta-carotene are mangoes, sweet potatoes, cantaloupe, peaches, carrots, apricots, butternut squash, and pumpkin. Bioflavonoids work together with vitamin C to improve overall health and heart health, reduce the risk of cancer, strengthen bones and teeth, and contribute to more rapid wound healing. Best sources of bioflavonoids are oranges, tangerines, peaches, pears, yellow pepper, grapefruit, clementines, nectarines, pineapple, lemons, apricots, papaya, and yellow raisins.

Red fruits and vegetables—from deep red to bright pink—contain lycopene and anthocyanins. Lycopene has been linked to a reduced cancer risk. Good sources of lycopene are watermelons, pink grapefruits, fresh tomatoes, and tomato-based products, such as spaghetti sauce, tomato paste, and tomato juice. Red fruits and vegetables that are good sources of anthocyanins include red raspberries, sweet cherries, strawberries, cranberries, beets, red apples, red cabbage, red onion, kidney beans, and red beans.

Even white vegetables—onions and garlic—contain an important phytochemical called allicin. Allicin has been linked to lowered cholesterol and blood pressure, as well as provide a boost to the body's infection-fighting ability. All vegetables in the onion family, including chives, scallions, and leeks, contain allicin.

See also: Dietary Guidelines for Americans; MyPlate.

FURTHER READING

Ambrose, Jeanne. "Take 5 at the Very Least." *Better Homes and Gardens*, June 2002, 282.
"5 A Day Works!" Centers for Disease Control and Prevention. Atlanta: U.S. Department of Health and Human Services, 2005. www.cdc.gov/nccdphp/dnpa/nutrition/health_professionals/programs/5aday_works.pdf.
Sugarman, Carole. "Eat Your Purples: Color Coding Is the Latest Approach to a Healthful Diet." *Washington Post*, June 13, 2001, F1.
www.5aday.gov

5-Factor Fitness

For those who dream of having the toned body of a celebrity in only five weeks, the 5-Factor Fitness diet seems like a dream come true. Harley Pasternak, trainer to big name stars like Halle Berry, Orlando Bloom, Lady Gaga, Katy Perry, Robert Pattinson, and many others, developed the diet filled with rules revolving around the number 5.

Those rules include eating five meals a day to boost metabolism; making sure each meal has five ingredients including a lean protein, whole grains, fiber, a healthy fat, and water or another sugar-free beverage; and working out five days a week with Pasternak's 5-Factor Fitness plan. His exercise program is made up of five-minute phases including a cardio warm-up, two phases of strength training, a fourth phase that focuses on the midsection, and a final cardio session and cool down. The author encourages dieters to follow the plan for five weeks and has gone on to market it in more than five different ways, from hardback and paperback editions to a Nintendo Wii version and a Microsoft Xbox 360 workout, along with personal training sessions, his appearances on television shows like Oprah and interviews in magazines like *People, Seventeen,* and *Men's Health.*

At age 35, Canadian-born Pasternak is considered one of the world's most successful fitness trainers with an A-list of clients that also includes famous

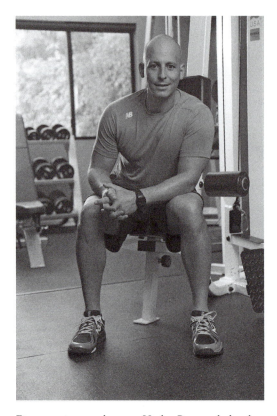

Fitness trainer-to-the-stars Harley Pasternak developed the 5-Factor Fitness, focused on the number 5. (PRNewsFoto/Shaklee)

musicians Kanye West, Common, and Alicia Keys. The first 5-Factor book was released in 2004 and landed on the *New York Times* best-seller list. It was followed by the *5-Factor World Diet*, making Pasternak a media darling.

The diet and fitness plan according to Pasternak is meant to accommodate real life and need not be followed rigidly. He even incorporates a "cheat" day into the mix. Using commonsense nutrition, Pasternak says the eating and exercise program is based on his research on interval training and the success of eating balanced meals. His diet not only closely follows the government's Recommended Dietary Allowance (RDA) for carbohydrate consumption but also encourages dieters to eat more lean proteins while limiting their fat intake to only 0.5 or 15 percent of the RDA's intake of healthy fats. He recommends chicken, fish, egg whites, cottage cheese, lean varieties of red meat, turkey, seafood, game meat, whey-protein shakes, or veggie meats made out of soy for protein sources.

The diet warns against carbohydrates that have a high glycemic index, which is the measure of how quickly a food once eaten increases blood sugar. Foods with a high glycemic index like white bread and table sugar break down quickly and create immediate increases in blood sugar. These same foods bring with them an increase in insulin that causes the body to store them as fat. Low glycemic foods, on the other hand, digest slowly and have less demand for insulin.

The diet also calls for a fiber-rich diet of plenty of fresh fruits and vegetables, which are filled with vitamins, fiber, and minerals. Dieters are encouraged to avoid saturated fats and trans fats and to substitute unsaturated fats like olive oil, avocado oil, or the majority of nut oils in their place. The fifth piece of diet advice centers on drinking water and avoiding any beverage with sugar or empty calories like juice, milk (except for skim), sports drinks, fancy coffees, or alcoholic drinks.

A sample daily meal plan on the 5-Factor Diet might include a breakfast of nonfat cottage cheese with berries or other fresh fruit, or a low-fat, whites-only omelet. A mid-morning snack of a protein shake or nonfat yogurt and fruit would be followed by a lunch of soup and salad or an open-face sandwich using lean meat on flourless bread or rice cakes. The afternoon snack might include nonfat cheese and fruit, or vegetables and a light hummus dip. Finally, dinner would include a lean protein, anything from chicken breast to fish or turkey with an additional complex carbohydrate such as a sweet potato, spaghetti squash, or grains like quinoa or wild rice.

Other commonsense tips include setting a one-serving limit (no seconds); downsizing the size of plates, bowls, and glasses so that portions automatically become smaller; cleaning all of the junk food and unhealthy snacks out of the house before starting the diet; and sitting down to a meal rather than eating while driving or while standing in the kitchen or sitting in front of the TV. Basically, beyond the 5-Factor hype, the diet is a fairly sound, sensible approach to eating less and exercising more.

See also: Carbohydrates; Exercise; Insulin.

FURTHER READING

"Get Fit & Fired Up! These Five Quick and Easy Moves Are Like a Shot of Caffeine for Your Brain and Body. After Just 15 Minutes You'll Feel Strong, Toned, and Energized." *Seventeen* 69, no. 5 (May 2010): 93.

Hagloch, Susan. "Starting on a Lighter Note: Get Slim and Trim with These 20 Diet/ Fitness Books." *Library Journal* 30, no. 1 (January 1, 2005): 144.

Pasternak, Harley. *5-Factor Fitness.* New York: G.P. Putnam's Sons, 2004.

Pergament, Danielle. "Confessions of a Celebrity Trainer." *Allure* (November 2012): 102.

Rubin, Courtney. "A Trainer to the Stars Who's a Star-To-Be." *The New York Times,* March 14, 2013, E8.

Shea, Courtney. "Buff like Harley: Lady Gaga, Halle Berry, Kanye West and Robert Downey Jr. Would All Be as Flabby as the Rest of Us if It Weren't for Celebrity Trainer Harley Pasternak." *Toronto Life*, July 2010, 56.

Food and Drug Administration (FDA)

The Food and Drug Administration (FDA) is that part of the U.S. Department of Health and Human Services charged with regulating a variety of products, from food ingredients to drugs and new medical devices. According to its Web site, www.fda.gov, "Stated most simply, FDA's mission is to promote and protect the public health by helping safe and effective products reach the market in a timely way, and monitoring products for continued safety after they are in use. Our work is a blending of law and science aimed at protecting consumers."

The FDA reviews new food products, such as artificial sweeteners, before they can be produced for sale. It also reviews and limits the health claims products and foods can make on their labeling.

See also: Nutrition Facts Label.

Food Guide Pyramid

The Food Guide Pyramid is a visual reminder of a balanced and varied diet, developed by the U.S. Department of Agriculture and replaced in 2011 by MyPlate. The foods at the bottom of the pyramid—breads and cereals, for example—should make up the bulk of your diet. The foods at the top—fats, oils, and sweets—should be eaten sparingly.

See also: Food and Drug Administration; MyPlate.

Food Safety Modernization Act

President Barack Obama signed the Food Safety Modernization Act into law on January 4, 2011. The first sweeping reform in food safety laws in 70 years, the act addresses the overall safety of food products. It affects manufacturers and suppliers of dietary supplement ingredients. Suppliers of these ingredients, such as vitamins, minerals, fish oils, and glucosamine, will be held to higher regulatory standards and requirements. The law, which goes into effect in phases over several years, will expand the U.S. Food and Drug Administration's enforcement authority over the industry, allowing it to announce recalls, and inspect facilities and record-keeping and require more comprehensive labeling of ingredients. Imports of foreign supplies must verify that they meet compliance standards.

See also: Food and Drug Administration.

FURTHER READING

Link, Connor. "Remember FSMA? Well, Now It Matters." *Nutrition Business Journal*, January 8, 2013.

French Women Don't Get Fat

Think lifestyle rather than diet. Think of eating for pleasure rather than meals filled with guilt. And think fresh, seasonal, and natural rather than processed or fast food, and you have a basic understanding of Mireille Guiliano's best-selling diet book, *French Women Don't Get Fat*. Published in 2010, the diet encourages readers to treat every meal as a special affair, changing courses, lighting candles, and focusing on the flavor by liberally using herbs and spices, rather than counting calories or relying on low-fat versions of things like butter and cream.

Guiliano focused her advice on what she calls the three Ps: pleasure, portion, and plan. That translates into slowing down and sitting down for each meal, preparing the food, serving realistic portions as a way to avoid overeating, and setting a nice table with linens or using dishes usually reserved for special occasions.

Three is a significant number throughout Guiliano's diet directions, starting with her advice to eat three meals per day including breakfast, lunch, and supper, and she is adamant that snacking is unhealthy and causes weight gain.

The idea of dinner as a three-course event is central to her theory, which she based on her experiences growing up in France. She also recommends that food choices, especially for dinner, should have three colors on the plate and include the three most important types of food: protein, carbohydrates, and fat. One other important three theme is her assertion that the first three mouthfuls of any meal are the most enjoyable, and there is nothing wrong with small portions or eating just a bite or taste. She encourages everyone not to feel guilty about leaving food on the plate.

Working with the premise that French women have an innate style and way of life that insulates them against the standard American diet or weight gain, the author sets out to share the mystique and what she identifies as a basic French philosophy: fool yourself. Equipment needed is a small scale to weigh some foods during what Guilianos called the critically important first three months.

The author starts dieters out with her "Magical Leek Soup," which she describes as a mild diuretic that is low in calories and high in nutrients. To jumpstart the diet, she suggests 48 hours of leek soup along with unlimited water. The first three months of the diet should also be devoted to self-reflection as a way to identify bad eating habits or other problems that add to weight gain. Guiliano recommends shopping like a French woman by avoiding prepared and processed foods and shopping several times a week to buy only what is needed for a day or two of meals. Other commonsense suggestions include keeping foods out of the house that you eat automatically, such as potato chips or sweets, and slowly reducing portion sizes until you are eating a sensible, small serving instead of the giant American "super-sized" helpings.

Another important tip focuses on seasonal menu planning. A sample spring menu might include strawberries for breakfast with yogurt or cereal and a slice of multigrain bread. Lunch would incorporate spring greens in a salad and a dish featuring asparagus, plus a fruited desert with cherries or another spring berry. Dinner might be pea soup, grilled spring lamb, and rhubarb compote, all vegetables and fruits available in season. A summer menu would include summer fruits like peaches and blueberries, as well as fresh vegetables such as tomatoes, fennel, and arugula.

The author explains that eating foods at their peak of freshness is an important way to fight boredom, which she suggests is a food-lover's worst enemy. Having a single taste experience in a meal forces the diner to overeat, using volume instead of taste and texture to get satisfaction from the food. She credits French women with an exceptional ability to use seasonings and fresh food to "fool yourself" into thinking that each meal is a rich, complicated affair when it is composed of just a few, fresh ingredients. A good example is ratatouille, a French summer classic that features tomatoes, zucchini, and eggplant, along with a few fresh spices.

Guiliano takes readers on a pleasant stroll through her book and sprinkles recipes here and there but never seems in a hurry to present any hard and fast rules, as do so many American diet books, such as Scarsdale or Atkins. For those who want a lifestyle choice filled with simple but delicious meals, this may be the diet of choice for them. A spinoff of the *French Women Don't Get Fat Diet* is called Le Forking, where dieters eat only foods that fit on their forks and are naturally eaten with a fork, leaving out anything that has to be cut up with a knife, scooped with a spoon, or picked up and eaten like fried chicken or pizza.

See also: Atkins Nutritional Approach; Calories.

FURTHER READING

Adriani, Lynn. "K.I.S.S. Low-Carb Goodbye: Balanced Diet, Exercise and Go Easy on the Fads." *Publishers Weekly* 252, no. 45 (November 14, 2005): 28(5).

Crosby, Jackie. "Let Them Lose Weight; A Paris-Based Nutrition Firm Is Coming to America, Marketing Its Weight-Loss Plans to Twin Cities Companies." *Minneapolis Star Tribune*, February 12, 2011, Business News, 1D.

"Eat Yourself Happy." *Prevention*, March 2013, 13.

Forman, Adrienne. "Resist the American Way by Eating Less, Moving More." *Environmental Nutrition* 28, no. 4 (April 2005): 2.

Guiliano, Mireille. *French Women Don't Get Fat: The Secret of Eating for Pleasure*. New York: Alfred A. Knopf, 2005.

http://go.galegroup.com/ps/i.do?id=Gale%7CA326575998&v=2.

Parnass, Alexandra. "Holiday Survival Guide: Expert Advice on How to Prevent Weight Gain, Banish Stress, and Look Your Best during Party Season." *Harper's Bazaar* no. 3541 (December 2006): 192.

"Study: Western Style Diet Can Be a Killer." *UPA NewsTrack*, April 17, 2013. General Reference Center Gold. Accessed November 6, 2013.

Gluten-Free

Gluten is a glue-like protein that is part of most grains including wheat, barley, and rye. In the world of modern, processed foods, it is also found in everything from deli meats and soy sauce to vitamins and chocolates. A decade ago there was very little discussion of gluten, and the only people eating a gluten-free diet were the handful of people who suffered from celiac disease.

Now, the number of people with celiac disease is 1 percent of the U.S. population or just more than 3 million people. However, research shows that some 18 million Americans may be suffering from non-celiac gluten sensitivity. According to the National Association for Celiac Awareness Foundation, this figure is six times the number of people who have been diagnosed with celiac disease. Celiac disease is an immune response to eating gluten that causes inflammation and eventual damage to the lining of the small intestine. This damage then prevents absorption of needed nutrients and can also cause diarrhea, bloating, and other physical symptoms. If left untreated, over time complications such as autoimmune diseases, osteoporosis, thyroid disease, and cancer can also develop.

It appears that the explosion of Americans dropping gluten from their diets is not just due to sensitivity to gluten or even a growing awareness of celiac disease, but instead a desire to easily lose weight. While influenced in part by celebrities like singer Miley Cyrus, actress Gwyneth Paltrow, and professional tennis player Novak Djokovic who attribute their current health and slim figures to being gluten-free, this growing number of Americans are motivated by the idea that gluten causes weight gain along with other autoimmune health problems.

GLUTEN-FREE WEIGHT LOSS

Statistics show that Americans are limiting how much gluten they eat, even though most do not have a diagnosis of celiac disease. Gluten-free food sales in the United States reached more than $2 billion in 2010 and are expected to top $5 billion by 2015, according to the figures from the National Association for Celiac Awareness. The gluten-free foods are being purchased by more than 30 percent of Americans who self-report gastrointestinal problems under the label of gluten sensitivity or gluten intolerance.

Health experts and nutritionists caution that going gluten-free is not a healthy weight loss plan, but they are fighting against pictures of gluten-free, thin stars like Gwyneth Paltrow, Victoria Beckham, and Miley Cyrus, who publically suggest the opposite. Nutritionists suggest that the initial weight loss on a gluten-free diet may be the result of changing eating habits by eliminating white flour, sugar, junk food, and a large amount of processed foods, all of which contain

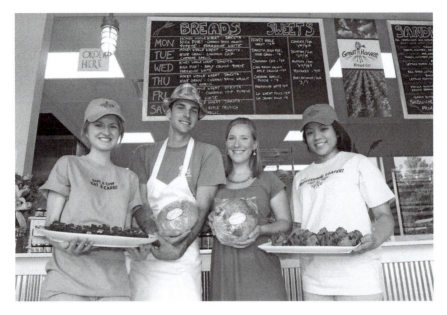

These workers in a Charlottesville, VA, Great Harvest Bread Co. store show some of the gluten-free products they sell. (AP Photo/The Daily Progress/Damien Dawson)

gluten. That initial weight loss coincides with a drop in overall calories rather than just the absence of gluten.

WHY GLUTEN-FREE?

While many American are turning against gluten, critics suggest that gluten-free is simply a marketing tool. On the other side of the argument, individuals like tennis professional Novak Djokovic exemplify those who are switching to a gluten-free diet. Djokovic has been ranked as the number-one tennis player in the world. The Serb native has risen to the top of the tennis world but used to suffer from all kinds of illnesses, everything from cramps and fatigue to colds and flu. Then, according to Djokovic, he changed his diet and removed gluten, and the illnesses disappeared. In 2012, Djokovic defeated tennis star Rafael Nadal in the Australian Open following a six-hour match and he has gone on to win at least six Grand Slam singles titles.

PROBLEMS WITH GLUTEN

What is all the fuss about gluten? When gluten is eaten by someone who is allergic, such as those with celiac disease or by someone who is sensitive to it, the gluten attacks the lining of the small intestine and begins to damage the tiny villi, small fingerlike growths that absorb nutrients from food. As the damage increases, the villi are unable to absorb needed nutrients leading to a number of problems including chronic diarrhea, anemia, malnutrition, headaches, fatigue, and skin rashes. Once a gluten-free diet is started, those with celiac disease should see an improvement in their health within several months. However, some people may need up to one year to fully recover, and there is a small percentage of people with extreme damage to their small intestine who do not improve. This is called refractory celiac disease and if that is diagnosed, other treatments may be needed to restore their ability to absorb nutrients.

Health professionals agree that most Americans would benefit from less gluten in their diets. Experts suggest replacing large amounts of bread, pasta, or other carbohydrate foods with fresh vegetables and fruits, lean meat, fish, and chicken. However, problems develop when gluten foods are switched with gluten-free processed foods that are often as high in saturated fat as the foods they replace. In fact, gluten-free foods may contain higher amounts of salt and sugar and have even more calories than their regular counterpart. Plus, many celiac sufferers resent the idea that anyone would go gluten-free just to lose weight. Those with celiac disease find it very challenging to eat gluten-free in a world filled with processed and fast foods.

GLUTEN-FREE FOOD CHOICES

What does gluten-free eating look like? Foods that do not contain gluten and are safe to eat include beans, unprocessed nuts and seeds, eggs, fresh meats, chicken, and fish that are not breaded or batter-coated or marinated, fresh fruits and vegetables, and the majority of dairy products. Grains safe to eat are those not mixed with additives. Other safe foods include corn and cornmeal; potato; sweet potato; flax; gluten-free flours like rice, soy, corn, potato, and coconut; millet; quinoa; and rice.

For individuals looking to avoid all gluten, it is important to avoid any foods or beverages that contain barley, rye, wheat, triticale—a cross between wheat and rye—bulgur, durum flour, graham and graham flour, semolina, and spelt. It is also wise to avoid most prepared foods since gluten is often included in them. Foods like deli lunchmeats, cakes, candies, cookies, crackers, gravies, sauces, beer, cereals, pastas, seasoned rice mixes, self-basting poultry, and prepared soups all need to be avoided.

Many college campuses are answering the call for gluten-free foods for their students, although cross-contamination is a big concern for individuals and food providers alike. Problems develop if equipment used in manufacturing or preparing food is exposed to a variety of products. Many labels include a statement that their product "may contain" things like wheat, dairy, eggs, or soy. For those who suffer from celiac disease, the statement that there may be wheat means they should completely avoid that product to be safe. Health care professionals suggest that before anyone decides to go gluten-free, they should discuss their concerns with their primary care physician.

LABELING

In response to concerns by gluten-free consumers, the Federal U.S. Food and Drug Administration (FDA) released new regulations at the end of 2013 that created standards for gluten-free food labels. This follows similar standards by Canada and the European Union. The FDA standards state that food manufacturers cannot call their product gluten-free unless it contains fewer than 20 parts per million of gluten, which researchers have determined is the safest level that can be consumed by people with celiac disease or other gluten-sensitivities. The ruling takes effect August 2014.

See also: Anemia; Carbohydrates; Celiac Disease.

FURTHER READING

Baker, Jeff. "Novak Djokovic's Gluten-Free Diet Is Effective for Weight Loss and Increased Energy." *The Oregonian,* October 27, 2013, www.oregonian.com.

"FDA Sets Gluten-Free Labeling Standard." *Environmental Nutrition* 36, no. 11 (November 2013): 1.

Neporent, Liz. "Gluten Free Diets No Help in Losing Weight." *ABC News,* June 25, 2013, www.abcnews.go.com/health/gluten-free-lead-weight-loss/story?id=19476263.

"What I Need to Know about Celiac Disease." *National Institute of Diabetes & Digestive & Kidney Diseases.* November 2007. http://www2.niddk.nih.gov.

Glycemic Index

The glycemic index is a measurement of how much foods cause blood sugar to rise in two or three hours after consuming them. Consuming carbohydrates causes the body to produce the hormone insulin. The glycemic index is one way to measure the amount of insulin that might be produced as a result of eating foods. This measurement is important for insulin-dependent diabetics who must inject sufficient insulin to cover a meal. It has also become of interest to advocates of a high-protein, low-carbohydrate diet who argue that excess insulin production can lead to other health problems.

Even so, the glycemic index reveals nothing about a food's nutritive value. For example, Skittles and whole wheat bread both have a relatively high glycemic index of around 70. (Glucose has a glycemic index of 100.) Yet that does not make them of equal value in any regard other than the accompanying rise in blood sugar.

See also: Carbohydrates; Insulin.

FURTHER READING

www.glycemicindex.com.

Ghrelin

Ghrelin is a new and promising discovery in the fight against obesity. Pronounced GRELL-in, this growth hormone has an effect on whether a person is hungry, raising hopes for a breakthrough in the treatment of obesity. And in a country where obesity is an epidemic, understanding how ghrelin works could lead to effective weight-loss drugs or drugs to promote weight gain in anorexics and cancer patients. Research published in the May 23, 2002, issue of the *New England Journal of Medicine* suggests that ghrelin may turn out to be one reason people feel hungry and why it's so hard for dieters to keep weight off.

Scientists know that part of the brain's hypothalamus controls food intake, but until recent years the only chemical substances known to turn it on have been found in the brain. New research now shows ghrelin's receptors are in the brain, but its primary site of production is in the stomach. This research suggests that the stomach pumps ghrelin into the bloodstream and the hormone then travels to the pituitary, a vastly different mechanism from other peptides that affect appetite. Those are made in the brain, do not travel into the bloodstream, and work only when injected directly into the appropriate brain regions.

Ghrelin, a peptide consisting of 28 amino acids, was first identified by Kenji Kangawa of the National Cardiovascular Center Research Institute in Osaka, Japan. The name uses the root "ghre," which means "growth" in Hindi and related languages, and the name's initial letters also refer to ghrelin's role as a growth hormone—releasing factor. Following its identification in 1999, doctors have started looking at ghrelin in the treatment of obesity as well as in wasting syndromes stemming from AIDS, cancer, heart disease, and a variety of other illnesses. Although the hormone's role in the body is not yet fully understood, recent studies show that people suffering from wasting illnesses actually manufacture more ghrelin than normal. But, surprisingly, the highest blood concentrations of ghrelin recorded are in people suffering from anorexia nervosa. Apparently while anorexics are starving themselves to death, blood analysis indicates large amounts of ghrelin are released as normal body mechanisms continually signal the need for food.

Another interesting aspect of the report found that after a group of 13 obese people dieted and lost some 17 percent of their body weight, their ghrelin levels were significantly higher throughout the day than before the weight loss when ghrelin levels would rise before meals but fall afterward. Scientists suggest this increase in ghrelin in people who have lost weight dieting may reflect the body's attempt to regain lost pounds, a mechanism that originally evolved to defend against starvation during humankind's early history when food supplies fluctuated erratically. Today in developed nations like the United States with an abundance of high-calorie foods, this early survival advantage may now contribute to obesity.

On the other hand, low ghrelin levels were noted in people who underwent gastric-bypass surgery. They experienced a drop in their ghrelin levels but did not appear to suffer any side effects. In fact, according to the study, people who undergo this surgery describe a generalized disinterest in food with a noticeable drop in ghrelin production. Researchers say that following bypass surgery, stomach cells that produce ghrelin are no longer exposed to food and ghrelin production may no longer be stimulated. During gastric-bypass surgery, surgeons sew much of the stomach shut, leaving room for a dieter to eat only a small amount of food.

Still, researchers are warning against overenthusiasm about ghrelin's prospects. They say similar hopes were raised years ago for leptin, a hormone that acts as an appetite suppressant. Yet after years of research, no useful medication was developed because researchers found that patients quickly developed a tolerance to leptin. Nonetheless, the discovery of ghrelin is a major advance in the understanding of what controls appetite, and this leaves researchers hungry to learn more.

See also: Anorexia Nervosa.

FURTHER READING

Cummings, David E., D. S. Weigle, R. S. Frayo, P. A. Breen, M. K. Ma, E. P. Dellinger, and J. Q. Purnell. "Plasma Ghrelin Levels after Diet-Induced Weight Loss or Gastric Bypass Surgery." *New England Journal of Medicine,* 346, no. 21 (May 23, 2002): 1623–30.

Doheny, Kathleen. "Hormone Ghrelin Raises Desire for High-Calorie Foods." *WebMD Health News,* June 22, 2010, www.webmd.com/diet/news/20100622/hormone-ghrelin-ups-desire-for-high-calorie-foods.

Fischman, Josh. "A Hungry Hormone." *U.S. News & World Report,* June 3, 2002, 53.

Flier, J. S., and E. Maratos-Flier. "The Stomach Speaks—Ghrelin and Weight Regulation." *New England Journal of Medicine* 346, no. 21 (May 23, 2002): 1662–63.

Lemonick, Michael D. "Lean and Hungrier: Is a Recently Discovered Hormone the Reason Why Folks Who Lose Weight Can't Keep It Off?" *Time,* June 3, 2002, 54.

"New Role for 'Hunger Hormone." MIT press release, October 15, 2013. Massachusetts Institute of Technology. www.newsoffice.mit.edu/2013/ghrelin-ptsd-1015.

Pinkney, Jonathan, and Gareth Williams. "Ghrelin Gets Hungry." *Lancet* 359, no. 9315 (April 20, 2002): 1360.

Travis, John. "The Hunger Hormone? An Appetite Stimulant Produced by the Stomach May Lead to Treatments for Obesity and Wasting Syndromes." *Science News* 161, no. 7 (February 16, 2002): 107–109.

Graham, Sylvester

Sylvester Graham (b. July 4, 1794, in West Suffield, Connecticut; d. September 11, 1851, in Northampton, Massachusetts) is considered one of America's first food faddists. Graham believed that a high-fiber, natural-food diet would remedy cholera, alcoholism, premature aging, violence, sexual abuses, and digestive ills. His early followers included the Kellogg brothers, who were famous for their religious colony and health sanitarium at Battle Creek, Michigan. Graham's fanaticism and zeal for natural food attracted early followers, like the Kelloggs; they became known as "Grahamites."

Like many other health reformers, Graham had an early history of bad health. He was the youngest of 17 children born to Massachusetts minister John Graham, who died when Sylvester was just two years old. According to records, Graham's

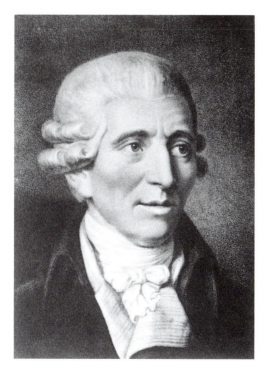

Nearly 200 years ago, Sylvester Graham was among the first to recommend a diet of raw foods, whole wheat, coarsely ground homemade bread and no alcohol. (Library of Congress, Prints and Photographs Division, Washington, D.C. [Library of Congress])

mother was "in a deranged state of mind" after her husband's death, so the court appointed a guardian for Sylvester and two older siblings. His health and education suffered as he was passed from relative to relative, finally settling years later in Newark, New Jersey, where he was eventually reunited with his mother and an older brother. It was at this time that he also began to prepare for the ministry. He studied at Amherst Academy but was expelled after one quarter. He then studied privately with a minister and was ordained in 1826, the year he married the woman who had previously nursed him through a nervous breakdown.

While Graham was interested in saving souls, he also lectured on the evils of alcohol for the Pennsylvania Society for Discouraging the Use of Ardent Spirits. This temperance group worked to moderate the per capita consumption of alcohol, but Graham from the first advocated total abstinence. Soon he was also talking about diet and sex as well as alcohol. During this time, he studied human physiology and diet. The cholera epidemic of 1832, the first of three cholera epidemics in the United States of the 19th century, gave Graham a renewed platform when he suggested that greasy, spicy meat, combined with "excessive lewdness," caused the cholera outbreak.

But his most famous advice was that thick, coarse bread, baked at home and eaten daily, should be the mainstay of every diet. He believed his bread, made from the whole of the wheat and coarsely ground, known as "dyspepsia or temperance bread," was best when eaten a day old. It was the early version of today's graham cracker and he was convinced of its healing powers. Graham also recommended hard mattresses, open bedroom windows, cold baths, and a raw-food, vegetarian diet as best, because it was closest to nature. Even though he realized that people were devoted to white bakery bread, he continued to condemn it as a horrible food choice. Graham's book, *Treatise on Bread*, sold for $4 a dozen and described the breadmaking process as the province of the loving wife and mother. Because he accused bakers of adulterating their products with additives, he was criticized by many, including well-known author Ralph Waldo Emerson, who publicly ridiculed Graham's diet.

The dietary world of the 1830s was filled with disease and bad health caused by consumption, chronic indigestion, and dyspepsia —a blanket term for constipation, stomachaches, headaches, and foul breath. Americans ate meat at every meal—some 180 pounds yearly per person—and foods were soaked in grease or gravy and washed down with whiskey. Long before the discovery of nutrition, fiber, vitamins, minerals, and cholesterol, Graham insisted that diet and health were directly connected. He believed that eating meat, particularly pork, led to sexual excess. Sexual excess then led to increased consumption of more rich foods and unhealthy meat, which, according to Graham, predisposed an individual to disease.

After the cholera epidemics subsided, Graham continued to lecture to mass audiences, traveling through Massachusetts, New York, New Jersey, Pennsylvania, Rhode Island, and Maine. Graham's talks were controversial; he continued to criticize the nation's diet, hygiene, and sexual practices. But it was this obsession with masturbation, what he called the "solitary vice," that eventually alienated many would-be sympathizers. In 1837, as his popularity faded, he moved to Northampton, Massachusetts, with his wife Sarah and their two children. He died there on September 11, 1851, at the age of 57.

In America, talk of "Grahamism" would continue for many years as followers such as abolitionists William Lloyd Garrison, Horace Greeley, and Henry Stanton remained firm believers in his health ideals. Ellen Harmon White, spiritual leader and founder of the Seventh-day Adventist Church and founder of Battle Creek, Michigan's Western Health Reform Institute, also continued to recommend Graham's ideas and diet following his death. Slowly but surely, the American medical and scientific communities would one day come to accept Graham's theory that diet and health were interrelated. Although he was ahead of his time, Graham's belief that eating too much salt, meat, and fat can cause health problems is now accepted nutritional wisdom.

See also: Vegetarian Diet.

FURTHER READING

Armstrong, David, and Elizabeth Metzger Armstrong. *The Great American Medicine Show: Being an Illustrated History of Hucksters, Healers, Health Evangelists, and Heroes from Plymouth Rock to the Present.* New York: Prentice Hall, 1991.

DiBacco, Thomas V. "Behind the Graham Cracker, a Health Food Tale: One Man's Battle to Make Americans Think about Nutrition." *Washington Post,* July 25, 1989, 3.

Dictionary of American Biography. Farmington Hills, MI: Gale Group, 2001.

Encyclopedia of World Biography. 2nd ed. Farmington, MI: Gale Group, 1998.

Farmer, Jean. "The Rev. Sylvester (Graham Cracker) Graham: America's Early Fiber Crusader." *Saturday Evening Post,* March 1985, 32–37.

Gordon, John Steele. "Sawdust Pudding." *American Heritage,* July–August 1996, 16–18.

Nissenbaum, Stephen. *Sex, Diet and Debility in Jacksonian America: Sylvester Graham and Health Reform.* Chicago: Dorsey Press, 1988.

Grapefruit Diet

A favorite with generations of dieters, the grapefruit diet has been around since at least the 1930s. This word-of-mouth plan calls for eating a few select vegetables, limited protein, plus the all-important serving of grapefruit or grapefruit juice with every meal. Over the years, countless dieters have been encouraged to believe that grapefruit contains a special fat-burning enzyme. Dozens of variations of the grapefruit diet exist, but they all contain that one special ingredient—grapefruit.

Typically the diet lasts two or three weeks. Breakfast consists of half a grape-fruit and black coffee. In several variations, breakfast also includes protein foods like bacon and eggs but no carbohydrates. Lunch includes half a grapefruit plus an egg, cucumber, dry melba toast, and plain tea or coffee. Again, some variations suggest meat with this meal. Dinner calls for the obligatory grapefruit eaten with half a head of lettuce, a tomato, two eggs, and coffee or tea.

Some variations on the grapefruit diet theme call for dinners that include meat or fish, cooked any way from broiled to fried, baked, or grilled. Every ver-sion of this diet is low in carbohydrates, and cutting out carbohydrates generally means a big reduction in daily calorie consumption; often less than 800 calo-ries consumed per day. Anyone eating so few calories per day will lose weight no matter what foods they eat. So, on the one hand, nutritionists praise the grapefruit as an excellent food choice, saying it has no fat, is low in sodium, is packed with vitamin C, is high in water and fiber, and the pink variety has beta-carotene.

But those same nutritionists laugh at the suggestion that grapefruit or its juice acts as a special catalyst for fat burning. Experts say the fat-burning properties of grapefruit are just part of the cultural diet mythology. Scientists add that there are no magical properties in grapefruit or any other citrus fruits to help it burn ex-traordinary amounts of calories. They suggest that dieters eat grapefruit but they should do it for the right reasons, because it is a healthy food choice.

See also: Calories.

FURTHER READING

"The Allure of Grapefruit for Weight Loss: What's Under the Skin?" *Environmental Nutri-tion* 34, no. i5 (2011):7 (1).
Brown, Jordana. "Get Ripped Grapefruit: the New Grapefruit Diet." *Flex* 27, no. i9 (2009):134 (1).

Healthy Eating Plate

Americans who eat the standard hamburger or hotdog on a white bread bun with French fries and a milk shake won't find anything critical of that meal on the U.S. Department of Agriculture's MyPlate. That's according to the creators of the Healthy Eating Plate, which uses the same plate concept as the USDA but offers what developers say is a more detailed and helpful roadmap for healthy eating. Created by nutritionists at the Harvard School of Public Health in part-nership with editors at Harvard Health Publications, the Healthy Eating Plate is one more tool for Americans to use in their efforts to wade through mountains of confusing nutrition information. This independent plate also comes without any input from the agricultural or food industries, something its supporters say does influence the MyPlate recommendations.

Based on the premise of quality not quantity, the Healthy Eating Plate is half filled with fruits and vegetables, while the other half is divided evenly between protein and whole grains. At first glance the government's MyPlate and the Healthy Eating Plate seem similar, but supporters of the Harvard version say that the USDA's nutrition advice lacks specifics and is misleading. They point to key differences in every area of the plate from the whole grains and proteins to vegetables, fruits, and oils or fats.

For example, critics say MyPlate does not differentiate between types of grains and the Healthy Eating Plate encourages consumers to choose whole grains and to avoid foods like white bread, white rice, and sugar. The Healthy Eating Plate also encourages a large variety of vegetables but cautions Americans to stay away from potatoes and especially French fries. The MyPlate does not distinguish between healthy vegetables and French fries.

Another key difference between the two plates is in the area of dairy foods. MyPlate recommends milk and other dairy foods be eaten at every meal, while the Healthy Eating Plate suggests water is the best beverage and encourages consumers to limit milk and dairy to only one or two servings each day.

When it comes to proteins, the Healthy Eating Plate suggests that consumers stick to fish, poultry, beans, or nuts and cautions against red meat or processed meats. MyPlate does not draw any distinctions between protein foods and could easily include a hamburger or hot dog or other processed meats, which can be high in fats and sodium. The USDA plate also fails to recommend healthy fats such as olive, canola, or other plant oils and places no limits on butter or trans fats. The Healthy Eating Plate specifically recommends no trans fats and encourages Americans to limit their red meat consumption to avoid the risk of colon cancer, weight gain, heart disease, and diabetes.

On the subject of diabetes, the Healthy Eating Plate suggests that consumers avoid sugary beverages and even juices to limit their risk of the disease. When it comes to caffeine, the Healthy Eating Plate does not limit caffeine for adults but it does agree with the American Academy of Pediatrics (AAP) that energy drinks, sports drinks, and sodas do contain caffeine and have no place in the diet of children and adolescents. In fact, according to the AAP, soft drinks are the largest source of caffeine for U.S. children.

In its role as a planning guide, the Healthy Eating Plate does not call for any specific number of calories or servings each day. The focus instead is on relative portions since each individual's nutritional needs and calorie intake will be different based on their age, gender, level of fitness, and size. It does, however, encourage people to consume fewer carbohydrates than typically found in the American diet and to be sure the carbs they eat are healthy choices.

Staying active is another important factor in weight loss or control and the Healthy Eating Plate encourages people to be active, while the USDA MyPlate fails to mention the importance of exercise or physical activity.

While critics of the USDA MyPlate say there are flaws in the program, scientists, nutrition experts, and others suggest that the two can work in partnership to help Americans create a healthier diet. MyPlate was created in 2011 to replace the USDA's earlier MyPyramid, which critics called vague and confusing. The USDA released MyPyramid in 2005 to answer complaints about the Food Guide Pyramid, which critics said was based on weak scientific evidence and failed to recognize the connection between diet and health. The Food Guide Pyramid when originally created by the USDA in 1992 was a very visible symbol of what the USDA called the elements of a healthy diet.

Since the creation of the Harvard School of Public Health's Plate and earlier Healthy Eating Pyramid, researchers have compared the two information sources. Study results continue to show that participants who scored highest using the Healthy Eating tools were less likely to develop major chronic diseases including lowered cardiovascular disease than their counterparts who followed the MyPyramid or MyPlate.

See also: MyPlate.

FURTHER READING

Belin, R. J., P. Greenland, M. Allison, L. Martin, J. M. Shikany, J. Larson, L. Tinker, B. V. Howard, D. Lloyd-Jones, L. Van Horn. "Diet Quality and the Risk of Cardiovascular Disease: The Women's Health Initiative (WHI)." *American Journal of Clinical Nutrition* 94, no. 1 (July 2011): 49–57. doi:10.3945/ajcn. 110.011221. Epub May 25, 2011.

"Healthy Eating Plate and Healthy Eating Pyramid." The Nutrition Source, Harvard School of Public Health. http://www.hsph.harvard.edu/nutritionsource/healthy-eating-plate/.

"Sports Drinks and Energy Drinks for Children and Adolescents: Are They Appropriate?" *Pediatrics* 127 (2011): 1182–89.

"State-Specific Trends in Fruit and Vegetable Consumption among Adults-United States 2000–2009." *MMWR Morbidity and Mortality Weekly Report* 59 (2010): 1125–30.

U.S. Department of Agriculture. "Development of 2010 Dietary Guidelines for Americans Consumer Messages and New Food Icon." USDA Center for Nutrition Policy and Promotion, June 2011. http://www.choosemyplate.gov/food-groups/downloads/MyPlate/ExecutiveSummaryOfFormativeResearch.pdf.

Healthy People 2020

In an effort to create a society where all people live long, healthy lives, the U.S. Department of Health and Human Services (HHS), along with other federal agencies and the Healthy People 2020 Advisory Committee, have joined together to create Healthy People 2020, a large-scale public health initiative to identify health priorities and then see those goals come to fruition. Each initiative, based on the accomplishments of the previous one, lasts one decade and is defined by a specific title.

The goal for Healthy People 2020 is "A Society in Which All People Live Long, Healthy Lives." Developed under the leadership of the Federal Interagency Workgroup (FIW), the main goals for the current initiative include working with U.S. citizens so that they can live lives free of preventable diseases, disability, and premature death. Goals also include achieving health equity, eliminating disparities in the health of all citizens, and creating both social and physical environments that promote healthy lives for all Americans.

This public health initiative follows the previous initiatives: Healthy People 1979: The Surgeon General's Report on Health Promotion and Disease Prevention; Healthy People 1990: Promoting Health/Preventing Disease: Objectives for the Nation; Healthy People 2000: National Health Promotion and Disease Prevention Objectives; and Healthy People 2010: Objectives for Improving Health.

The most recent update to 30 years of work by the HHS was released in December 2010. In its discussion on nutrition, physical activity, and obesity, a leading health indicator, the report overview says, "Most Americans, however, do not eat a healthful diet and are not physically active at levels needed to maintain proper health." Citing a Centers for Disease Control and Prevention study, it says that fewer than one-in-three adults and an even lower proportion of adolescents eat the recommended amount of vegetables each day. Compounding this is the fact that a majority of adults (81.6%) and adolescents (81.8%) do not get the recommended amount of physical activity, as outlined in the HHS *Physical Activity Guidelines for Americans*.

The overview continues to say that approximately one-third (34%) of American adults and one-in-six children and adolescents (16.2%) are obese. "Obesity-related conditions include heart disease, stroke, and type 2 diabetes, which are among the leading causes of death. In addition to grave health consequences, overweight and obesity significantly increase medical costs and pose a staggering burden on the U.S. medical care delivery system," the report states.

HHS Secretary Kathleen Sebelius called the launch of the newest Healthy People initiative a challenge and opportunity to avoid preventable diseases from occurring in the first place. According to HHS officials, more than 8,000 comments were considered while drafting the Healthy People 2020 objectives, and those comments lead to the addition of new topics for consideration. These include Alzheimer's disease; genomics; global health; lesbian, gay, bisexual, and transgender health; blood disorders; and blood safety.

Medical and health experts from across the country, a range of federal, state, and local government officials plus a consortium of more than 2,000 organizations and the general public were invited to provide feedback for the newest initiative. HHS officials said that the act of setting national objectives and monitoring progress toward achieving them continues to be a catalyst for action. At the same time, the HHS announced a newly redesigned Web site for users to explore their resources.

While recognizing that health and behaviors that promote good health can be influenced by a number of factors, the Healthy People 2020 initiative was expanded to include prevention, education, plus social and physical interventions on the local, state, and national level. The framework also draws attention to issues that can create disparities in services such as race and ethnicity, socioeconomic status, gender, age, sexual orientation, disabilities, and urban versus rural living. Key partners working on the Healthy People 2020 initiative to disseminate public health information include the Nationwide Health Information Network and the ONC-Coordinated Federal Health IT Strategic Plan.

The need for a strong public health system has been a priority among government services; however, following the attacks of September 11, 2001, the additional anthrax attacks, and natural disasters like Hurricane Katrina and Superstorm Sandy, the government placed an additional urgency on the importance of preparing for national health emergencies. The government continues to award millions of dollars in grants to programs at the national, state, and local level to support these objectives.

The Healthy People initiatives for each decade are measured by data collected by the National Center for Health Statistics (NCHS) working with the Centers for Disease Control and Prevention (CDC). The CDC tracks progress toward the various objectives, while the NCHS partners with the HHS to update data and release it when the CDC makes it available. A drop in the number of people dying from heart disease and cancer was among important changes in the nation's health noted by the Health People 2000. Statistics also showed a minor reduction in the number of Americans who smoked in the Healthy People 2010 data. Unfortunately, the 2010 results also showed significant increases in obesity rates for all age groups. Due to those results, the HHS made it clear that curbing obesity is now a priority in Healthy People 2020.

See also: Exercise; Obesity.

FURTHER READING

"Healthy People 2020." Centers for Disease Control and Prevention, July 23, 2013. http://www.cdc.gov/dhdsp/hp2020.htm.

"HHS Announces the Nation's New Health Promotion and Disease Prevention Agenda." *HHS News,* U.S. Department of Health and Human Services. December 2, 2010. http://www.healthypeople.gov/2020/about/DefaultPressRelease.pdf.

Koh, Howard K. "A 2020 Vision for Healthy People." *New England Journal of Medicine* 362, no. 18 (May 6, 2010): 1653–56.

"Nutrition, Physical Activity, and Obesity." *Healthy People 2020*. HealthyPeople.gov. June 6, 2013. http://www.healthypeople.gov/2020/LHI/nutrition.aspx.
Slade-Sawyer, Penelope. "Healthy People 2020 Inspires People to Improve Health of Communities." *Nation's Health* 41, no. 4 (May/June 2011): 515.

Herbal Diet Teas

Herbal teas for dieters contain senna, aloe, buckthorn, and other plant-derived laxatives that, when consumed in excessive amounts can cause diarrhea, vomiting, nausea, stomach cramps, chronic constipation, and, in severe cases, death. By 1997, the Food and Drug Administration (FDA) had received a number of "adverse event" reports about dieter's teas, including information on the deaths of four young women where the teas may have been a contributing factor. Those four deaths involved women with a history of the eating disorders: anorexia nervosa and bulimia.

Based on that information, the FDA now advises consumers to carefully follow package directions when using dieter's teas or any other dietary supplements containing senna, aloe, or other laxatives. The agency also encourages anyone experiencing persistent diarrhea, abdominal cramps, or other bowel problems to see a doctor. Although the agency has not required manufacturers to place a warning on the products' label, detailing the potential side effects, some manufacturers are voluntarily doing so.

Herbal diet teas are often purchased in health food stores or through mail-order catalogs. Green tea and green tea extract have also become increasingly popular in recent years. Green tea has a higher level of antioxidants than some other teas, and it also contains caffeine. While many weight loss formulas contain a green tea extract, the effectiveness of green tea has not been proven.

Herbal teas' popularity comes from the mistaken consumer belief that increased bowel movements would prevent absorption of calories, would stop weight gain, and would even encourage weight loss. However, a special report from the FDA's Food Advisory Committee concluded that studies show using laxatives to cause diarrhea does not work and does not reduce the body's absorption of calories in any significant way.

With words like "dieter's," "diet," "trim," or "slim" in their names, it is easy to understand how consumers would expect weight loss from drinking the teas. Plus, package labeling often promotes the tea as a natural bowel cleanser and may include information about other weight-loss practices. Unfortunately, nutritionists suspect the diet teas are also very attractive to people with anorexia or bulimia because they act quickly and can be extremely effective as a laxative.

FDA reports show three types of problems most often associated with dieter's teas. Short-term problems like stomach cramps, nausea, vomiting, and diarrhea are most likely to occur in a first-time user who drinks more than the recommended amount. More serious chronic problems include ongoing diarrhea, pain, and constipation due to laxative dependency. In one report to the FDA, a person who admitted using herbal products with laxatives for decades eventually required surgery to remove their colon when it stopped functioning. People who develop chronic problems have often used these products for years.

Finally, the FDA lists severe side effects such as fainting, dehydration, and electrolyte disorders, which bring with them low blood potassium, a condition that can cause paralysis, irregular heartbeat, and, in some cases, death. Severe problems with these products may develop when consumers drastically reduce their food intake or when they are already in poor nutritional health because they have an eating disorder.

So while a cup of herbal tea may feel soothing to the soul, people drinking dieter's teas must be careful to follow directions. Otherwise it can be dangerous to their health.

See also: Anorexia Nervosa; Bulimia Nervosa; Food and Drug Administration (FDA).

FURTHER READING

Bender, Michele. "Are Herbal Weight-Loss Teas Safe for Me to Drink?" *Cosmopolitan*, January 2001, 89.
Danitz, Tiffany, Karen Riley, and Michael Rust. "Read the Leaves before Drinking: Health Risks of Herbal Teas." *Insight on the News*, May 20, 1996, 42.
Fraser, Laura. "The Dangers of Natural Diet Aids." *Glamour*, March 1996, 62–65.

Herbalife

Herbalife, a company started in 1980 by a 19-year-old high school dropout, Mark Hughes, whose mother died from a diet pill overdose, has been as controversial as it has been successful. The company slogan, "Lose weight now/Ask me how," became a familiar sight on buttons in the early 1980s, but by 1985 regulators from the Food and Drug Administration (FDA) were asking different questions concerning some of the ingredients in the Herbalife products. That same year the California Attorney General's office investigated Herbalife, alleging that the company supported some of its products with false medical claims and that the multilevel marketing operation could be an "illegal pyramid scheme." The company settled with the state of California for $850,000, without admitting fault.

Herbalife uses a multilevel sales approach, in which independent distributors handle all the pills, powders, juices, and other products. To earn money, distributors must sell Herbalife to retail customers, but they also take a percentage of the sales from other distributors they recruit to sell the product. Those recruits, in turn, recruit others. Sales from the diet shakes and vitamin supplements reached $427 million by 1985. Today Herbalife does business in 49 countries and has yearly sales of about $880 million.

Right from the start, Hughes, the consummate salesman, insisted that his products would help people lose weight—from 10 to 29 pounds per month. And he told distributors and customers that Herbalife could cure a wide variety of ailments, from asthma to baldness or venereal disease, all while boosting energy levels. The original diet, known as the Slim and Trim Plan, included a variety of Herbalife pills and powders along with one 1,000-calorie meal per day, supplemented with two low-calorie skim milk shakes that contained the company's own protein powder. The daily assortment of herbal vitamins and minerals included vitamin B_6, lecithin, senna leaves, kelp, chickweed, and dandelion.

However, back in 1982, trouble first began for the company when the FDA received numerous reports of adverse reactions to Herbalife products. Those reactions ranged from constipation, diarrhea, and nausea to headaches and allergic reactions. The government maintained that Herbalife products contained powerful laxatives and diuretics. The FDA then sent Herbalife a "Notice of Adverse Findings," in which it stated that one of the company's products contained the ingredients mandrake and pokeroot, both considered unsafe by the FDA for food use. Mandrake, used at one time as a suicide drug by American Indians, and pokeroot were voluntarily removed from Herbalife formulas.

Besides side effects, questions were raised about unknown ingredients and about how the products were tested and determined fit for human consumption. Hughes said in an article in *People* that he tests products on himself. For years, Hughes also refused to have Herbalife products analyzed by medical experts outside the company and insisted that product nutrition was sound. He suggested that a study of those products was unnecessary, since Herbalife helped more people lose weight than any other institution in the world.

Hughes, the 44-year-old founder of Herbalife, was found dead in his Malibu beachfront mansion in 2000. He died after accidentally mixing alcohol and the antidepressant and sleeping aid Doxepin. Today, Herbalife continues to offer a wide range of products for weight loss as well as for skin and hair care and cosmetics. In April 2002, two venture-capital firms acquired the company for approximately $685 million.

See also: Food and Drug Administration (FDA).

FURTHER READING

Carey, John. "Selling Herbalife's Way." *Newsweek*, April 8, 1985, 89.
Carlson, P. "Despite Critics and Lawsuits, Herbalife Has Made Mark Hughes Wealthy If Not Healthy." *People*, April 29, 1985, 78–80.

Contemporary Newsmakers 1985. Detroit: Gale Research, 1985.

"Herbalife Founder Dies." *Los Angeles Business Journal* 22, no. 22 (May 29, 2000): 49.

Rakoff, David. "Death Be Not a Punch Line: Vitamin King Takes Pill and Dies." *New York Times Magazine*, January 7, 2001, 3.

High-Protein Diets

High-protein diets, although extremely popular with Americans, have not been proven effective for long-term weight loss. Like other fad diets, nutritionists say these diets pose potential health threats for people who follow them for more than a short period of time. Critics point to popular diets such as the Atkins, Zone, Protein Power, and Sugar Busters! diets as examples of high-protein eating plans.

The diets emphasize foods high in saturated fat, like meat and eggs, and limit high-carbohydrate foods such as cereals, grains, fruits, and vegetables. Concerns from groups like the American Heart Association (AHA) center on the fact that most Americans already eat more protein than their bodies need. Too much protein is not healthy when it comes to the human body. If too much is eaten, the excess is converted to fat and waste. Plus, breaking down that excess strains the kidneys and liver and can increase the risk of osteoporosis. And, according to the AHA and other health organizations, eating too much protein can also increase the possibility of coronary heart disease, diabetes, stroke, and several types of cancer.

According to the USDA, the average American consumes about 90 grams of protein daily, significantly more than the 50 grams per day average the USDA recommends for healthy adults. The AHA guidelines, similar to the USDA recommendations, urge most adults to consume less than 30 percent of their total daily calories from fat and less than 10 percent of that from saturated fat. Most high-protein diets cannot meet these goals based on their suggested food choices.

The theory behind high-protein diets is that our bodies inefficiently burn carbohydrates, turning too many into fat. By eating fewer carbohydrates foods, these diets suggest that someone will reduce fat production and lose weight. But scientists say carbohydrates are the body's most efficient fuel and, when they are lacking, muscle gets burned for food or worse, ketosis develops. Ketosis is a toxic condition that occurs when ketones are released into the bloodstream. It can be triggered by starvation or untreated diabetes and it brings with it nausea, dehydration, constipation, or diarrhea. Prolonged ketosis may lead to kidney disease, gallstones, and even, in severe situations, cardiac complications. There is considerable disagreement among health organizations and high-protein diet advocates about the benefits and risks of ketosis resulting from high-protein eating programs.

High-protein diets can also fail to provide essential vitamins, minerals, fiber, and other nutritional elements that come from fruits, vegetables, whole grains, and nonfat dairy products because they severely limit these food groups. Many programs, such as the Atkins diet, do recommend vitamin supplements for participants. Health groups like the AHA criticize high-protein diets, saying they work for the same reason all diets work; they limit calories. Fewer calories from any source, whether it's protein, fat, or carbohydrates, will cause weight loss.

In 2001, the AHA issued a strong recommendation against high-protein weight-loss programs, including the Atkins diet, Protein Power, the Zone, and Sugar Busters!, citing a lack of credible scientific evidence of long-term weight loss for these programs and the possibility of increased risk for those dieters with diabetes and heart disease. The report noted that high-protein weight-loss programs are "especially risky for patients with diabetes," because they can speed the progression of kidney disease even if followed for a short time. Like the U.S. Dietary Guidelines, the AHA's newest guidelines recommend a diet low in fat and high in fruits, vegetables, whole grains, and low-fat dairy products.

See also: Atkins Nutritional Approach; Carbohydrate Addict's Diet; Ketones/Ketosis; Sugar Busters!; The Zone.

FURTHER READING

Albertson, Ellen. "Walking the Protein Tightrope." *Better Homes and Gardens*, April 1999, 118.

Norris, Eileen. "High-Protein Diets: Where's the Beef?" *Harvard Health Letter*, 22, no. 3 (January 1997): 1–4.

Squires, Sally. "Heart Association Skewers Atkins Diet; High Protein Plans Called Unproven, Risky." *Washington Post*, October 9, 2001, F1.

Hudson, Jennifer

Jennifer Hudson (b. September 12, 1981, in Chicago, IL) became the spokesperson for Weight Watchers in 2010. She is an award-winning singer, actress, and is considered one of American's style icons, appearing on the cover of *Vogue* magazine as only the third African American woman to do so.

Hudson first found fame as a contestant on *American Idol* in 2004, and although she did not win that year's contest, she became a superstar with her breakout role as Effie in the Broadway musical *Dreamgirls* in 2006. Hudson and her voluptuous figure was a feature on the red carpet as she won both a Golden Globe and the Academy Award for Best Supporting Actress for her role.

After the birth of her first child, David, in 2009, Hudson turned to Weight Watchers International and began what would total an 80-pound weight

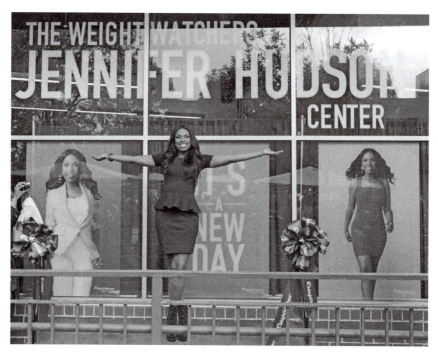

Award-winning singer and actress Jennifer Hudson became a Weight Watchers spokes-person after she managed to lose 80 pounds after the birth of her son. The company opened the Weight Watchers Jennifer Hudson Center in Chicago in 2011. (AP Photo/M. Spencer Green)

loss. In honor of her achievements and her success in keeping the weight off, the company opened the Weight Watchers Jennifer Hudson Center in a Chicago neighborhood in 2011. According to a statement released by the company, this was the first time they have named a building for a spokesperson. Company officials referred to the center as a symbol of Weight Watchers commitment to Hudson, her healthy lifestyle, and to Hudson's hometown.

During the center's opening, Hudson called it a way to give back to her community. Hudson said, "Weight Watchers has helped make my new lifestyle a reality by teaching me the tools I need to be successful." She said she hopes the center can inspire others to find a healthy way to lose weight. Weight Watchers officials also announced they would donate a portion of the center's proceeds to Hudson's foundation, the Julian D. King Gift Foundation.

Hudson started the foundation to honor her nephew Julian, who along with Hudson's mother and brother was murdered in 2008 by her former brother-in-law. The foundation celebrates children who are successful in school and through fund-raising events uses those proceeds to support and encourage the children to continue their educations.

The star has spoken candidly about her weight loss and her time as a plus-size singer and actress in Hollywood. In several interviews she discussed how she had to learn an entirely new and healthy way to eat. She had decided to try the Weight Watchers system of points because she wanted a flexible plan that would accommodate her busy lifestyle and constant travel. She also focused on portion control, something she had never been introduced to as a child.

Earlier attempts by the singer to lose weight had ended in failure. Hudson described how she had tried a number of fad diets including detox-style plans where she would eat only grilled chicken, brown rice, and vegetables. Her yo-yo dieting contributed to her losing the same weight over and over again. It wasn't until 2009 when she joined the Weight Watchers program and began working with a counselor that she was able to examine her eating and find healthy alternatives for fast food and other less healthy choices.

See also: Celebrity Endorsements.

FURTHER READING

Dunn, Jancee. "I'm Getting Used to My New Self: Jennifer Hudson Is on a Confidence Roll, with a Body She Loves, a New Fashion Line and Cool TV and Movie Roles. Four Years after Her Family Tragedy, She's Planning a Bright Christmas." *Redbook*, December 2012, 116.

Sangweni, Yolanda. "Jennifer Hudson Opens Her Own Weight Watchers Center. *Essence.com*, September 28, 2011. http://www.essence.com/2011/09/28/jennifer-hudson-weight-watchers-center-chicago/SO AD

Stedman, Alex. "Hudson Turns Tragedy to Philanthropy: The Julian D. King Foundation Honors Late Nephew." *Variety*, November 12, 2012, 100.

Truesdell, Jeff. "Jennifer Hudson Family Murder Trial: Her Fight for Justice." *People Weekly* 77, no. 18 (April 30, 2012): 66.

Human Chorionic Gonadotropin (HCG)

Human chorionic gonadotropin (HCG) is a hormone produced during pregnancy. HCG levels are used to determine if a woman is pregnant. Home pregnancy kits can easily measure those levels. During the early 1970s, HCG was a popular component of a low-calorie weight-loss plan. But in 1974, the Food and Drug Administration (FDA) issued a statement that expressed growing concern about the continued use of HCG in weight-loss clinics around the country, saying there was no evidence that the drug was effective in treating obesity. Clinics that offered HCG as part of a weight-loss plan often coupled it with a 500-calorie diet. Diets that are low in calories will cause weight loss, no matter what foods are eaten or supplements taken.

The FDA also announced that the drug HCG must bear a label saying it is worthless for weight loss. The report stressed that although no injuries had been noted among patients taking the hormone, any active drug can have unexpected adverse reactions. The FDA later issued an alert on the dangers of contaminated HCG reportedly being used by athletes and bodybuilders to counter the effects of steroids. Doctors legitimately prescribe HCG to treat cases of undescended testicles in men or infertility in women.

See also: Food and Drug Administration (FDA); Obesity.

FURTHER READING

Ballin, J.C., and P.L. White. "Fallacy and Hazard: Human Chorionic Gonadotropin Diet and Weight Reduction." *Journal of the American Medical Association* 230, no. 5 (November 4, 1974): 693.

"Disclaimer Ordered on Drug Used in Antifat Clinics." *New York Times*, December 15, 1974, 55.

Haupt, Angela. "HCG Diet Dangers: Is Fast Weight Loss Worth the Risk?" *U.S. New & World Report*, March 14, 2011. http://health.usnews.com/health-news/diet-fitness/diet/articles/2011/03/14/hcg-diet-dangers-is-fast-weight-loss-worth-the-risk.

Prince, Rayma. "FDA Issues Alert on Phony, Contaminated HCG." *Drug Topics* 132, no. 1 (1988): 40.

Insulin

Insulin is a hormone required to convert sugars and starches from the food we eat into the energy we need. Diabetes is a condition in which the body no longer or inadequately produces insulin. People with Type 1, or insulin-dependent, diabetes must take daily insulin injections—often multiple injections—to stay alive. People with Type 2 diabetes use a variety of controls, including diet, exercise, oral medications, and, sometimes, injections of insulin.

Not until 1920 did a Canadian doctor, Frederick Banting, first conceive of the production of insulin. The first patient treated with insulin was a 14-year-old Canadian boy. Today, there are more than 20 kinds of insulin available—some act very quickly or peak at different times, and some last all day long. There are also different ways to deliver insulin—syringes, insulin pens, and insulin pumps.

Researchers are also making progress in solving the riddle of diabetes. Research into prevention of Type 1 diabetes is under way, as are efforts to transplant insulin-producing cells into the bodies of Type 1 diabetics. Other researchers, meanwhile, are finding new ways to help people who have the condition to control it.

See also: Diabetes.

FURTHER READING

www.diabetes.org.

Internet Dieting

Online support for dieters is easy to find these days. Nearly every major weight loss program, such as Weight Watchers, Jenny Craig, Nutrisystem, and more offer online programs that include online support through chats or community boards, ways to order products and apps to help with counting calories or calculating calories used.

Internet-based diet plans offer the advantage of providing information and support 24/7, as well as a level of discretion or anonymity that weigh-ins and other community-based programs can't provide.

Costs of Internet diet programs vary, depending on the level of services to which a user subscribes. Some plans offer free encouragement and menu planning, while others require that users purchase some level of meal plans, nutrition bars, or shakes, for example.

See also: Weight Watchers.

FURTHER READING

"Best Diet Websites." Good Housekeeping. http://www.goodhousekeeping.com/health/diet-plans/best-diet-websites.

Depillis, Lydia. "Internet Killed the Dieting Star: Why Weight Watchers Is Floundering." *The Washington Post*, August 4, 2013. www.washingtonpost.com/blogs/wonkblog/wp/2013/08/04/internet-killed-the-dieting-star-why-weight-watchers-is-floundering/.

Stroup, Katherine. "Desktop Dieting: Is the Internet the Answer to Losing Those Extra Pounds?" *Newsweek*, May 20, 2002, 70.

www.ediets.com.
www.jennycraig.com.
www.nutrisystem.com.
www.richardsimmons.com.
www.weightwatchers.com.

Jenny Craig

Jenny Craig, Inc., is a weight-loss program combining personalized support with a variety of prepackaged meals. At Jenny in Center programs, a dieter meets weekly with a consultant, reviews the past week, plans the menu for the upcoming week, and generally receives support. Jenny Craig also offers its Internet-based program, Jenny Anywhere.

Jenny Craig's programs include additional support on exercise, and manuals with strategies for losing weight and maintaining weight loss. The company also offers foods, which the Web site says are "specifically chosen for slow, steady weight loss, with calories levels ranging from 1,200 to 2,300 calories per day." The Jenny's Cuisine line includes breakfast, lunch, dinner, and snack items.

Jenny Craig was founded in 1983, by Jenny and Sid Craig. They opened their first Jenny Craig Centre in Australia when Jenny was 50 and Sid was 51. Jenny

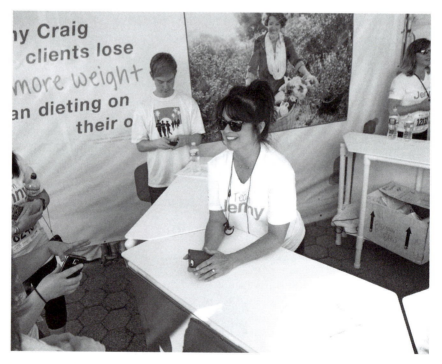

The weight-loss program Jenny Craig has had its celebrity ambassadors for the brand. Shown here is Valerie Bertinelli at an American Heart Association event. (Michael Loccisano/Getty Images)

Craig became interested in weight control after she gained 45 pounds during her pregnancy. Her biography on the Web site notes that Craig's mother had been overweight after having children and died of an obesity-related stroke at age 49. "In an effort to avoid a similar situation, Jenny joined a local gym and shed her excess pounds using a two-pronged approach of healthy eating and exercise." That combination of nutrition, physical activity, and lifestyle changes is the underpinning of the Jenny Craig program. With her husband, marketing specialist Sid Craig, the couple grew Jenny Craig, Inc., from that one center to one of the largest weight-loss programs.

In May 2002, a private investor group acquired Jenny Craig, Inc. Sid and Jenny Craig were part of that investor group. The company has been sold again, most recently in November 2013, when North Castle Partners acquired Jenny Craig from Nestlé. North Castle plans to join Jenny Craig with Curves International, a chain of women's fitness centers, creating a one-of-a-kind wellness company.

See also: Internet Dieting; Weight Watchers.

FURTHER READING

Press release: "New Study Results Find That Jenny Craig Helps People with Type 2 Diabetes Manage Their Weight Better than Usual Care." April 23, 2014. http://www .marketwatch.com/story/new-study-results-find-that-jenny-craig-helps-people-with-type-2-diabetes-manage-their-weight-better-than-usual-care-2014-04-23.

Thompson, Stephanie. "Two Ad Pitches for Weight Loss Gain More Heft; Weight Watchers and Jenny Craig Stress Personalized Diet Programs." *Advertising Age*, December 4, 2000, 3.

www.jennycraig.com.

Ketones/Ketosis

Ketones or ketone bodies are created by the liver when it converts fats into chemicals for the body to use as fuel. Ketosis is an abnormal increase of ketone bodies in the bloodstream, triggered by starvation or by a low- to no-carbohydrate diet. During digestion, the liver converts carbohydrates into the simple sugar glucose, an important fuel for most body functions. Proteins replace themselves as needed and any excess protein also becomes glucose.

Ketosis occurs when there is a shortage of carbohydrates for fuel, which triggers the production of large amounts of ketone bodies to compensate for the lack of glucose. Problems develop because the tissue in the brain and in the muscles used for rapid movement cannot use ketone bodies as efficiently as they use glucose for fuel. A low-carbohydrate diet forces the brain to use ketones for its fuel. This change in fuel slows thinking and reaction times.

The symptoms of ketosis include unpleasant odor or bad breath, nausea, dehydration, constipation, and diarrhea. Severe and prolonged ketosis may lead to kidney disease, gallstones, gout, or cardiac complications. Advocates of high-protein, low-carbohydrate diets, such as the Scarsdale Medical Diet and the Atkins Nutritional Approach, acknowledge that dieters following their eating programs will experience ketosis. However, they claim that the condition can enhance the effectiveness of a low-carbohydrate diet.

According to the U.S. Department of Agriculture, a number of factors contribute to weight loss for people following a low-carbohydrate diet. The factors include water weight loss, decreased appetite, and the unpleasant symptoms of ketosis along with the elimination of carbohydrates as a food group, which creates a corresponding decrease in calorie consumption. Doctors have successfully prescribed ketogenic diets for people afflicted with epilepsy. Those ketogenic diets slow down all brain functions, making it less likely the brain will react to the triggers that set off an epileptic episode.

See also: Atkins Nutritional Approach; MyPlate; Scarsdale Diet.

FURTHER READING

"Fad Diets." *The Nurse Practitioner* 25, no. 10 (October 2000): 1s18.
Merriam-Webster's Medical Dictionary. Spring-field, MA: Merriam-Webster, Inc., 1995.
Tarnower, Herman, and Samm Sinclair Baker. *The Complete Scarsdale Medical Diet.* New York: Rawson, Wade Publishers, Inc., 1978.

Let's Move

Childhood obesity numbers have tripled over the past several decades and now one in three children in America are overweight or obese. When Barack Obama was elected president in 2008, his wife, Michelle, began what she called a national conversation about the health and well-being of the country's children. However, it was more than just policy and talking heads, the First Lady has been determined to bring healthy nutrition and physical activity to the forefront of her discussion.

Let's Move, part of that discussion, is a key weapon in the First Lady's fight against obesity and the health problems associated with it. This comprehensive initiative, described as a way to put together strategies and common sense, looks at the problem from several angles. Information is a huge component of Let's Move; information for parents to help them make healthy choices for their children. Let's Move is also behind the effort to get healthier foods into school lunch

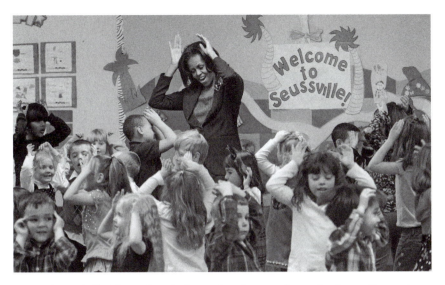

First Lady Michelle Obama does the bunny hop dance with preschoolers in Concord, NH, as part of her Let's Move initiative in 2012. (AP Photo/Jim Cole)

programs across the country, and Obama has met with private sector companies and used her bully pulpit to urge manufacturers and stores to improve the quality of the food they sell to U.S. consumers.

Empowering parents and caregivers and providing healthy food in schools are two of the five pillars of the Let's Move initiative. The other three components include creating a healthy start for children, improving access to healthy, affordable foods for everyone, and increasing physical activity for everyone too. To coincide with the First Lady's efforts, the President signed a Presidential Memorandum that called for a Task Force on Childhood Obesity. The task force, whose members were drawn from 12 different government agencies, were then asked to review every government program and policy that related to childhood nutrition and physical activity and to create a plan to improve how federal resources are used to support the First Lady's goal.

After several years of a comprehensive effort that included improvements in the content of school lunches, a focus on family gardens led by the First Lady who planted her own garden on the White House Lawn, and the roll out of Let's Move and its associated Let's Move Cities and Towns, Let's Move Faith and Communities, and the Let's Move Outside Junior Rangers, there was tentative good news. Figures released by the Centers for Disease Control and Prevention (CDC) in 2013 reported that after decades of growing obesity rates, especially in low-income communities, the numbers have started to go down. Government officials suggest that the decline may be coming from this multipronged approach; improvements in the food being marketed, better labeling of packaged foods, more information for families on healthy eating habits, encouragement to improve physical activity and community-wide support for Let's Move and other health programs, and that the combination worked together to create change.

The Let's Move program also lists other suggestions on its Web site to encourage kids to eat healthier and to move more. Those tips include making sure children get 60 minutes of vigorous play every day, serving fruit and or vegetables with every meal, drinking water or low-fat milk instead of sugary sweetened soda's or other drinks, increasing the variety of vegetables served and finding different, delicious ways to prepare them, substituting healthier ingredients such as whole grains or lean meats instead of fast food or junk food, and sitting down to eat meals as a family. Other suggestions include supporting a community garden, making sure family members have regular check-ups with a health care provider that includes a Body Mass Index (BMI) check, or working toward a Presidential Active Lifestyle Award (PALA). The award is given to those who commit to an activity five days each week for six weeks.

The Let's Move initiative continues to seek volunteers as it asks everyone to play a role in solving the national problem of childhood obesity.

See also: Obama, Michelle; Obesity.

FURTHER READING

Canale, Larry. "Get Up and Dance: or Run, Walk, Climb, and Somersault—Just Keep Moving! A Model Community Shows the Way." *Odyssey* 23, no. 2 (February 2014): 38.

Gibi, Kathleen. "Let's Move! Cities, Towns and Counties: Program Paves Way to National Partnerships." *Parks & Recreation* 48, no. 10 (October 2013): 37.

Let's Move! http://www.letsmove.gov/.

"Nutrition Improving in U.S. Schools." *Nutraceuticals World* 16, no. 8 (October 2013): 16. http://www.nutraceuticalsworld.com/.

"Retailers Pledge to Bring Relief to 'Food Deserts.'" *MMR (Mass Market Retailer)* 29, no. i1 (January 9, 2012): 41.

Life Choice Diet

The Life Choice diet by Dr. Dean Ornish is a low-fat, vegetarian eating plan that focuses on beans, fruits, vegetables, and whole grains, and recommends that dieters consume only 10 percent of their calories from fat. Ornish, director of the Preventive Medicine Research Institute in Sausalito, California, also encourages regular exercise, stress-management techniques, and group support as key components in his plan. Ornish wrote his best-selling book,

Dr. Dean Ornish's Program for Reversing Heart Disease: The Only System Scientifically Proven to Reverse Heart Disease without Drugs or Surgery, in 1990. The system was developed from Ornish's study data, which showed that program participants who followed his plan had a reduction in overall heart blockages after a relatively short time. The data also showed that his heart patients lost an average of 22 pounds, even though they had not been trying to lose weight during the treatment period.

Ornish published the Life Choice diet in 1993, geared toward people without significant heart disease who wanted to lose weight and improve their health. The book, *Eat More, Weigh Less: Dr. Dean Ornish's Life Choice Program for Losing Weight Safely While Eating Abundantly*, immediately sold half a million copies. According to the author, the Life Choice diet is based on the type of food a person eats rather than the amount of food. This, he said, creates a sense of abundance rather than deprivation. The diet book also echoes the Ornish heart treatment plan by outlining a diet made up primarily of fruits, vegetables, grains, and beans with only 10 percent of calories from mostly polyunsaturated fat. In the book, Ornish explains that the human body needs about 4 to 6 percent of its calories as fat to synthesize essential fatty acids. The Life Choice diet's 10 percent fat goal is less than what is routinely recommended. In fact, a typical 2,000-calorie-a day diet that follows the Dietary Guidelines for Americans and the American Heart Association's guidelines of less than 30 percent of calories from fat per day means eating up to 67 grams of fat daily. By contrast, the Life Choice diet, with only 10 percent fat, means participants eat a mere 22 fat grams a day. The program is now called the Ornish Spectrum.

The Life Choice diet's simple guidelines are not a list of dos and don'ts. Rather, Ornish suggests a spectrum of foods grouped from most beneficial to least beneficial, based mainly on fat and cholesterol content. Group 1 foods, those that are most beneficial, include whole grains from barley to couscous, oats, brown rice, and soybeans, to name just a few. Good-for-you-vegetables range from A to Z: asparagus and artichokes, kale, leeks, potatoes, squash, turnips, and zucchini. Legumes like adzuki beans, black beans, lentils, all kinds of soy products, plus tempeh and tofu are also Group 1 choices. And Ornish encourages dieters to eat a wide variety of fruits, including apples, berries, dates, figs, and all kinds of melons.

Next, in Group 2, are foods that should be eaten in moderation: nonfat dairy products such as skim milk, nonfat yogurt, and egg whites, plus nonfat or very low-fat commercially available products, including whole-grain breakfast cereals, nonfat mayonnaise and salad dressings, and fat-free crackers. Ornish also names a variety of Pritikin products, developed by Nathan Pritikin and the Pritikin Longevity Center, in this category. Group 3 foods to be eaten sparingly are things like oils, low-fat dairy products, fish, maple syrup, and honey. Group 4 foods, to be avoided when possible, include poultry, all shellfish, and refined sugar products. Group 5 foods, products which are not considered healthful, range from all beef and pork products to fried chicken, coconut oil, egg yolks, cream, whole milk foods, salt, and alcohol, plus any commercially available product with more than 2 grams of fat per serving. A typical day on the Ornish diet would feature a breakfast menu with buckwheat pancakes, nonfat yogurt, sliced bananas, kiwi, and fresh strawberries, plus orange juice. Lunch might be tomato and lentil soup, a zucchini salad, and a pear. A dinner entrée might be sweet and sour vegetables with tofu, broccoli, and teriyaki sauce; brown rice pilaf; a green salad with no-fat dressing; and fruit.

While recognizing that these foods sound strange and unfamiliar to many people, Ornish recommends them as part of what he calls comprehensive changes rather than only moderate changes. According to Ornish, big or comprehensive changes disrupt old routines, which, in turn, make change easier. For example, if people who usually eat 8 ounces of steak reduce that to just 4 ounces, they feel cheated. They may ultimately find it easier not to eat any steak at all, to eat something totally different. While Ornish acknowledges that big change is stressful at first, in the long run he maintains that it is easier when people abandon their old habits and then form new ones.

Ornish also suggests in his book that conventional dieting doesn't work when the diet tells people what *not* to do and what *not* to eat. He contrasts his approach, saying it allows dieters to make informed and intelligent choices from the options, selections, and preferences he outlines. With a spectrum of choices, he writes, "Each person will see they have the authority to decide what is right for them." He also criticizes some weight-loss regimes, which might do more harm than good, especially high-protein diets like the Atkins diet that recommends increasing consumption of meats and eggs while reducing carbohydrates and fiber. Health organizations, including the American Heart Association, warn dieters not to eat excessive animal protein with its accompanying saturated fat, saying studies show that it leads to overweight, heart disease, and other illnesses.

See also: Atkins Nutritional Approach; Dietary Guidelines for Americans; Ornish, Dean; Pritikin, Nathan.

FURTHER READING

Brink, Susan. "The Low-Fat Life." *U.S. News & World Report,* July 12, 1999, 56.
Condor, Bob. "Lifestyle Changes Can Go Right to the Heart." *Chicago Tribune*, February 13, 2000, 3.
Cowley, Geoffrey. "Healer of Hearts." *Newsweek*, March 16, 1998, 50–57.
Gavalas, Elaine. "The Great Diet Debate." *Better Nutrition*, May 2000, 32–36.
Lindley, Sarah. "Heart Smart: Natural Remedies for a Healthy Heart." *Vegetarian Times*, May 1997, 58–66.
Ornish, Dean. *Eat More, Weigh Less: Dr. Dean Ornish's Life Choice Program for Losing Weight Safely while Eating Abundantly.* New York: HarperCollins, 1993.
Thomson, Bill. "The Second Act of Dean Ornish." *Natural Health*, November–December 1998, 112–19.

Liposuction

Liposuction is a surgical procedure to remove pockets of fat from your body. A narrow tube is inserted into a fat layer beneath the skin, and the fat cells are broken up and suctioned out. Typically, liposuction is used to sculpt the abdomen, hips, buttocks, thighs, knees, upper arms, chin, cheeks, and neck. According to the American Society of Plastic Surgery, in general, liposuction costs about $3,000. However, surgeon and hospital fees, anesthesia and prescriptions, medical tests and supportive clothing can add to the cost.

Liposuction was the most common cosmetic surgery in the country in 2013, according to the American Society of Aesthetic Plastic Surgeons. That year, there were 363,912 liposuction procedures performed, an increase of 16.3 percent over the year before.

Recent advances in liposuction, such as laser and ultrasound-assisted lipoplasty (UAL), have made the procedure less rough and the recovery a little easier. However, despite its popularity, the decision to have surgery shouldn't be taken lightly. The American Society of Plastic Surgeons emphasizes that liposuction is not a weight-control method, but a body-contouring option for areas that are "not responsive to diet and exercise."

Liposuction has distinct risks—including death. According to the Food and Drug Administration, different studies assess the risk differently. One found the risk of death due to liposuction is as low as 3 deaths for every 100,000 liposuction operations performed, but others have determined it can be as high as between 20 and 100 deaths per 100,000 liposuction procedures. The risk may increase if other surgical procedures are performed at the same time. The FDA notes that one study compared the death rate from liposuction procedures to that of car accidents (16 per 100,000).

Liposuction does not remove cellulite. Nor can a physician guarantee results. Sometimes, the area where the fat was removed may look dimply, a "cottage cheese" effect. Excess skin may stay loose and sag. Fat deposits may develop in new places, and if you gain more than 10 pounds after surgery, the fat may come back to haunt the same area, as well.

The American Society of Plastic Surgeons, which offers a Web-based clearing-house at *www.plasticsurgery.org*, suggests that the best candidates "are normal-weight people with firm, elastic skin who have pockets of excess fat in certain areas. You should be physically healthy, psychologically stable and realistic in your expectations. Your age is not a major consideration; however, older patients may have diminished skin elasticity and may not achieve the same results as a younger patient with tighter skin." The site notes that the risks increase for people with medical problems, especially heart or lung disease or poor blood circulation.

The surgeons' site details the different kinds of liposuction procedures, and prospective patients should discuss the options and their expectations with their physician. It also suggests getting help at home for a day or two following surgery. Liposuction can be performed in an office-based center, an outpatient surgery center, or a hospital. Smaller procedures can be done in the first two; the hospital is a more appropriate setting if more fat is to be removed or if other procedures are being done at the same time. How long the surgery takes depends on how much fat is being removed and how many areas are being sculpted. According to *www. plastic-surgery.org*, following surgery, "You may still experience some pain, burning, swelling, bleeding and temporary numbness." Most people can return to work within a few days and begin to feel better in the next week or so. A noticeable difference in the way you look occurs about four to six weeks after surgery when the swelling has gone down, but it can take about three months for the full effect to emerge.

See also: Obesity Surgery.

FURTHER READING

"The American Society for Aesthetic Plastic Surgery Reports Americans Spent Largest Amount on Cosmetic Surgery since the Great Recession of 2008," press release, March 20, 2014. http://www.surgery.org/media/news-releases/the-american-society-for-aesthetic-plastic-surgery-reports-americans-spent-largest-amount-on-cosmetic-surger.

"Boom (and Busts) for Plastic Surgeons." *U.S. News & World Report*, June 25, 2001, 10.

Diclementi, Deborah. "Pressure to Be Perfect: Since 1996, the Number of Teens Having Plastic Surgery Has Nearly Doubled. Is that a Healthy Choice—or a Dangerous Trend?" *Teen People*, April 1, 2001, 200.

Fitzgerald, Susan, and Marian Uhlman. "A Popular Surgery, a Young Life Lost." *Philadelphia Inquirer*, August 5, 2001, A1.

Gerhart, Ann. "Nipped in the Bud: More and More Young Women Choose Surgical 'Perfection.'" *Washington Post*, June 23, 1999, C1.

Gutman, Matt. "Liposuction Tragedy: Mother's Death Highlights Dangers of Plastic Surgery." *Good Morning America*, ABC News, June 21, 2011. http://abcnews.go.com/Health/liposuction-tragedy-mothers-death-highlights-dangers-plastic-surgery/story?id=13890319.

Henig, Robin Marantz. "The High Cost of Thinness." *New York Times Magazine*, February 28, 1988, 41.

Lamendola, Bob. "Liposuction Deaths End Surgeon's Career." *Health News Florida*, August 1, 2013.

"Liposuction: What Are the Risks or Complications?" FDA.gov. http://www.fda.gov/MedicalDevices/ProductsandMedicalProcedures/SurgeryandLifeSupport/Liposuction/ucm256139.htm.

"Liposuction Rated as Most Popular Procedure for Second Year." *Women's Health Weekly*, February 28, 2002, 11.

Patrick, Stephanie. "Doctors Pioneer Gentler Liposuction." *Dallas Business Journal* 24, no. 49 (July 20, 2001): 3.

www.plasticsurgery.org.

Liquid Protein Diets

Liquid protein diets are not a new concept. Protein formula products, both liquid and powdered, were popular as long ago as the 1930s. But this form of fad dieting almost completely disappeared during its most sensational period in the late 1970s, when at least 58 deaths were linked to the use of liquid protein diets. At that time, an investigation by the Food and Drug Administration (FDA) and the federal Centers for Disease Control and Prevention (CDC) revealed a number of deaths from what they called irreversible abnormal heart rhythms. Those who died had used the liquid protein diets for several months and had lost large amounts of weight. Although publicity concerning the deaths and a warning issued by the FDA almost wiped out the market, by changing ingredients, names, and advertising, liquid diet drinks are once again a moneymaker for the $3 billion-a-year weight-loss industry.

Many of those 58 deaths occurred during the diet's two-week period known as refeeding, when dieters stopped eating the liquid protein and started eating conventional foods. Doctors suspect the deaths occurred when large increases in food intake produced changes in metabolic rates and electrolyte balance, which in turn caused the fatal arrhythmias. The women who died were in their mid-20s to mid-30s; most had been on the liquid protein diets for months and had started eating small amounts of solid food again. In studying those deaths, a Harvard Medical School doctor said in a 1978 *New York Times* interview that he believed the patients had been dangerously depleted of essential nutrients, such as potassium and other minerals. This loss of important minerals, in his opinion, contributed to the heart damage seen in the victims.

There are two basic categories of liquid protein diets: the aforementioned draconian regimes, also known as very-low-calorie diets, now modified to be administered under medical supervision; and the over-the-counter cans or powders designed to replace a meal or two per day. Those over-the-counter liquid replacement meals date back to the early 1930s when Dr. Stoll's Diet Aid, the Natural Reducing Food, was sold to women through beauty parlors. Dr. Stoll's was the most famous reducing drink of its day. Directions called for dieters to combine a cup of water with a teaspoon of the protein powder made from milk chocolate, starch, and an extract of roasted whole wheat and bran. Although there were no statistics on the success or failure of Dr. Stoll's Diet Aid, this product was the first in a growing list of popular over-the-counter liquid diet drinks.

In 1959, Metrecal became a household name; thanks to the doctors at the Rockefeller Institute. They developed their diet drink to resemble breast milk by including a precise balance of protein, fat, and carbohydrate. That new formula made Metrecal a commercial success. During the 1970s, hospitals began offering medically supervised liquid protein plans like Optifast to obese patients. Following the supervised diets came over-the-counter choices with names like

Prolinn, GroLean, and Cherrmino. These liquid protein products began innocently enough through the work of Harvard Medical School professor George Cahill, Jr., and his colleague, Dr. George Blackburn. The two were among others studying the problem of malnutrition and the detrimental effects of fasting among postoperative patients. Their solution was to feed people small amounts of pure protein following surgery. Their successful strategy caught the attention of osteopath Dr. Robert Linn. In 1976, Linn took the idea of liquid protein replacement as the main focus of his own diet program and he explained it all in his best-selling diet book, *The Last Chance Diet*. The book sold more than 2 million copies and laid out his simple plan: take in just enough protein to keep the body going without breaking down lean muscle tissue. For a time, dieters could live off their own fat and lose as much as 10 pounds per week. And it was easy, just drink 6 to 8 ounces of liquid protein daily, either straight or mixed with diet soda, and drink plenty of water.

Blackburn's harsh response to Linn's protein diet was quoted in a 1977 *Newsweek* article. He called the Linn diet program "amateurish and totally without credence." Blackburn maintained that insufficient research had been done on the effectiveness of this type of diet, especially problems with long-term maintenance and the need for specific vitamins and minerals. In his book Linn did urge dieters to consult a doctor who could then prescribe the needed supplemental vitamins and minerals. But because the product was sold over the counter, users rarely saw a doctor before starting on the diet. As a result, many suffered from a lack of potassium, a deficiency known to lead to kidney damage or potentially fatal abnormal heart rhythms or arrhythmias.

A study released in 1977 by the FDA noted that three well-known brands of liquid protein contained protein of "extremely poor" quality. Some of the early liquid protein diets were made from ground-up livestock bones and ears. Linn's first liquid diet, Prolinn, contained beef hide. He later switched his main ingredient to pigskin and named it EMF, or Enzymatic Modular Food. Linn admitted that there were problems with his early formula; diarrhea was one of the main side effects.

Health groups like the American Dietetic Association say current liquid protein products contain more and better protein, some carbohydrates, and more vitamins and minerals than their 1970 counterparts. Today's liquid diets are still designed to replace solid food entirely for weeks at a time, but now they are handled through hospitals or doctors' offices so that health professionals can check blood pressure, heart function, urine content, and potassium and electrolyte levels. Another common problem with very-low-calorie diets is that dieters risk losing valuable lean muscle if they take weight off too quickly. That problem can be avoided by limiting participants to only those patients who are truly obese, weighing in at over 20 to 30 percent of their ideal weight. Nutrition education and behavior modification training with a psychological component is also part of current very-low-calorie diet programs.

Since 1984 the FDA has required that all very-low-calorie protein diets, meaning diets that provide fewer than 400 calories a day, carry a warning that they can cause serious illness and need to be followed under medical supervision. The initial warning that followed the 58 deaths in 1978 affected nearly all liquid protein products. But newer regulations only require warnings on protein products that provide more than half of a person's calories and are promoted for use in losing weight or as a food supplement. So diet drinks like Slim-Fast protein powder, introduced in 1978, have been able to escape the need for the FDA warning label by recommending that users also eat one sensible meal each day. That way the drinks do not fall into the very-low-calorie range. For example, three Slim-Fast shakes a day provide 660 calories; a snack and sensible dinner add to that for a total of 1,200 or so calories per day. Famous Slim-Fast users include former New York City mayor Ed Koch, baseball manager Tommy Lasorda, and singer Mel Tormé.

When celebrities lose large amounts of weight, it adds glamour along with an aura of success to the liquid diet programs, but success is far from guaranteed once the pounds are gone. Unfortunately, clinical studies now show that as many as 90 percent of the people who lose 25 pounds or more on any diet gain them back within two years. Medically supervised plans like Optifast have claimed for years that about two-thirds of the patients who complete their programs keep the majority of pounds off for at least 18 months. Still, health agencies like the American Dietetic Association continue to caution consumers about the risks of liquid protein diets, especially their poor long-term results. And doctors say evidence shows that a high percentage of patients treated by liquid protein diets alone regain weight almost as quickly as they lose it. This is caused by the body's metabolic rate. When dieters lose a lot of lean body mass, their resting metabolic rate slows, and a lowered metabolism makes it that much more difficult to keep off pounds without the help of a daily exercise program—a vital part of any long-term weight-loss plan.

For example, in 1988 celebrity Oprah Winfrey lost 67 pounds using the Optifast liquid protein diet. But after one year the star was 17 pounds heavier and went on to regain most of the lost weight. It wasn't until several years later that Winfrey incorporated daily exercise into her weight-loss effort. Following her use of Optifast, she vowed she would never again reveal her weight or go on a diet. Oprah's televised Optifast weight loss in 1988 created an initial national frenzy, along with a huge growth in the liquid diet industry, which saw profits of $200 million that year alone. Few Americans had tried liquid diets since the tragic deaths of the 1970s but Winfrey's success gave the industry a needed boost. After the actress regained the pounds, liquid diet drinks came under sharp review by the Federal Trade Commission (FTC). And in 1991 the FTC charged Optifast, Medifast, and Ultrafast with deceptive advertising. The three reached a settlement with the FTC after the companies agreed to stop using what the FTC alleged were deceptive claims about the long-term results and the safety of liquid diets.

Today, liquid diet drinks continue to have the support of some medical professionals who call the programs a successful alternative to high-risk gastric-bypass surgery for very obese patients. While the gastric-bypass surgery reduces the stomach's capacity for food, limiting the amount of food an individual can eat, liquid protein diets take away all food decisions. These rigidly structured programs begin with a fasting period of three months or more, when patients eat only the protein shakes and take in from 400 to 800 calories a day. After patients lose anywhere from 3 to 10 pounds a week and reach their target weight, they begin to reintroduce solid foods, lean meats, salads, or vegetables. Last is the maintenance stage when dieters make their own food choices, a difficult phase according to patients, many of whom haven't learned to eat well-balanced, nutritious meals. Yet doctors say liquid meal replacement is a good option for people who have problems with portion control as long as solid food choices include lots of fruits and vegetables and complex carbohydrates to provide plenty of fiber and phytochemicals. And while the specialists recognize that the risks of liquid diets include heart irregularities and sudden death, they believe medically supervised liquid protein plans can work for people who desperately need to lose weight but have failed for years on other diets.

See also: Overnight Diet; Slim-Fast.

FURTHER READING

Beck, Melinda. "The Losing Formula: Liquid Diets Take Pounds Off Fast. But a Quick Fix Can Be Risky and Doesn't Ensure Long-Term Success." *Newsweek*, April 30, 1990, 52–58.

Cowley, Susan Cheever, and Patricia J. Seth. "No-Food Diet: Liquid-Protein Regimen." *Newsweek*, July 11, 1977, 74.

Deveny, Kathleen. "Liquid Diet Plans Are Staging a Comeback." *Wall Street Journal*, September 7, 1993, B5.

Langway, Lynn. "Feasting on Fat." *Newsweek*, December 5, 1977, 83.

Larkin, Howard. "Liquid Diets Suffer Another Blow to Their Image." *American Medical News* 34, no. 42 (November 11, 1991): 22.

Mitgang, Lee. "Liquid Protein Dies a Natural Death." *New York Times*, October 15, 1978, 64.

Rhodes, Maura. "America's Top 6 Fad Diets." *Good Housekeeping*, July 1996, 100–103.

Sachs, Andrea. "Drinking Yourself Skinny: Liquid Diets Are Back in Vogue, but Are They Safe?" *Time*, December 19, 1988, 68.

Schmeck, Harold, Jr. "FDA Still Seeking Specific Health Hazard in Liquid Protein Products." *New York Times*, May 16, 1978, 16.

Silberner, Joanne, Pamela Sherrid, and Francesca Lunzer Kritz. "The Real Skinny on Liquid Diets." *U.S. News & World Report*, October 28, 1991, 90.

"Three Liquid Diet Marketers Told to Alter Ad Claims." *New York Times*, October 17, 1991, D2.

Wadden, Thomas A., Theodore B. Van Itallie, and George L. Blackburn. "Responsible and Irresponsible Use of Very-Low-Calorie Diets in the Treatment of Obesity." *Journal of the American Medical Association* 263, no. 1 (January 5, 1990): 83–86.

Macrobiotics

Macrobiotics is a diet considered by followers to be a spiritual and social philosophy of living and eating. Macrobiotic principles stem from the ancient Asian philosophy of yin and yang. Its name comes from the Greek words *macro*, meaning "great," and *bios*, meaning "life." The basic diet, developed by Japanese philosopher George Ohsawa, calls for followers to eat whole foods native to one's environment and to gradually stop eating refined and processed foods.

The diet attempts to balance the intake of yin and yang foods to establish a harmony in the body, which will produce good health. Yin foods include vegetables, grains, beans, and seaweed. Animals and animal products are labeled as yang and include salt, fish, and fowl. Macrobiotic followers aim for a balance of five parts yin to one part yang in their diet. So a macrobiotic eating plan would include 50 to 60 percent of calories from whole grains, including brown rice, barley, millet, oats, corn, rye, wheat, and buckwheat. Fresh vegetables would be 25 to 30 percent of the diet and soybean products, such as tofu and tempeh, along with seaweed that might make up 5 to 10 percent of foods eaten. Preparation of the food is an important aspect of macrobiotics. Followers believe that vegetables should be lightly steamed, boiled, or sautéed in vegetable oil. Rice must be pressure-cooked, and gas is the only acceptable cooking fuel. Wood utensils are allowed, while plastic ones are to be avoided. Pots should be made of glass, ceramic, or stainless steel. Electric stoves as well as copper, aluminum, and Teflon pots should be avoided.

During the 1960s, the diet was known as "the brown rice diet," and was identified largely with hippies, dropouts, and the drug culture. In 1971 the American Medical Association condemned macrobiotics, labeling it "a major public health problem" that posed a serious hazard to the health of individuals. While the diet is hardly conventional, over the years it has gained support. Recent studies show the diet can decrease the risks for heart disease and some forms of cancer, according to Harvard nutritionist Dr. Frederick Stare. Stare equated macrobiotics to a typical vegetarian diet even as early as 1978 in a *New York Times* interview. Despite some benefits, serious problems can occur with strict interpretations of this diet. Those following it can become deficient in protein, vitamin B_{12}, vitamin D, calcium, iron, and riboflavin. Experts say adding eggs and dairy products or other forms of supplementation to a macrobiotic diet can alleviate those problems.

See also: Ohsawa, George; Vegetarian Diet; Vitamins.

FURTHER READING

Bruder, Jessica. "The Picky Eater Who Came to Dinner." *The New York Times*, June 29, 2012, ST1.

Kastner, M. *Alternative Healing: The Complete A to Z Guide to over 160 Different Alternative Therapies*. La Mesa, CA: Halcyon Publishing, 1993.

Sifton, D. W. *The PDR Family Guide to Natural Medicines and Healing Therapies*. New York: Three Rivers Press, 1999.

Wells, Patricia. "Macrobiotics: A Principle, Not a Diet." *New York Times,* July 19, 1978, C1–C9.

Woodham, A., and D. Peters. *Encyclopedia of Healing Therapies*. 1st ed. New York: Dorling Kindersley, 1997.

Malnutrition

Malnutrition results from an improper diet. In its extreme, malnutrition can lead to starvation. Poverty is the leading cause of malnutrition, but people in wealthy and developed countries may suffer from malnutrition and undernourishment as well. People who are malnourished are generally weak and lethargic. Following the U.S. recession of 2008, research suggests that hunger and food insecurity are increasing in homes with little money and where adults have lost their jobs or been laid off. Statistics from the U.S. Department of Agriculture (USDA) Economic Research Service show that some 15 percent of U.S. families at some point during the year missed meals due to a lack of money. Many families are also eating cheap, less healthy foods, a choice that can lead to malnutrition and other health-related problems. The situation is even worse worldwide as statistics show there are 52 million children in the world suffering from acute malnutrition due to poverty, war, and famine.

Specific deficiencies in a diet result in particular problems: anemia is the most common in developed countries. Anemia results from an iron deficiency. Other dietary problems are less common: night blindness can be a result of a vitamin A deficiency; rickets can be due to a lack of vitamin D or adequate sunlight; and scurvy can result from too little vitamin C in the diet.

According to the *Miller-Keane Medical Dictionary*, "Ignorance of the basic principles of nutrition is probably almost as great a cause of undernourishment as poverty. Misplaced faith in vitamin pills as a substitute for food, for example, can cause undernourishment if carried to extremes. So can overreliance on excessively processed foods."

People who severely cut back their food intake, who eat a very limited diet, or who take megadoses of vitamins to offset the reduction in food could be susceptible to malnutrition. Most commonly, however, malnutrition remains a problem in countries where lack of access to nutritious food and poverty are continuing problems.

See also: Vitamins.

FURTHER READING

"Georgie Takes a United Front against Food Insecurity and Obesity." The Center for Disease Control and Prevention National Center for Chronic Disease Prevention and Health Promotion, November, 2010. http://www.cdc.gov/obesity/downloads/field/field_factsheet_georgia.pdf.

"Getting the Full Picture on Food Poverty." *The Guardian (London)*, April 25, 2014, Regional News, 37.

Johnson, Steven Ross. "Hunger as a Health Issue; Food Insecurity Adds to Health System's Costs; October Summit Seeks Solutions." *Modern Healthcare* 43, no. 39 (September 30, 2013): 0012.

Master Cleanse Diet

Looking for a diet where you never feel hungry, where your body is cleansed of toxins and you drop pounds instantly? Looking for a diet that has been around for decades and can wipe the floor with any juice fast out there? Then consider the Master Cleanse, also known as the lemonade diet or the maple syrup diet. Developed and released in a type of user's guide in 1976 by Stanley Burroughs, the plan is a fasting and cleansing program. Burroughs actually created it back in 1940 but waited 36 years to release it. The program was later revised in 1993 and has been offered as a kit on Amazon.

The diet is rumored to have helped Beyonce Knowles lose 20 pounds for her role in *Dream Girls* and once used by Gwyneth Paltrow to keep her razor thin figure. The cleanse is simple and requires dieters to drink 6 to 12 glasses every day of a homemade lemonade made of lemons, maple syrup, sea salt, cayenne pepper, senna tea, and some eight gallons of purified water. The daily lemonade routine is followed each evening by an herbal laxative tea and then a quart of salt water in the morning. The Master Cleanse is recommended for only 10 days, followed by a return to regular eating that requires up to four days to safely accomplish.

Supporters of the diet suggest the lemon juice breaks up waste in the colon, while the maple syrup provides energy in the form of sugar along with a number of minerals and vitamins. The cayenne cuts through the mucus and dilates blood vessels to warm the body and the laxative tea at night helps clean the intestines.

There are detox symptoms to be aware of including irritability, aches, and pains along with cravings. Nutritionists also caution that liquid fasts will not help anyone who struggles with eating in moderation. Health care professionals suggest there is evidence that fasts like the Master Cleanse can trigger worse eating problems in those susceptible to more serious disorders like bulimia or anorexia nervosa.

While a cleanse diet creates a sudden weight loss, those pounds come from water and muscle, not fat. Plus, once the dieter begins eating regular food the weight returns. Nutritionists caution that these extreme diets are an unhealthy quick fix and not sustainable for any period of time. They do not allow the dieter

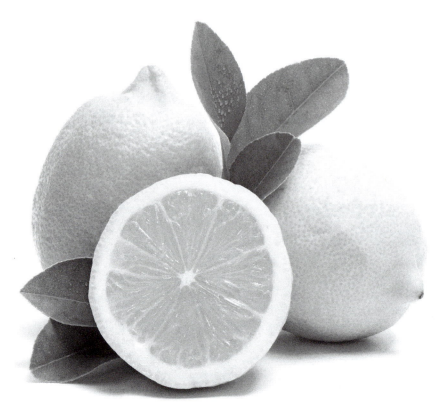

Cleanse diets typically involve limiting food intake and drinking large amounts of liquid. The Master Cleanse recipe includes lemonade made with maple syrup, cayenne pepper, senna tea, and sea salt to be used for no more than 10 days. (Christian Jung/Dreamstime .com)

to develop regular or healthy eating habits and with the diet's complete lack of protein, it is impossible to exercise while following it, especially since much of the weight loss may come from muscle.

The cleanse diets severely limit calories each day, the Master Cleanse provides only 650 calories, which is a great deal less than the 1,800 or 2,000 recommended by any other weight loss group such as Weight Watchers, or by the federal gov-ernment in their Dietary Guidelines for Americans and the DASH diet.

See also: DASH Diet; Dietary Guidelines for Americans; Weight Watchers.

FURTHER READING

Gaffey, Caitlin. "Do You Need to Detox? Overindulged This Holiday Season? Here, the Pros and Cons of the New Cleansing Diets." *Harper's Bazaar* no. 3554 (January 2008): 58.
Glickman, Peter. *The Master Cleanse Coach.* New York: Peter Glickman, Inc., 2013.

Rubin, Courtney. "Cleansing's Dirty Secret: Touted for Myriad Health Benefits, Chic Juice Diets Are All the Rage, but in Their Quest to Detox and Lose Weight, Some Women, Call Them Juicerexies, Are Hitting the Bottle to Dangerous Degrees." *Marie Claire* 20, no. 5 (May 2013): S148(2).

Rubin, Tina. "Mastering the Master Cleanse: After 34 Years, It's Still among the Most Popular Cleanse Programs Around." *Better Nutrition* 72, no. 9 (September 2010): 22(4).

Steingarten, Jeffrey. "Mr. Clean." *Vogue* 202, no. 5 (May 2012): 198.

Woloshyn, Tom. *The Complete Master Cleanse: A Step-by-Step Guide to the Benefits of the Lemonade Diet.* Berkeley, CA: Ulysses Press, 2007.

McDougall Program

The McDougall Program, developed by Dr. John McDougall, is a low-fat, starch-based, vegetarian diet designed to promote weight loss along with other lasting health benefits. It's a complete reversal of high protein plans like Atkins, South Beach, and Dukan diets. With a focus on education, the McDougall plan emphasizes nutrition, exercise, and disease prevention. And, according to its founder, successful participants can do everything from lowering their blood pressure, cholesterol, and blood sugar to rebalancing their hormones and reducing their risk of future health problems. Under his close supervision, McDougall says, patients have been able to safely reduce or discontinue their medications for such illnesses as high blood pressure, diabetes, arthritis, and stomach pain, and to avoid what he calls unnecessary surgeries.

McDougall personally cares for all participants during the 10-day live-in program, which features a complete medical evaluation and health assessment. The personalized program of diet and exercise includes a low-fat, vegan diet made up of 80 percent complex carbohydrates along with activities like walking and swimming. And, according to McDougall, most overweight people who follow his plan lose 6 to 15 pounds of fat a month while eating as much as they want of approved complex-carbohydrate foods. His weight-loss program is also available through his best-selling books, *The McDougall Plan* (1983), *The McDougall Program: 12 Days to Dynamic Health* (1990), and *The McDougall Program for Maximum Weight Loss* (1994). His most recent publication, *The Starch Solution: Eat the Foods You Love, Regain Your Health and Lose the Weight for Good!* (2013) was co-written with his wife, Mary. They make the argument that starch foods are healthy and can prevent disease as well as help dieters lose weight.

For decades, the cornerstone of the McDougall Program is a diet of starchy plant foods from beans and corn to pastas, potatoes, and rice. This approved list of carbohydrate foods also includes unfamiliar grains like quinoa, bulgur, and triticale wheat; exotic fruits such as kiwi, kumquat, mango, papaya, quince, and guava; and unique vegetables like kohlrabi, jicama, adzuki beans, arugula, Swiss chard, and turban squash. Typical breakfast menus might be oatmeal, seven-grain cereal, cold breakfast cereals that meet low-fat requirements, whole wheat or oil-free bagels with fruit spread, plus fresh fruit or fruit juices and herbal teas. Lunches range from pita bread stuffed with beans and vegetables, baked potato salad, pasta salad, to various soups made with beans, legumes, or grains.

Dinner selections include bean burrito casserole, Cajun rice with tossed green salad, gingered vegetable soup with seasoned potatoes, a simple pasta with meatless marinara sauce, or pasta primavera with cauliflower. Dessert recipes in McDougall's book center around fruit and range from frozen fruit sorbet to easy fruit pudding or something he calls quick apple pie. Beverages consist mainly of water, herbal or iced teas, or fruit juices, and he recommends against caffeine-laden drinks like coffee or soda.

McDougall developed his diet program in response to research, which he believed proved American health problems were due in large part to their typical high-fat, animal-based diet. He said he also experienced firsthand the connection between diet and health during his early years as a doctor at a Hawaiian sugarcane plantation. In his book, McDougall wrote that he treated several generations of workers and their families, from immigrant grandparents to American, third-generation children. He discovered that the older workers were often the healthiest, living on a traditional diet of rice and vegetables, foods low in cholesterol and high in fiber. Each generation that followed became more Americanized, eating richer foods like meats, eggs, dairy products, and processed foods. According to McDougall, those children and grandchildren suffered more chronic diseases like obesity, heart disease, hypertension, and diabetes than their elders.

For heart disease patients, McDougall's program eliminates all animal foods, even nonfat dairy products. He also limits high-fat plant foods like coconut, avocado, tofu, and nuts, and suggests that the health benefits of dietary oils, even olive oil, do not outweigh the problems they cause. McDougall's program for heart patients is similar to the low-fat, vegetarian eating plan developed by Dr. Dean Ornish. The Ornish program, known as the Life Choice diet, focuses on beans, fruits, vegetables, and whole grains, and recommends that dieters get only 10 percent of their calories from fat.

In 2000, McDougall joined other diet doctors Robert Atkins, Barry Sears, and Dean Ornish for the USDA-sponsored Great Nutrition Debate. Agriculture Secretary Dan Glickman said the USDA sponsored the debate to sort out what the secretary called conflicting information and claims about weight loss and diet. During the panel discussion, McDougall had harsh words for popular high-protein diets, which he said are often based on gimmicks or the mistaken belief that eating large amounts of protein foods will magically prompt weight loss.

McDougall said the end result, of what he called "the make yourself sick diets," is only a short-term weight loss. But because Americans are desperate to lose weight, he said diets based on protein foods, like beef roasts, hams, butter-drenched lobsters, or crispy bacon, appeal to those who don't want to give up the foods they love—an example of wanting to have their steak and eat it too. McDougall joins other health organizations, including the American Dietetic Association, the

American Heart Association, and the American Cancer Society, in recommending that Americans change from a diet full of animal products and saturated fat to a vegetarian diet of nutrient-rich and heart-healthy plant foods.

See also: Atkins Nutritional Approach; Barnard, Neal; Life Choice Diet; Ornish, Dean; Sears, Barry.

FURTHER READING

Errico-Cox, Lisa A. "The McDougall Program for Women: What Every Woman Needs to Know to Be Healthy for Life." *Library Journal* 124, no. 1 (January 1999): 141.
Gavalas, Elaine. "The Great Diet Debate." *Better Nutrition*, May 2000, 32.
Lindley, Sarah. "Heart Smart: Natural Remedies for a Healthy Heart." *Vegetarian Times*, May 1997, 58–64.
McDougall, John. *The McDougall Plan*. New York: New Century Publishing, 1983.
McDougall, John. *The McDougall Program for Maximum Weight Loss*. New York: Dutton/Penguin Books, 1994.
McDougall, John. *The McDougall Program: 12 Days to Dynamic Health*. New York: Dutton/Penguin Books, 1990.
McDougall, John. *The Starch Solution: Eat the Foods You Love, Regain Your Health, and Lose the Weight for Good!* Emmaus, PA: Rodale, 2013.
Parker-Pope, Tara. "Nutrition Advice from the China Study." *The New York Times*, January 7, 2011. http://well.blogs.nytimes.com/2011/01/07/nutrition-advice-from-the-china-study/comment-page-5/.
Wiley, Carol. "Dear Diary. . . : A Week of Weight Loss at the McDougall Program." *Vegetarian Times*, May 1990, 48–55.

Meridia

Meridia (sibutramine) was a prescription drug for weight loss that acted upon the central nervous system by regulating the brain's appetite-control center. It was taken off the market in October 2010 because of the risk of cardiovascular events.

See also: Dietary Supplement Health and Education Act (DSHEA); Food and Drug Administration (FDA).

FURTHER READING

Czarnecki, Joanne, and Shelley Drozd. "Rating the Fat-Fighters." *Men's Health,* January 1999, 60.
Gleick, Elizabeth. "Available from a Doctor Near You." *Time International,* October 25, 1999, 65.
Shute, Nancy. "FDA Approves New Diet Drug." *U.S. News & World Report,* December 8, 1997, 38.

"Sibutramine Could Sustain Weight Loss, but Question of Safety Remains." *Obesity, Fitness & Wellness Week*, January 13, 2001, 2.

Wilhelm, Carolyn. "Growing the Market for Anti-Obesity Drugs." *Chemical Market Reporter* 257, no. 20 (May 15, 2000): 23.

Metabolife

Metabolife 356 was one of the best-selling herbal dietary supplements in the United States and the brainchild of San Diego businessman and former police officer Michael J. Ellis. In 2001, the ephedra-based Metabolife line of products accounted for 36 percent of diet pill sales in U.S. drugstores, according to a statement from Eric Larsen, vice president of sales at Metabolife International, Inc., reported in the February 2002 issue of *Chain Drug Review*. But the company was rocked by a series of legal problems and filed for Chapter 11 bankruptcy in 2005. The bankruptcy filing followed a serious drop in sales and at least a billion dollars in legal claims over the company's Metabolife 356 containing ephedra. The FDA had banned the sale of dietary supplements containing ephedra in 2004. Later, a 2006 appeals court upheld its decision, further sealing Metabolife's fate

Metabolife 356 was born, according to the company's Web site, www.metabolife.com, when Ellis developed an herbal blend to boost his ailing father's energy level. Company lore states that the formula was so successful that Joseph Ellis made his son promise to market the herbal combination so that others could reap its benefits.

Ephedra is chemically identical to ephedrine, a synthetic compound used in asthma medicine. They are amphetamine-like compounds, powerful stimulants that act on the central nervous system and the heart. They can cause rapid or irregular heartbeats, hypertension, strokes, and seizures, along with psychological side effects such as depression, nervousness, and insomnia.

Since early 1990, the FDA had issued numerous warnings to consumers of diet products and supplements containing ephedra, ephedrine, or ma huang. Court documents show that Metabolife founder Ellis was convicted in 1990 on charges linking him to an illegal meth lab. His arrest and conviction were detailed in a 1999 *Washington Post* article. The story states that, following his conviction and while on probation, Ellis launched his first ephedra-based product. Called Fosslip, it contained 18 vitamins, minerals, and herbal extracts, including caffeine and ephedra. It was designed for weight lifters but sales were disappointing. In 1995, Ellis renamed the formula Metabolife 356 and marketed it strictly as a weight-loss aid. The *Washington Post* reported that sales for the company grew from less than $2 million in 1996 to $600 million in 1998. Ideasphere, Inc., a rival maker of dietary supplements, purchased Metabolife's non-ephedra-containing assets in 2007.

See also: Dietary Supplement Health and Education Act (DSHEA); Ephedra/ Ephedrine; Vitamins.

FURTHER READING

Babcock, Charles R. "Stimulant Propels Diet Empire: Herbal Coalition Fights FDA's Proposed Safety Regulation." *Washington Post,* May 24, 1999, A1.

"Be Wary of Chinese Herbs, American-Style." *Environmental Nutrition,* April 2000, 8.

Cowley, Geoffrey, and Jamie Reno. "Mad about Metabolife: Some Call It a Dieter's Dream; Others Say It's a Health Hazard. But Americans Can't Get Enough of This Herbal Weight-Loss Remedy." *Newsweek,* October 4, 1999, 52–53.

Crabtree, Penni. "Little Pill, Big Trouble." *SignOnSanDiego.com,* July 20, 2003. http:// legacy.utsandiego.com/news/business/20030720-9999_mz1b20metabo.html.

"Criminal Investigation Sought for Diet Supplement Seller." *USA Today,* August 15, 2002. http://usatoday30.usatoday.com/news/health/2002–08–15-ephedra_x.htm.

Fessenden, Ford. "Hearings to Begin on Makers of a Popular Diet Product." *The New York Times,* July 22, 2003. http://www.nytimes.com/2003/07/22/us/hearings-to-begin-on-makers-of-a-popular-diet-product.html.

Gugliotta, Guy. "A Neutral Comment, a Company's Tough Reaction." *Washington Post,* July 23, 2000, A16.

"No Category Is More Faddish than Weight Loss." *Chain Drug Review* 24, no. 4 (February 18, 2002): 48.

Wallace, Phil. "Jury Decides for Plaintiffs in Metabolife Product Case." *Food Chemical News* 44, no. 41 (November 25, 2002): 15.

Webb, Marion. "Metabolife to Appeal Court's Defamation Ruling." *San Diego Business Journal* 20, no. 47 (November 22, 1999): 4.

MyPlate

The Food Guide Pyramid is no more. In its place, the government unveiled in 2011 a simpler image, a plate divided into basic food groups. Visible on the government Web site, the new icon is split into four sections including vegetable, grain, fruit, and protein servings with the dairy off to the side. The U.S. Department of Agriculture (USDA) officials describe MyPlate as a visible reminder for Americans to think about what goes on their plate and to make healthy food choices. For years, many nutritionists criticized the earlier program, which was symbolized by a food pyramid, first released in 1992, calling it difficult to understand. The plate is seen as a simpler concept that places a great deal of emphasis on fruits and vegetables.

The MyPlate logo and program were created by the USDA with input from First Lady Michelle Obama, her anti-obesity staff, other federal health officials, and focus groups of American citizens. Mrs. Obama is well known for her official support of good nutrition and exercise, especially her Let's Move campaign

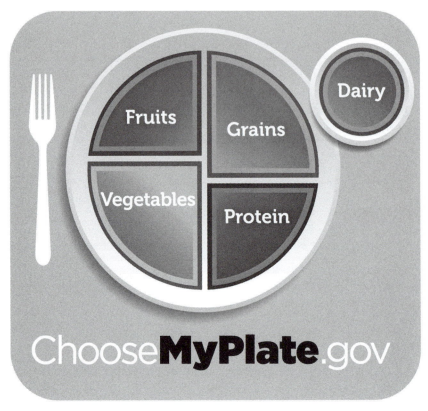

MyPlate replaced the old Food Guide Pyramid as the government's symbol for nutritional guidance in 2011. It's a visual cue for how to fill your plate with a variety of healthy foods. (USDA Center for Nutrition Policy and Promotion (CNPP))

to end childhood obesity. In replacing the pyramid graphic, the new design follows a long history of the government nutrition education, which began in 1894 when the USDA released its first nutritional guidelines. The original food groups included meat and milk, cereals, fruits and vegetables, fats and fatty foods, and sugars and sugary foods.

With food rationing during World War II, butter and sugar were in short supply, and to assist citizens in getting the right amounts of vitamins and minerals the government released recommended dietary allowances known as RDAs. Those suggested guidelines were changed again after World War II ended and the basic four groups became dairy, meats, fruits and vegetables, and grains. This remained unchanged until the 1970s when the USDA included another food category that contained fats, sweets, and alcoholic beverages; all items it recommended should be eaten in moderation.

The new MyPlate graphic shows a plate with 20 percent of grains, 30 percent vegetables, and an equal 30 percent fruits, then the final 20 percent of protein foods. The dairy products are represented by a small circle to the side to illustrate a glass or serving of low-fat, nonfat, or reduced-fat milk, yogurt, or cheeses.

Recommendations for the grain category include whole grains and refined grains. The MyPlate suggests that individuals have at least half of their grains from whole grains, instead of refined grains. Examples of whole grains might include brown rice, whole cornmeal, oatmeal, whole-wheat pasta, and whole-wheat flour. The vegetable group is divided into five subgroups: dark green vegetables, orange vegetables, dry beans and peas, starchy vegetables, and other vegetables.

The fruits—fresh, canned, frozen, and dried—range from apples, apricots, bananas, and berries to plums, prunes, and raisins. The protein group includes all kinds of meats from beef, pork, and lamb to venison and rabbit, poultry, eggs, fish and seafood, nuts and seeds, and dry beans and peas. The smaller dairy category is made up of nonfat, low-fat, and reduced-fat dairy foods such as milk, yogurt, cheese, and ice cream.

Like other sites dealing with health, MyPlate recommends at least 30 minutes of moderate or vigorous activity or exercise each day that increases the heart rate. Choices for exercise range from moderate activities like briskly walking or bicycling to vigorous exercise such as running, jogging, or aerobic exercise. The information developed for MyPlate is based on the 2010 Dietary Guidelines for Americans which describe a healthy diet as one that features fruits, vegetables, low-fat dairy products, whole grains, and lean meats, and is low in saturated fats.

While the USDA supports MyPlate, there are some health professionals who suggest it falls short of giving Americans a complete picture of good nutrition and instead includes a serving of political or food industry pressure. For example, officials with the Harvard School of Public Health and the Harvard Medical School developed their own Healthy Eating Plate to underscore the problems with the USDA version. With respect to grains, the Healthy Eating Plate encourages consumers to limit refined grains and exclusively eat whole grains for maximum good health and to lower the risk of heart disease or diabetes.

See also: Let's Move; Obesity.

FURTHER READING

Davis, Carole, and Etta Sallo. "Dietary Recommendations and How They Have Changed over Time." In *America's Eating Habits: Changes and Consequences*. U.S. Department of Agriculture, May 1999. http://www.ers.usda.gov/publications/aib750b_1_-1.pdf.

"Healthy Eating Plate." Harvard Health Publications, Harvard Medical School, Harvard University. http://www.health.harvard.edu/plate/healthy-eating-plate. Accessed January 27, 2014.

Sweet, Lynn. "Michelle Obama Hypes Icon Switch: Bye Food Pyramid, Hello Food Plate." *The Scoop from Washington (blog)*, Chicago Sun-Times, June 2, 2011. http://blogs.sun

times.com/sweet/2011/06/michelle_obama_hypes_icon_swit._html. Accessed January 27, 2014.

U.S. Department of Agriculture. "Choose MyPlate.gov." http://www.choosemyplate.gov. Accessed January 27, 2014.

U.S. Department of Agriculture and U.S. Department of Health and Human Services. *Dietary Guidelines for Americans, 2010.* 7th ed. Washington, DC. U.S. Government Printing Office, December 2010.

National Weight Control Registry

The National Weight Control Registry is a database of people who have been successful at losing large amounts of weight and being able to maintain that weight loss. It was founded in 1993 as a collaborative venture between researchers at the University of Colorado and the University of Pittsburgh. By identifying such a large group of people who have been successful at maintaining weight loss (60% of registrants have lost an average of 60 pounds and have kept it off for five years), researchers are able to draw some conclusions about actions and motivations.

The registry contains names of more than 10,000 people from the United States who have lost a significant amount of weight and have kept it off for some time. Registrants must be at least 18. It's free to register and names of registrants are kept confidential. New registrants are asked to fill out questionnaires when first enrolling and all participants are sent annual questionnaires. The Web site mentions some of the characteristics these registrants share:

Successful weight losers report making substantial changes in eating and exercise habits to lose weight and to maintain their losses. On average, registrants' report consuming about 1400 kcal/day (24 percent calories from fat) and expending about 400 kcal/day in physical exercise. Walking is the most frequently cited physical activity. . . . Two-thirds of these successful weight losers were overweight as children and 60 percent report a family history of obesity. About 50 percent of participants lost weight on their own without any type of formal program or help.

See also: Exercise; Obesity.

FURTHER READING

Alderman, Lesley. "For a Frugal Dieter, Weight Loss on a Sliding Scale." *The New York Times,* July 4, 2009, B6.

"Data on Weight Loss Reported by Researchers at University of Colorado." *Obesity, Fitness & Wellness Week*, October 5, 2013, 306.

http://www.uchsc.edu/nutrition/nwcr.htm.

Nutrisystem

Nutrisystem is a weight-loss and weight-maintenance program that comes with its own low-calorie, portion-controlled food. Dieters choose from more than 150 prepackaged meals and snacks for a daily calorie count of about 1,000.

In 2014, the company introduced Nutrisystem My Way—a program tailored to the individual's metabolism, along with its Fast 5™ kit, a one-week kick start that can help customers lose five pounds in their first week of dieting—backed by a money-back guarantee. Fast 5 includes seven days of breakfasts, lunches, and dinners, plus all-new shakes with formulations for men and women.

According to the press release announcing the new program, "'A third-party's clinical test, sponsored by Nutrisystem, supports the effectiveness of Fast 5,' explained Dr. Anthony Fabricatore, a clinical psychologist who heads up Nutrisystem's Research and Development team. 'Getting a quick jump out of the gate can be very motivating as individuals move into their tailored Nutrisystem My Way

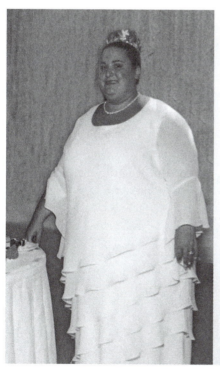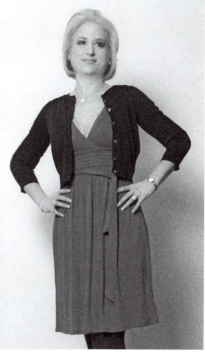

Since it was incorporated in 1972, Nutrisystem has grown by featuring many of its success stories, such as this one from 2007 with Danielle Carter, who lost 246 pounds using Nutrisystem products and ideas. (AP Photo/PRNewsFoto/Nutrisystem, Inc.)

program. Research from multiple lifestyle programs shows that achieving early weight loss is a reliable predictor of longer-term success.'" The program continues with a customer meal plan based on an individual's metabolism. Customers are given a personalized meal plan and exercise suggestions to help them burn fat efficiently and boost fat metabolism. Consumers are encouraged to check in periodically with a Nutrisystem counselor as their metabolic needs change in response to weight loss.

The celebrity spokeswoman in 2013 was actor Melissa Joan Hart, who credited Nutrisystem with helping her lose 30 pounds after the birth of her third son.

The Nutrisystem program is divided into two sections: weight loss, followed by weight maintenance. Participants can choose menu options for breakfast, lunch, dinner, dessert and snack items, and protein drinks. The participant buys 28 days' worth of food that is delivered right to the participant's home. In addition, some items, such as fresh fruit and vegetables and whole grain bread, will need to be purchased at the grocery store. Through its Web site, www.nutrisystem.com, the company offers live counseling online or via telephone, as well as a 13-week online program to help users reassess their relationship with food. This move from bricks-and-mortar centers was designed to make weight-loss efforts more private and to draw more men.

Incorporated in 1972 and taken public in 1981, Nutrisystem was developed by Harold Katz, a Philadelphia native who got the idea for the program from his mother after she had tried every kind of diet from pills to low-calorie foods to behavioral counseling. Katz put together a program geared for the individual, a departure from other early diet programs like Weight Watchers that worked with groups.

As a publicly traded company, Nutrisystem reports its earnings on a quarterly basis. While the company showed growth in 2013, it has not always had an easy road. In 1991, when it was called Nutri/System, the company faced nearly 200 lawsuits charging that the diet had caused gallbladder damage in users due to rapid weight loss without medical supervision. The franchiser eventually won all of the 18 suits that went to trial and settled hundreds more, according to a 1993 article in the *Wall Street Journal*.

In 1997, Nutri/System ran into a public relations problem because it had been dispensing the drug fen-phen to dieters. The company stopped doing so just before the U.S. Food and Drug Administration withdrew phentermine from the market, but it created the NutriRx Phen-Pro program, a combination drug with Prozac. Prozac maker Eli-Lilly Company did not endorse the combination.

Other recent advertising strategies include a 2001 agreement signed with QVC, giving it exclusive rights to promote Nutri/System's weight-loss products on its television programs in the United States.

See also: Fen-Phen; Jenny Craig; Weight Watchers.

FURTHER READING

Davis, Riccardo A. "Weight of One Lawsuit Off, Nutri/System Gains Another." *Philadelphia Business Journal* 10, no. 28 (September 16, 1991): 12.

Donahue, Peggy Jo. "Inside America's Hottest Diet Programs." *Prevention*, February 1990, 55.

Farhi, Paul. "Three Diet Firms Agree to Stop Disputed Ads." *The Washington Post*, September 30, 1993, D11.

"Feeding Frenzy." *Time*, May 17, 1993, 21–22.

Goldman, Kevin. "Ads Dished Up for Nutri/System Dieters." *Wall Street Journal*, May 7, 1993, B8.

Janofsky, Michael. "Nutri/System's Shrinking May Put Jenny Craig on a Gravy Train." *New York Times*, May 28, 1993, D4.

Key, Peter. "*Nutrisystem.com* Looks to Fatten Up." *Philadelphia Business Journal* 19, no. 9 (April 7, 2000): 3.

"Nutrisystem Expands Science Advisory Board." Nutrisystem press release, February 12, 2014. http://www.prnewswire.com/news-releases/nutrisystem-expands-science-advisory-board-245258711.html.

"Nutrisystem Introduces Nutrisystem My Way with All-New Fast 5™ Kit." Nutrisystem press release, December 10, 2013. http://www.prnewswire.com/news-releases/nutrisystem-introduces-nutrisystem-my-way-with-all-new-fast-5-kit-235246361.html.

Rosenberg, Hilary. "Nutri/System after the Fall." *Financial World*, August 15, 1983, 38–40.

Waters, Craig. "Slim Pickings, Harold Katz and Nutri-System Inc." *INC.*, May 1985, 94–100.

www.nutrisystem.com.

Nutrition Facts Label

Since the government passed the National Label Education Act in 1990, packaged foods in the United States are required to have a Nutrition Facts label. In March 2014, the Food and Drug Administration (FDA) proposed updates to the Nutrition Fact label to provide consumers more information about the foods they consume. These labels provide information on certain nutrients and are one of the best sources of understanding the quality of your diet. The labels must contain information about calories, fat, carbohydrates, fiber, sodium, cholesterol, and vitamin and mineral content of the food. The new labels, which feature a refreshed design, also include information about added sugars, and they update the daily values for nutrients, such as sodium, dietary fiber, and Vitamin D. The new labels also feature the calorie count more prominently, and serving sizes are updated. For example, foods that are typically consumed in one sitting will require the nutrition facts about the entire package contents. A 20-ounce bottle of soda, for example, will include the calorie content and other information for the whole package. Earlier nutrition labels may have stated that the soda bottle contained

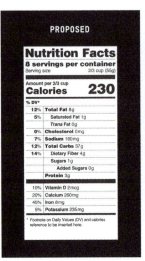

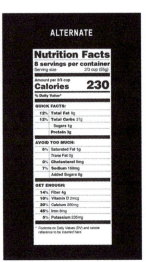

The Food and Drug Administration is proposing a revised food nutrition label that makes the calorie listing more prominent, includes information about added sugars, and adapts serving sizes, among other changes. (AP Photo/FDA)

more than one serving. In its press release announcing the change, the FDA wrote, "This way, people would be able to easily understand how many calories and nutrients they are getting if they eat or drink the entire package at one time."

The 2014 changes are the first major changes since the Nutrition Facts labels were introduced, other than the change in 2006, when the labels were changed to include trans fats. As part of the Affordable Care Act, the FDA has been directed to create similar labeling for restaurants, fast-food places, and vending machines.

Here is what is on a Nutrition Facts label.

CALORIES

A calorie is a measure of heat needed to raise 1 kilogram of water by 1 degree Celsius. Since food "stokes the furnace" of our bodies, foods have assigned calorie values. Fat and alcohol are high in calories. Foods high in both sugars and fat contain many calories but often are low in vitamins, minerals, or fiber. There are numerous calorie counters readily available—online and often in cookbooks. If you reduce your caloric intake, you'll lose weight. If you increase the amount of calories you consume, you'll gain weight. But that doesn't mean that a low-calorie diet is the best way to lose weight. That's how those awful grapefruit and black-coffee diets originated. Sure, if you starve yourself for a week, you'll lose weight. But if you return to your old eating habits, you'll put the weight right back on again. A pound equals 3,500 calories. So to lose a pound in, say, a week, you'll either have to eat 3,500 calories less or have to burn off 3,500 calories in exercise, or some combination of the two.

Exercise burns calories. For example, walking briskly can burn off about 100 calories per mile. Bicycling for a half hour at nearly 10 mph will burn about 195 calories. The specific number depends on the person's weight and the intensity of the activity. A variety of interactive exercise counters, available on the Internet, allow you to plug in your weight, age, and change variables such as the length of time and intensity of the activity.

The following formula will help you determine the approximate number of calories you need per day to maintain your body weight. Moderately active males should multiply their weight in pounds by 15. For example, if you weigh 170 pounds, you need about 2,500 calories per day. Moderately active females should multiply their weight by 12. A 130-pound female needs about 1,560 calories per day. However, the number of calories needed per day decreases as the level of activity decreases. Relatively inactive men should multiply their weight by 13 pounds and women in that category should multiply their weight by 10. So that 170-pound man who is relatively inactive needs only 2,210 calories and the 130-pound inactive woman needs only 1,300 calories to maintain body weight.

The information on nutrition labels is based on 2,000 calorie-per-day values. Keep that in mind if the caloric intake you need to maintain your weight is significantly higher or lower.

CALORIES FROM FAT

Numerous health and government authorities, including the U.S. Surgeon General, the National Academy of Sciences, the American Heart Association, and the American Dietetic Association, recommend reducing dietary fat to 30 percent or less of total calories. However, that doesn't mean you have to pass by all high-fat food products. For example, peanut butter with sugar added has 190 calories in a two-tablespoon serving. Of those, 130 calories are from fat— 68 percent. Add that peanut butter to two slices of whole wheat bread, which have 120 calories and 20 calories from fat, and the equation is different: now the fat is down to about 48 percent. It's still higher than the recommendation, but by adding a glass of skim milk and an apple, you start to bring it down a healthy level.

TOTAL FAT

This is measured in grams. For someone eating a 2,000-calorie-per-day diet, daily fat intake should not exceed 65 grams. Fatty foods are always high in calories. Despite its bad image, though, fat isn't all bad. Some fat is needed because fats supply energy and help the body absorb fat-soluble vitamins A, D, E, and K. Fats contain both saturated and unsaturated fatty acids. Saturated fat raises blood cholesterol more than other forms of fat. Limiting saturated fats to less than 10 percent of calories will help lower your blood cholesterol level. High levels of saturated fats and cholesterol in the diet are linked to increased blood cholesterol levels and a greater risk for heart disease.

While polyunsaturated and monounsaturated fats could help lower blood cholesterol levels, the recommendation still holds that total fat account for no more than 30 percent of daily calorie intake.

CHOLESTEROL

Your body makes cholesterol, but it is also obtained from food. Animal products, such as egg yolks, higher-fat milk products, poultry, fish, and meat, are high in cholesterol—and usually also in saturated fats. The daily intake of cholesterol should be 300 milligrams. There are two kinds of cholesterol: LDL, the so-called bad cholesterol, and HDL, or good cholesterol. LDL stands for low-density lipoproteins. If there's too much LDL cholesterol in the bloodstream, it can build up within the walls of the arteries and contribute to the formation of plaque, which can ultimately clog the arteries. That blockage could affect the flow of blood to the heart, and cause a heart attack, or to the brain, and result in a stroke. Doctors can measure the level of LDL in the blood—ideally it should be below 130.

High-density lipoprotein (HDL) is the "good" cholesterol because experts believe HDLs can carry cholesterol away from the arteries and to the liver, where it's passed from the body. HDL levels typically range from 40 to 50 mg/dL for men and 50 to 60 mg/dL for women. Levels below 35 mg/dL are abnormally low and pose a risk factor for cardiac problems. Low HDL levels can be caused by cigarette smoking, obesity, and physical inactivity.

SODIUM

Sodium is a trace mineral that helps maintain body fluid balance. Salt is an excellent source of sodium. One-quarter teaspoon, the typical serving, provides 540 milligrams of sodium, or 25 percent of the daily recommended allowance. Milk and processed foods are other sources. Sodium intake should stay below 2,400 milligrams. That might sound like a lot, but realize how quickly these sources add up. A frozen turkey pot pie, single serving, contains about 29 percent of the recommended daily intake. Hot dogs typically have at least 21 percent of the daily total of sodium per hot dog. Even a tablespoon of ketchup has 190 milligrams of sodium or 8 percent of the daily value. Lower sodium intake could help people avoid or control high blood pressure—a risk factor in heart disease and strokes. If you eat many processed, packaged foods and are exceeding the sodium intake, start looking for ways to duplicate the foods you like while cooking them fresh. Many herbs and spices have no sodium and can add tremendous flavor to foods. These include garlic, basil, pepper, parsley, chives, vinegar, sage, cinnamon, nutmeg, and cloves.

TOTAL CARBOHYDRATES

Carbohydrates provide energy for the brain, central nervous system, and muscle cells. They are found largely in sugars, fruits, vegetables, and cereals and grains. Meats generally have no carbohydrates. Carbohydrates can be classified as simple, such as sugars, or complex, such as breads and pastas, which are broken down into sugars in the body. Someone with a 2,000-calorie-per-day diet should limit carbohydrates to 300 grams. Someone with a 2,500-calorie-per-day diet can consume up to 375 grams of carbohydrates. A medium-baked potato with skin has 51 grams of carbohydrates. An apple has about 21 grams of carbohydrates, a tablespoon of sugar has 12 grams, and a slice of pie can pack 60 or more grams of carbohydrates.

Carbohydrates are divided into three kinds: monosaccharides or simple sugars, such as glucose and fructose; disaccharides—composed of two monosaccharides— such as maltose, sucrose, and lactose; and polysaccharides, which are starches and glycogen.

On the Nutrition Facts label, total carbohydrates include starch, sugars, sugar alcohols, and dietary fiber.

DIETARY FIBER

Fiber helps the body digest food. Soluble fiber, combined with a low-fat diet, may reduce levels of "bad cholesterol." The Recommended Dietary Allowance for fiber is 25 grams. Generally, grains, such as oat, wheat, and rice products, are good sources of fiber, as are some vegetables. But some foods that might seem as though they would be high in fiber, such as cereals, in fact have very little. High-sugar cereals often have just 1 gram of fiber; a high-fiber hot wheat cereal could have 5 grams; and a 100 percent bran cereal could have up to 8 grams or more. Some fruits such as an apple (3.5 grams), a banana (2.4 grams), three prunes (3 grams), and a half grapefruit (3.1 grams) also have high fiber content.

SUGAR

Sugars in foods are the monosaccharides and disaccharides described previously. In some foods, carbohydrate makeup is almost entirely sugar. For example, a tablespoon of fruit preserves, sweetened only with fruit juices, derives 9 of its 10 grams of carbohydrates from sugar. Breads and pastas, on the other hand, have much high polysaccharide contents. One pita bread pocket, for example, has 2 grams of sugar out of its 24 grams of total carbohydrates. Looking at the Nutrition Facts label becomes especially important if you're seeking to cut down on the simple sugars. Take breakfast cereals, for example. Let's look at two boxes of General Mills cereal designed to appeal to children. One is Kix; the other Apple Cinnamon Cheerios. Both have 120 calories per serving and similar carbohydrate totals. But of the 25 carbohydrate grams in Apple Cinnamon Cheerios,

13 are sugar and 11 are "other," and there's 1 gram of dietary fiber. Of the 26 carbohydrate grams in Kix, only 3 are sugar and 22 are "other." There's also 1 gram of dietary fiber there.

The proposed new labels will also include an entry for added sugars so that consumers can understand the difference between naturally occurring sugars, in foods such as yogurt or dairy-based desserts, and the sugars that are added to these foods. Added sugars contribute an average of 16 percent of the total calories in American diets. The FDA is defining "added sugars" as sugars that are added during the processing or packaging of foods or the addition of naturally occurring sugars that are isolated from a whole food and concentrated (such as fruit juice concentrates).

PROTEIN

Protein is actually a combination of 22 amino acids. Your body makes 13 of these amino acids on its own. These are called nonessential amino acids. But nine of the amino acids—essential amino acids—must come from the foods you eat. Protein builds up and maintains the tissues in your body. Protein comprises much of your muscles, your organs, even some hormones. Protein also makes hemoglobin, the part of the red blood cells that carries oxygen around the body. Protein also makes antibodies that help fight off infections and disease. Protein is found in meat, chicken, fish, eggs, nuts, dairy products, and legumes.

VITAMINS AND MINERALS

These are expressed on Nutrition Facts labels as the percentage of the recommended dietary allowance (RDA). If you're eating a varied diet most days, and not severely limiting your calories, chances are good that you do not need additional vitamin or mineral supplements.

The proposed changes to the Nutrition Facts label will require manufacturers to add Vitamin D and potassium to the label. Calcium and iron will stay on the new Nutrition Facts labels, but Vitamins A and C will no longer be required, as deficiencies related to these vitamins are uncommon.

Some foods are enriched with additional nutrients. For example, enriched flour and bread contain added thiamine, riboflavin, niacin, and iron; skim milk, low-fat milk, and margarine are usually enriched with vitamin A; and milk is usually enriched with vitamins A and D. The ingredient list on packaging will let you know which nutrients are in the food. In a nutshell, vitamin A is found in fruits and dark-green and deep-yellow vegetables, such as carrots, pumpkins, and spinach. Vitamin A is important to your vision and healthy skin. Vitamin B actually refers to a group of vitamins—B_1, B_2, B_3, B_5, B_6, B_7, B_9, B_{12}. These vitamins play a role in making red blood cells, which carry oxygen to all the parts of your body. In other words, the B vitamins help with energy. Fish, beef, pork, chicken, whole wheat grains, green leafy vegetables, dried beans, and enriched breads and cereals are sources of vitamin B. Vitamin C strengthens bones and muscles and also has some infection-fighting capabilities. However, large doses can result in kidney problems. Good natural sources of vitamin C are citrus fruits, strawberries, melons, sweet potatoes, cabbage, broccoli, tomatoes, and peppers. Vitamin D contributes to strong healthy bones and teeth and it also helps the body absorb calcium. You can get vitamin D through fortified milk products, egg yolks, and fish. Another great source for vitamin D is sunshine. Vitamin E helps form red blood cells, muscles, and other tissues throughout the body. Vitamin E also helps your body store vitamin A. It's found in vegetable oils and dark-green leafy vegetables, nuts, poultry and seafood, and wheat germ and fortified cereals. Vitamin K is essential for blood clotting. It's also found in dark-green vegetables, whole grains, potatoes, cabbage, and cheese.

CALCIUM

Calcium warrants special attention because new research is pointing to an even more crucial role than previously thought and because calcium requirements are highest for young people whose bones are developing. Calcium is used in building bone mass and also plays a role in the proper functioning of the heart, muscles, and nerves maintaining blood flow. The recommended daily allowance for calcium for 14- to 18-year-olds is 1,300 mg/day, and for adults between 19 and 50 years, it is 1,000 mg/day. Adequate calcium can also reduce the risk of osteoporosis, a weakening of the bones that can occur late in adulthood. Calcium is found naturally in dairy products and in dark-green leafy vegetables.

IRON

Iron is a trace mineral found in red meat, liver, fish, green leafy vegetables, enriched bread, and some dried fruits such as prunes, apricots, and raisins. Recommended iron intake for girls aged 14–18 is 15 milligrams per day, increasing to 18 milligrams per day for women between the ages of 19 and 50. The recommended amount for teenage boys aged 14–18 is 11 milligrams per day, decreasing to 8 milligrams per day after age 19. The level of iron required for women stays the same until menopause. Blood loss, such as menstrual cycles, is a major cause of iron deficiency. Low iron levels can result in iron-deficiency anemia. Iron supplements can be taken, and you can eat more foods that are higher in iron content. Vitamin C can help iron absorption, while coffee, tea, wheat bran, eggs, and soy inhibit iron absorption. Medications such as antacids, for example, can also interfere with iron absorption.

Iron demands are typically highest for pregnant women at 27 milligrams per day.

See also: Calories; Carbohydrates; Dietary Guidelines for Americans.

FURTHER READING

Cha, Ariana Eunjung, and Thompson, Krissah. "Food Labels to Get First Makeover with New Emphasis on Calories, Sugar." *The Washington Post*, February 27, 2014.

Neistat, Casey. "Calorie Detective." *The New York Times*, February 12, 2013.

Tavernise, Sabrina. "New F.D.A. Nutrition Labels Would Make 'Serving Sizes' Reflect Actual Servings." *The New York Times*, February 27, 2014, A14.

White House press release, Office of the First Lady. "The White House and FDA Announce Proposed Updates to Nutrition Facts Label." February 27, 2014.

Obama, Michelle

Michelle Obama (b. January 17, 1964, in Chicago, IL) has acted as this nation's First Lady since her husband, Barack Obama, was elected in 2008 as the President of the United States. The Obama's are the first African American family to live in the White House, and Mrs. Obama is a popular speaker, an educated woman, and a devoted mother and wife. Most importantly, as First Lady Mrs. Obama has chosen to focus on diet and health, and her many ideas and programs are aimed at trying to improve the nutrition of U.S. families significantly, while at the same time change the way food manufacturers and companies look at the quality of what they provide American consumers.

Mrs. Obama, a Harvard Law School graduate, left her job as an executive at the University of Chicago Medical Center to join her husband in the White House and is best known for her initiative to promote healthy eating and exercise, especially among children. Her signature campaign called "Let's Move" is aimed at reducing the nation's childhood obesity rates. As part of that effort, she has praised community vegetable gardens and received a lot of attention for planting an organic garden on the White House lawn. She also advocates exercise and movement by exercising at numerous public appearances.

As the nation battles an epidemic of obesity, Mrs. Obama continues to push for improvements in the nutritional quality of public school meals, and while she does not propose specific legislation, the attention she focused on that issue was a positive force in the passage of the Hunger-Free Kids Act, a bill that provides increased federal funding for school breakfasts and lunches. Through her Let's Move campaign, Mrs. Obama continues to encourage food service companies that stock the nation's school cafeterias to lower levels of fats and sugars in their foods and to increase the amount of whole grains and fresh fruits and vegetables they make available to the schools.

The First Lady has welcomed private businesses into her healthy eating conversation, inviting major retailers including Walmart, Walgreens, and Supervalu to remove trans fats, salt, and sugar from their processed foods. Following those discussions, Walmart officials announced that they now require suppliers to eliminate all trans fat and reduce salt content in their foods by 25 percent and set a 2015 deadline for those proposed changes. Walmart is a giant force in the retail marketplace, and when it announces a health initiative, other stores usually follow suit.

On the government side of nutrition education, Mrs. Obama worked with officials from the Agriculture Department to redesign the official food pyramid. The newly created alternative is called MyPlate, and features an icon of a plate that shows five food groups and suggested proportions for good nutrition. The MyPlate program is part of the 2010 Dietary Guidelines for Americans, which include information to assist U.S. consumers in making more nutritious meal choices.

Supporters of the First Lady say her decision to focus on nutrition, healthy eating, and exercise is a way to combine positive strategies with common sense. The five main pillars of Mrs. Obama's Let's Move initiative include creating a healthy start for children; empowering parents and caregivers; providing healthy food in schools; improving access to healthy, affordable foods; and increasing physical activity.

There are a few preliminary statistics on benefits to Mrs. Obama's Let's Move campaign. One study released in the fall of 2013 suggests that the antiobesity message may be starting to make a difference. The study was published in the September issue of the journal *Pediatrics*, and analyzed date from tens of thousands of children in grades 6 through 10. In that study researchers measured fruit and vegetable consumption as well as physical activity. Supporters of the First Lady say they expect to see more of a downward trend in obesity rates as her public health message continues to increase awareness of the importance of good nutrition and exercise for individuals and families.

See also: Let's Move; MyPlate; Obesity.

FURTHER READING

"America's Move to Raise a Healthier Generation of Kids." Letsmove.gov, December 20, 2012. http://www.letsmove.gov.

Burros, Marian. "Obamas to Plant Vegetable Garden at White House." *The New York Times*, March 20, 2009, A1.

Burros, Marian. "Promoting Healthy Eating, with 31 Other First Ladies." *The New York Times*, September 25, 2010, A15.

"First Lady Michelle Obama." White House, December 9, 2013. http://www.whitehouse.gov/administration/first-lady-michelle-obama.

Nixon, Ron. "New Rules for School Meals Aim at Reducing Obesity." *The New York Times*, January 25, 2012, A22.

O'Connor, Anahad. "Teenagers are Shifting Food Habits, Study Finds." *The New York Times*, September 16, 2013, A12.

Steinhauer, Jennifer. "Michelle Obama Promotes Healthy Eating with a Grass-Roots Campaign." *The New York Times*, June 19, 2013, A17.

Obesity

Obesity is defined as having a body mass index (BMI) of over 30. The obesity rate in the United States continues to rise alarmingly. According to a March 2014 article in the *Journal of the American Medical Association*, more than one-third of the adults in the United States are obese. In 2000, the rate was 19.8 percent, and in 1991, it was 12 percent. Obesity places people at risk for other conditions such as hypertension, Type 2 diabetes, coronary heart disease, stroke, and some cancers.

Obesity rates vary throughout the country, with the Midwest (29.5%) and South (29.4%) having a higher prevalence of obesity and the Northeast (25.3%) and West (25.1%) having lower rates, according to the Centers for Disease Control and Prevention (CDC).

In 2012, the lowest rate of self-reported obesity among adults in the United States was in Colorado (20.5%), while the highest was in Louisiana (34.7%). At the time, 13 states—Alabama, Arkansas, Indiana, Iowa, Kentucky, Louisiana, Michigan, Mississippi, Ohio, Oklahoma, South Carolina, Tennessee, and West Virginia—had a prevalence equal to or greater than 30 percent, according to the CDC.

The government's Healthy People 2020 initiative calls obesity a leading health indicator, and the updated initiative calls for a 10 percent reduction in the percentage of people in the United States—from 33.9 percent to 30.5 percent. Healthy People 2020 also calls for cutting the prevalence of obesity among children (through age 19) from 16.1 percent to 14.5 percent, a 10 percent reduction.

The Healthy People 2010 initiative had similar goals. At that time, 11 percent of children and adolescents and 23 percent of adults were obese. The hoped-for decreases did not occur, and the rates of obesity in both groups went up in the decade in-between.

The 2020 objectives aim to reach these goals through several different ways: providing access to healthier food, especially in school meals; increase the consumption of fruit, vegetables, and whole grains in American diets; encourage physicians to measure BMI routinely; and increase the amount of counseling and education on nutrition and diet.

The Healthy People 2020 report notes, "Obesity is a problem throughout the population. However, among adults, the prevalence is highest for middle-aged people and for non-Hispanic black and Mexican American women. Among children and adolescents, the prevalence of obesity is highest among older and Mexican American children and non-Hispanic black girls. The association of income with obesity varies by age, gender, and race/ethnicity."

Total costs related to obesity, calculated by direct medical costs and lost productivity, totaled an estimated $147 billion in 2008, up from $99 billion in 1995. The medical costs for people who are obese were $1,429 higher than those of normal weight.

See also: Body Mass Index; Childhood Obesity; Healthy People 2020.

FURTHER READING

"Clinical Guidelines on the Identification, Evaluation, and Treatment of Overweight and Obesity in Adults: The Evidence Report." National Instititutes of Health. NIH Publication No. 98–4083, September 1998. http://www.nhlbi.nih.gov/guidelines/obesity/ob_gdlns.pdf.

Finkelstein, Eric A., Justin G. Trogdon, Joel M. Cohen, William Dietz. "Annual Medical Spending Attributable to Obesity: Payer- and Service-Specific Estimates." *Health Affairs* 28, no.5 (July 27, 2009): 822–31. http://content.healthaffairs.org/content/28/5/w822.full.pdf.

Kaplan, Karen. "Weight Discrimination Worsens Health for People Who Are Overweight or Obese." *Los Angeles Times*, March 4, 2011. http://articles.latimes.com/2011/mar/04/news/la-heb-obesity-discrimination-health-declines-20110304.

Ogden, Cynthia, Margaret D. Carroll, Brian K. Kit, Katherine M. Flegal. "Prevalence of Childhood and Adult Obesity in the United States, 2011–2012." *The Journal of the American Medical Association* 311, no. 8 (February 26, 2014): 806–14.

www.cdc.gov/obesity/data/adult.html.

www.healthypeople.gov.

Obesity Surgery

Obesity surgery, also called bariatric surgery, is the last resort for severely obese people who have tried weight-loss and exercise programs and have repeatedly failed. The different procedures include gastric-bypass surgery, the lap band procedure, vertical banded gastroplasty, and jejunoileal bypass. The theory behind all types of obesity surgery is simple: if the volume the stomach holds can be reduced, bypassed, or shortened, people will not be able to consume or, in some cases, to absorb as many calories. With obesity surgery the volume of food the stomach can hold is typically reduced from about four cups to about a half a cup. But these procedures are not a magic solution. There is a long-term failure rate of up to 50 percent, additional surgery is necessary in some cases, and many patients face daily complications like intolerance to foods high in fats, lactose intolerance, vomiting, diarrhea, and intestinal discomfort. Statistics show that the number of bariatric or obesity surgeries in the United States has plateaued since 2003 at some 113,000 cases per year. However, even though there has been no growth in the number of Americans having the surgery each year, the cost to the economy is estimated at $1.5 billion annually.

Gastric-bypass surgery, developed in the 1960s, is a procedure in which surgeons sew the stomach shut to a fraction of its original size, and then reattach that portion directly to the small intestine, limiting room for food and time for absorption. Patients must be carefully screened physically and psychologically for the operation, which is suggested only for people with 100 or more pounds to lose, and always as a last resort. The operation can be risky; stomach perforations, infection, allergic reaction to anesthesia, or excessive bleeding or blood clots in the lungs, and heart attacks are among the serious or even fatal complications. And because the surgery can affect absorption in the intestine, all gastric-bypass patients have to take vitamins for the rest of their lives.

After the procedure, patients need to follow a lifelong diet, exercise, and behavior modification program, keeping in mind how important their food choices are now that they can literally fill up on a single piece of bread. Once patients return to eating solid food, poor choices leave them without necessary nutrients and can even make them physically ill. Foods to avoid include carbonated beverages, popcorn, nuts, fried foods, red meat, and sugar, meaning no pie, cookies, or cake. Still, some surgery patients experience a 10- to 20-pound weight gain once the new stomach stretches a bit, while others who do not adopt the necessary lifestyle and dietary changes find themselves returning to their weight prior to the operation.

The American Society for Metabolic and Bariatric Surgery (ASMBS) reports that up to 5 patients in 1,000 die from gastric-bypass surgery. On the other hand, complications from obesity, such as diabetes, high blood pressure, and arthritis, cost consumers millions of dollars in related health care costs each year. Major complications for adolescent patients are being studied as some 10,000 teenagers have undergone bariatric weight-loss surgery in the past decade.

The less invasive lap band procedure (short for laparoscopic adjustable gastric band), approved in June 2001 by the Food and Drug Administration (FDA), is intended for people with smaller weight-loss requirements and involves the surgeon wrapping a band around the top part of the stomach to restrict how much food it can hold. The procedure is cheaper and faster than gastric-bypass surgery, and requires a shorter hospital stay. Lap band surgery takes less than an hour and requires an overnight stay, compared to the more extensive bypass surgery that lasts two to three hours and requires a three-day hospital recuperation. The adjustable silicon band with a balloon at the end, used in the lap band procedure, can be adjusted or even removed if the patient experiences serious side effects, a reversal not possible with the gastric-bypass procedure.

Other obesity surgery procedures include vertical banded gastroplasty, where an artificial pouch is created using staples in a different section of the stomach. Plastic mesh is sutured into part of the pouch to prevent it from dilating. In this surgery, like the gastric-bypass operation, the food enters the small intestine farther along than it would enter normally, reducing the time available for absorption of nutrients and calories. Jujunoileal bypass, now rarely performed, involves shortening the small intestine. This procedure has a high occurrence of serious complications, such as chronic diarrhea and liver disease, and is thought to be the least effective of any of the procedures. It is rarely performed now and has been replaced by safer procedures.

Following obesity surgery, most patients are restricted to a liquid diet for up to three weeks. Patients then graduate to a diet of puréed food for about a month or two until they can tolerate solid food. High-fat food is especially hard to digest and causes diarrhea. Patients must also be careful not to eat too quickly or to ingest too much food or they can experience nausea, vomiting, and intestinal "dumping," when undigested food is shunted too quickly into the small intestine, causing pain, diarrhea, and dizziness.

Meanwhile, researchers continue to study the complex system of brain and body chemicals that govern weight and appetite. Exciting new studies on the growth hormone ghrelin have some scientists suggesting that an effective weight-loss drug is closer than ever before. The development and use of obesity drugs came under close scrutiny in 1997 when the FDA ordered the withdrawal of the drug combination fen-phen when it was discovered to have dangerous effects on the heart. Still, doctors say it may be a long time before obesity surgery becomes obsolete and at this time it remains the best option for some patients who have tried everything else and failed.

See also: Fen-Phen; Ghrelin; Obesity.

FURTHER READING

Abouzeid, Nehme E. "Insane Growth in Inquiries about Surgeries for Obesity." *Boston Business Journal* 21, no. 39 (November 2, 2001): 39–40.

Crawford, Dan, and Jeff Bell. "This Lap Band Is No Opening Act at Polaris." *Business First-Columbus* 17, no. 48 (July 20, 2001): A3.

Davidson, Tish. "Obesity Surgery." In *Gale Encyclopedia of Medicine*. 1st ed., edited by Jacqueline L. Longe and Deidre S. Blanchfield, 2079–80. Detroit: Gale Research, Inc., 1999.

Desloge, Rich. "Appetite for Thinness." *St. Louis Business Journal* 21, no. 46 (July 20, 2001): 8.

Haire, Pat. "Extreme Measures: Gastric-Bypass Surgery Is the Last Resort of the Overweight, but Iris Starr Says the Results More than Justify the Risks." *Sarasota Magazine*, November 2001, 211–16.

"Largest Safety Study on Teen Weight Loss Surgery Finds Few Complications." *Pediatrics Week*, November 23, 2013, 180.

Lemonick, Michael D. "Lean and Hungrier: Is a Recently Discovered Hormone the Reason Why Folks Who Lose Weight Can't Keep It Off?" *Time*, June 3, 2002, 54.

Livingston, E. H. "The Incidence of Bariatric Surgery Has Plateaued in the U.S." *American Journal of Surgery* 200, no. 3 (September 2010): 378–85. doi:10.1016/j.amjsurg.2009.11.007.

Ohsawa, George

George Ohsawa (b. October 18, 1893, in Kyoto, Japan; d. April 23, 1966, in Tokyo, Japan) is credited with introducing macrobiotics to the West. He was born Yukikazu Sakurazawa to Magotaro and Setsuko Sakurazawa. As a young man he attended a commercial high school to prepare for a career in business, a placement that exposed him to Western culture and opened his thinking to Western ideas.

At age 18, Sakurazawa was diagnosed with tuberculosis, a fatal disease at that time. During his illness he turned to the writings of Sagen Ishizuka. A Japanese army doctor, Ishizuka had established his theory of nutrition and medicine based on the traditional Asian diet, which he tied to the Western medical sciences of chemistry, biology, and physiology. Ishizuka's diet theories were published in two books, *Chemical Theory of Longevity*, in 1896, and *Diet for Health*, in 1898.

Sakurazawa responded well to Ishizuka's diet and regained his health. He then went on to become president of the Shoku-Yo-Kai, an association founded by Ishizuka before his death in 1910. In the years that followed, Sakurazawa became a prolific author, devoting his life to writing about the teachings of Ishizuka and lecturing around the world. He also began to develop his own ideas that expanded on Ishizuka's earlier work by incorporating the concepts of yin and yang into his 12 principles of macrobiotics. Yin and yang represent the two basic universal tendencies in Asian philosophy. According to Ishizuka, health problems were caused by the imbalance of yin and yang. Ohsawa carried this connection further when he linked yin with potassium and yang with sodium.

After World War II, Sakurazawa, to further his work in the West, changed his name to George Ohsawa and officially named his philosophy *Macrobiotics*, or "all-embracing life." After years of world travel, he and his wife, Lima Ohsawa, moved to New York in 1959 to join Michio Kushi and a small group of followers. Kushi, a teacher and founder of the East West Foundation and the Kushi Institute, originally met Ohsawa through the World Federalist Movement, an American peace movement and the precursor to the United Nations. It was through this organization that Ohsawa arranged for Kushi to go to the United States, and Kushi then used that opportunity to introduce macrobiotics in North America.

During his life, Ohsawa wrote more than 300 books and pamphlets in languages from Japanese and French to English and German. He also published a monthly magazine for more than 40 years. Ohsawa died at the age of 74 in 1966. The George Ohsawa Macrobiotics Foundation, Inc., a nonprofit organization, was founded in 1961 by Kushi and Herman Aihara, and continues to educate the general public about the principles and health benefits of a macrobiotic diet.

Macrobiotics calls for people to balance their overall intake of yin and yang foods and, by doing so, to establish a harmony within the body. Yin foods are thought to be foods like vegetables, grains, beans, and seaweed. Animals and animal products are considered yang foods. In later years, Kushi liberalized the diet by emphasizing a more relaxed approach to food, a shift away from the strict, cereal-based diet espoused by Ohsawa. Kushi also encouraged less salt or sodium in the diet. Contemporary critics say the current macrobiotic diet can improve health mostly because those who follow it stop eating refined foods, and cut back substantially on meat, milk, and other animal products, although it is not considered a completely vegetarian diet. They suggest that followers improve not because of the foods they take in, but because of the foods they leave out.

See also: Macrobiotics; Vegetarian Diet.

FURTHER READING

Kotzsch, Ronald E. *Macrobiotics: Yesterday and Today.* Tokyo: Japanese Publications, 1985.

Kushi, Michio. *Diet for a Strong Heart: Michio Kushi's Macrobiotic Dietary Guidelines.* New York: St. Martin's Griffin, 2003.

Melton, J. Gordon, Jerome Clark, and Aidan A. Kelly. *New Age Encyclopedia.* Detroit: Gale Research Inc., 1990.

Ohsawa, George. *Zen Macrobiotics: The Art of Rejuvenation and Longevity.* Reprint. Chico, CA: George Ohsawa Macrobiotic Foundation, 1995.

Wells, Patricia. "Macrobiotics: A Principle, Not a Diet." *New York Times,* July 19, 1978, C1–C9.

Ornish, Dean

Dr. Dean Ornish (b. July 16, 1953, in Dallas) is an innovative physician who has developed a scientifically proven system to reverse heart disease without drugs or surgery, replacing those invasive techniques with a very-low-fat diet, exercise, and stress management. And unlike many diet book authors, Ornish has published research findings about his program in medical journals such as the *Journal of the American Medical Association* and the *American Journal of Cardiology*.

In 2013 Ornish signed an exclusive agreement with Healthways, a global well-being improvement company that focuses on disease management, to offer his program for reversing heart disease to Healthways customers. This followed the announcement in 2011 by Medicare of the inclusion of the Ornish heart disease program in a new benefit category known as "intensive cardiac rehabilitation." In describing the Ornish heart program, Dr. Mehmet Oz and other celebrity doctors have applauded Ornish for his use of science and nutrition.

The doctor, whose best-selling books include *Dr. Dean Ornish's Program for Reversing Heart Disease: The Only System Scientifically Proven to Reverse Heart Disease without Drugs or Surgery* (1990); *Eat More, Weigh Less: Dr. Dean Ornish's Life Choice Program for Losing Weight Safely While Eating* (1993); *Stress, Diet and Your Heart* (1982), first gained attention from the medical community in 1989 when he released data showing a reduction in overall heart blockages in his patients. What was unusual was that the improvement came not from the standard treatment of drugs or surgery, but instead from a high-fiber, low-fat, vegetarian diet along with stress-management techniques. Founder and president of the

Preventive Medicine Research Institute of the University of California at San Francisco, Ornish champions what other cardiologists at first labeled "radical" ideas. Many in the medical establishment still continue to insist Americans will never find a soy and plant diet acceptable. He has served since 1995 as a clinical professor of medicine at the University of California, San Francisco.

During his career, Ornish has been honored many times including his appointment to the White House Commission on Complementary and Alternative Medicine Policy during the administration of former president Bill Clinton. Ornish was also appointed in 2011 by President Barack Obama to the Advisory Group on Prevention, Health Promotion, and Integrative and Public Health.

Ornish attended Baylor College of Medicine in Houston, and it was there that Ornish said he began questioning the standard treatment for heart patients. At the time, the Baylor-affiliated Texas Medical Center was a world leader in coronary-bypass operations. Yet years later Ornish told *Discover* that "having a bypass without changing your lifestyle is like trying to mop up the floor around an overflowing sink without turning off the faucet." In 1977 Ornish conducted his first medical experiment, a study titled "The Effects of Stress Management and a Low-Cholesterol Diet on Heart Disease." That study showed that after only 30 days on his plan, subjects said their chest pain was somewhat alleviated and more blood was flowing to their hearts. After graduating from Baylor, Ornish started his internship and residency at Massachusetts General Hospital, a Harvard University affiliate. By the time Ornish left Harvard, in 1984 he had completed his internship and residency, conducted more original research, and published his first book, *Stress, Diet and Your Heart*.

In the summer of 1984 Ornish moved to San Francisco and established the Preventive Medicine Research Institute with Shirley E. Brown, whom he later married. The institute is based in Sausalito and is affiliated with the University of California at San Francisco. National recognition came in 1988 and 1989 following another Ornish study, the results of which he presented at a meeting of the American Heart Association and which eventually won him grants from the National Institutes of Health among other major research organizations.

His work continued to achieve mainstream success when the Mutual of Omaha Insurance Company in 1993 agreed to provide full reimbursement to patients enrolled in Ornish's program for reversing heart disease. In the spring of 2000, the Health Care Financing Administration announced a demonstration project involving the Ornish program as an alternative to conventional medical treatments for selected Medicare patients. Meanwhile, dozens of health insurers now reimburse the cost of Dr. Ornish's program for selected patients. Today the idea of a low-fat diet is more acceptable to mainstream cardiologists who recommend that patients make food choices based on the U.S. Department of Agriculture, MyPlate, which is rich in fruits, vegetables, and whole grains.

Ornish admits that there is nothing new about his approach that, in fact, is similar to the low-fat food plan developed in the 1970s by the late Nathan Pritikin, the California inventor, author, and founder of the Pritikin Longevity Centers. Dr. John McDougall is another physician who developed a low-fat, vegetarian eating program, similar to the Ornish plan. McDougall established the St. Helena Health Center in 1987, located in California's Napa Valley.

Ornish broke more new ground in his research. In the 1998 book *Love and Survival: The Scientific Basis for the Healing Power of Intimacy*, he offers readers clinical and anecdotal evidence as well as research findings to support his newest theory that having deeply intimate, loving relationships can be invaluable in preventing and treating heart disease. The book classifies love broadly from the love of a mate to the love of family, friends, and God. But the overall message, along with his dedication to Molly, whom he married in 1998, remains that love and intimacy are among the most powerful factors in determining a person's health or illness.

See also: Life Choice Diet; McDougall Program; MyPlate; Pritikin Program for Diet and Exercise; Vegetarian Diet.

FURTHER READING

Brink, Susan. "The Low-Fat Life." *U.S. News & World Report*, July 12, 1999, 56.

Condor, Bob. "Lifestyle Changes Can Go Right to the Heart." *Chicago Tribune*, February 13, 2000, 3.

Cowley, Geoffrey. "Healer of Hearts." *Newsweek*, March 16, 1998, 50–57.

"Dean Ornish." *Contemporary Authors Online*. Detroit: Gale Group, 2001.

Grady, Denise. "Can Heart Disease Be Reversed?" *Discover*, March 1987, 54–66.

"Healthways and Dr. Dean Ornish Join Forces to Bring Proven Treatment for Reversing Chronic Disease to Millions." *Healthways*, July 23, 2013. http://phx.corporate-ir.net/phoenix.zhtml?c=91592&p=irol-newsArticle_pf&ID=1840093.

Ornish, Dean. "Healing Broken Hearts." *Nutrition Action Healthletter* 26, no. 5 (June 1999): 1.

Perlmutter, Cathy. "Heal Your Heart With Love: America's Favorite Doctor Dean Ornish Gives Advice on Preventing Heart Attacks." *Prevention*, August 1998, 118–25.

Osteoporosis

Osteoporosis is a skeletal disease, in which bones lose mass and density, pores enlarge, and bones become fragile. The National Osteoporosis Foundation estimates that the disease continues to cause more than 1.5 million bone fractures each year in the United States. The disease is four times more common in women than in men due to differences in bone density. Lack of exercise and low calcium

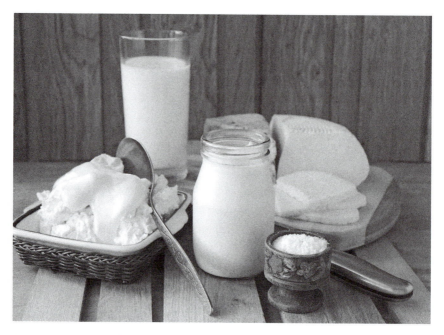

Dairy foods that are rich in calcium, as well as weight-bearing exercises, are important in the prevention of osteoporosis. (Victoria Shuba/Dreamstime.com)

intake during childhood, adolescence, and early adulthood are all risk factors for the disease. In a 2004 first-ever Surgeon General's Report on bone health and osteoporosis, Tommy G. Thompson reminded Americans that lifestyle changes and a focus on prevention through exercise and healthy nutrition, combined with early diagnosis and treatment millions of Americans can avoid the damaging impact of osteoporosis and other bone diseases.

The Surgeon General's Report followed a declaration in 2002 by former president George W. Bush that 2002–2011 was the Decade of the Bone and Joint. The designation brought the United States into alignment with other countries in committing resources to study and treat bone disease and arthritis. As part of this effort, the U.S. Department of Health and Human Services also developed goals that were included in its Healthy People 2010 initiative to focus on osteoporosis and its prevention and treatment.

See also: Calcium; Exercise.

FURTHER READING

Office of the Surgeon General (US). *Bone Health and Osteoporosis: A Report of the Surgeon General.* Rockville, MD: Office of the Surgeon General (US), 2004. http://www.ncbi.nlm.nih.gov/books/NBK45518.

"Osteoporosis." *Centers for Disease Control and Prevention.* Page last reviewed May 30, 2013. http://www.cdc.gov/nchs/fastats/osteoporosis.htm.

Overeaters Anonymous

Overeaters Anonymous (OA) is not a diet club; it doesn't advertise and there are no weigh-ins, no special frozen meals, and no recipes to swap. Modeled after the Alcoholics Anonymous program, OA is an organization for people who eat compulsively. According to the group, OA now serves more than 54,000 members in 80 countries. Groups meet in church basements, community rooms, private homes, anywhere they can gather to share their experiences and strength, and hope for recovery from what can be a crippling addiction to food. Figures released by OA show some 7,000 group meetings worldwide.

Given the growing number of weight-focused reality television shows such as *The Biggest Loser,* it is no surprise that OA has also been included in popular media in the situation comedy, *Mike & Molly.* In the show the characters discover each other at an OA meeting and begin a relationship that eventually leads to marriage.

Overeaters Anonymous looks at compulsive overeating as a physical, emotional, and spiritual disease. OA members include an eclectic group, from those who are extremely overweight, morbidly obese, of average weight or moderately overweight, to those who are underweight or those who cannot control their compulsive eating. Symptoms that members experience are as varied as the individuals. Those symptoms include obsession with body weight, size, and shape; eating binges or grazing; preoccupation with reducing diets; starving; laxative, or diuretic abuse; excessive exercise; inducing vomiting after eating; inability to stop eating certain foods after taking the first bite; vulnerability to quick weight-loss or fad diets; constant preoccupation with food.

While not a diet club, members often lose weight when they gain control over their overeating. Participants are treated much like recovering alcoholics; OA offers its members support in dealing with their problem one day at a time through the implementation of an eating plan under the guidance of an experienced sponsor. However, OA does not endorse, recommend, or distribute any specific diet or food plan; instead, anyone seeking nutritional guidance to lose weight is advised to talk to a doctor. Those members who don't find success in achieving their weight-loss goals may still experience recovery in other parts of their lives.

The individual eating plans are as diverse as each member and each plan is based on an honest appraisal of past experiences, current individual needs, and knowledge of "trigger foods" or situations that may contribute to an episode of overeating. The sponsor, a veteran member, helps new members work out a food plan and stick with it as part of the sponsor's commitment or obligation to OA. Critics of the organization say the rigid food plans, rules for sponsorship, and other techniques for avoiding "trigger" foods may actually reinforce obsessive food behavior, which can be a problem for a compulsive overeater.

Founded in 1960, the program is based on the 12 steps and 12 traditions of Alcoholics Anonymous. The Traditions describe attitudes early members thought were important to group survival. Anonymity is considered by OA to be the foundation of all of the other traditions, which include common welfare comes first since personal recovery depends on OA unity; group leaders are trusted servants but they do not govern; God is the ultimate authority; the only requirement for membership is a desire to stop eating compulsively; each group should carry its message to any compulsive overeater still suffering from an addiction to food; every OA group should be fully self-supporting and should decline outside contributions; and the OA public relations policy must be based on attraction rather than promotion.

The 12 steps, considered the heart of the OA recovery program, originated in Alcoholics Anonymous but were adapted for use with food addiction. Those steps include that members recognize they were powerless over food until they came to believe a greater power could restore their health. OA members are also expected to make a list of all persons they harmed and try to make amends; to take personal inventory and, when wrong, promptly admit it; pray for knowledge of God's will and also admit to God the exact nature of any wrongdoing. Members are required to ask God to remove any shortcomings and they should have a spiritual awakening as a result of the steps. This will make it possible to carry their message to other compulsive overeaters.

Like other 12-step groups, OA stresses that talk of spirituality has nothing to do with any structured religion. According to the OA Web site, the group "does not practice any religion in the meetings." Persons of all faiths are welcome: agnostics, Catholics, atheists, Jews, and Protestants. Recovery and spiritual growth are said to depend only upon any member's willingness to practice the principles and rules of the program on a daily basis.

While weight-loss groups like Weight Watchers or TOPS have regular weigh-ins and pounds are an important part of the discussion, OA members often talk about a variety of issues, since many join as a last resort to solving emotional troubles that go far beyond coping with excess pounds. So members place their faith and trust in the group itself, which underscores why member anonymity is so important. This reassures members that anything shared with the group will be held in the strictest confidence and will not be discussed outside of the meetings. OA says another important aspect of anonymity is that all members are considered equal in the program: outside status, wealth, or social standing has no bearing.

See also: *Biggest Loser, The*; TOPS, Take Off Pounds Sensibly; Weight Watchers.

FURTHER READING

Fletcher, Anne M. "Inside America's Hottest Diet Programs." *Prevention*, May 1990, 46.

Kaplan, Lee M. "Weight-Loss programs." *Weigh Less, Live Longer (Harvard Special Health Report)*, September 2006, 29.

"Overeaters Anonymous WSO Convention 2013 Offers Message of Hope with Rock 'N Recovery." *Mental Health Weekly Digest*, July 22, 2013, 140.

Seligman, Jean. "Helping Fight Extra Helpings: Food Junkies Are Turning to OA to Kick Their Habit." *Newsweek*, December 5, 1988, 78.

Wilson, Gail O. "Overeaters Anonymous Offers Help, Hope and Recovery." *Alcoholism & Addiction Magazine*, October 1989, 34.

Overnight Diet

Sleep yourself thin? A diet called the overnight diet claims that dieters can lose weight while they sleep—2 pounds overnight, according to Dr. Caroline Apovian, an obesity doctor at Boston Medical Center and the author of *The Overnight Diet* (2013).

The diet involves using high-protein smoothies that kick start the metabolism, allowing the dieter to lose up to 9 pounds by the end of the first week—without exercise necessary. The plan combines six days of high-protein foods, one day of liquid diet and plenty of sleep—which should help stave off hunger pangs.

Critics of the plan say such significant weight loss can only be caused by a drop in water weight, and Apovian doesn't entirely disagree. She says that the fast drop in water weight can help the dieter substitute lean, high-protein foods. Critics also say they're skeptical of any plan that doesn't require physical activity as a long-term way to sustain weight loss.

See also: Liquid Protein Diets.

FURTHER READING

Apovian, Caroline. *The Overnight Diet. The Proven Plan for Fast, Permanent Weight Loss*. New York: Hachette Book Group, 2013.

Caba, Justin. "'The Overnight Diet' Supposedly Helps You Lose Weight While You Sleep." *Medical Daily*, April 23, 2013. www.medicaldaily.com/overnight-diet-supposedly-helps-you-lose-weight-while-you-sleep-video-245206.

Davis, Linsey. "'Overnight Diet' Promises Weight Loss While You Sleep." *ABC News*, April 8, 2013. www.abcnews.go.com/blogs/health/2013/04/08/overnight-diet-promises-weight-loss-while-you-sleep/.

www.drcarolineapovian.com.

P90X

Are you a 96-pound weakling or the last one picked for teams and the first one picked on by bullies? Or are you one of those people doing the same weight-lifting routine you did in high school some 30 years later? If so, the fitness DVD called P90X is aimed directly at you. With more than 4 million copies sold since its debut in 2005, the workout is considered the cool kid on the block in the home fitness market. Celebrities from all walks of life have embraced it like Senator and vice presidential candidate Paul Ryan, who, during the 2012 presidential campaign, posed for *Time* curling barbells during a P90X workout.

Created by Tony Horton, who calls P90X the most successful fitness product in history, the program is designed as an alternative to the classic gym equipment and cardiovascular machine workouts popular for decades in gyms and fitness centers. Equipment needs for P90X are minimal, not much more than exercise bands or dumbbells, a chin-up bar and a DVD player. In fact, even critics of the program agree that while there is nothing new in the workouts, anyone who participates six days a week for three months will lose weight and build muscle.

The workouts are based on the classic fitness principles of variety, intensity, and consistency. Horton suggests what sets his DVD apart is the winning combination of sequence, pace, and variety. According to Horton there are four main principles or elements that make the program so successful. He calls his first principle one of "muscle confusion." The former celebrity trainer points to all the people who have been going to gyms for years and doing the same routines but who see poor results. He argues that mixing up exercise and intensity in his P90X program burns more calories, protects from injury, and keeps exercisers motivated.

The second principle of P90X is the idea of focusing on fitness weaknesses with the goal of improving those areas the most. Horton suggests selecting an exercise or fitness routine that is a struggle and then committing to improve fitness and flexibility in that area. Once that initial aversion is overcome, improvement can be dramatic and can become a real motivation to exercise more. The third principle according to Horton is for individuals to push themselves beyond their discomfort threshold. In fact, Horton calls the desire to exercise the secret to becoming fit.

Horton's final principle for success is to exercise to maintain health and flexibility rather than for vanity. He suggests yoga is an important type of exercise, which, he maintains, provides resistance, balance, and helps build stamina. He cautions that weight loss and muscle definition should not be the reason to exercise, and that inner strength and mindfulness are better long-term goals.

Not surprisingly, the popularity of the DVD had led to a market in pirated copies that the company, Beachbody, estimates have totaled over $75 million worth of sales each year. The California-based company is taking an aggressive stance with illegal copies and has hired lawyers and investigators to track and stop the illegal copying through sting operations and legal action. The company admits

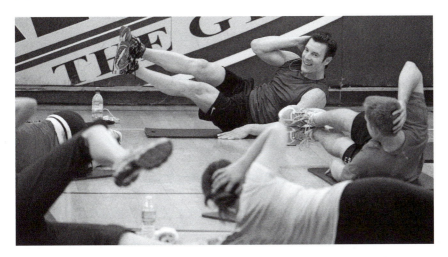

Fitness instructor Tony Horton developed P90X and other workout programs that are sold on DVDs. Here, he is teaching a class in Washington, DC. (The Washington Post/ Getty Images)

that price conscious consumers who are looking for a good deal online can be tricked into buying the fake programs without even knowing they are purchasing something illegal. Statistics show that other companies, including Nike, have followed Beachbody's example and are taking a hard line against counterfeiters and are asking the government for help. Statistics show the number of seizures of counterfeit merchandise by U.S. customs officials has increased and now is more than four times greater than it was just 10 years ago. Businesses are also asking Congress to consider legislation that will block "pirate" Web sites, especially any outside the United States to protect unwitting American consumers.

The additional P90X diet program, part of the entire package sold by Beachbody, calls for meals of lean protein, whole grains, fruits, and vegetables and has been compared to the paleo style of eating that focuses on proteins and few carbohydrates. However, as users progress through the P90X program, the diet shifts and lowers the protein ratio and raises the carbohydrate ratio. Beachbody and Horton have also released a follow-up to P90X named P90X2 in late 2011. The sequel was developed with assistance from Harvard-trained doctor Marcus Elliott, who specializes in assisting elite athletes.

See also: Paleo Diet.

FURTHER READING

Crowe, Deborah. "No Infomercial? No Sweat for New Workout Program: Beachbody Aims P90X2 at Previous Customers to Pump Sales." *Los Angeles Business Journal* 33, no. 49 (December 5, 2011): 13.

Hyson, Sean. "X Man: Tony Horton, the Trainer behind P90X, Breaks Down the Most Successful Fitness Product in History." *Men's Fitness* 28, no. 2 (March 2012): 22.

Kita, Joseph. "The Power of P90X." *Men's Health*, December 18, 2010, http://www.men shealth.com/fitness/p90x.

Lee, Alfred. "Fitness Company Sweats Copycats: Beachbody Brings in Muscle on DVD Counterfeiters." *Los Angeles Business Journal* (August 8, 2011): 1, http://www.labusi nessjournal.com.

Paleo Diet

The Paleo diet offers a plan to lose weight and regain health by eating like the early caveman or Neanderthals and lays the blame for many chronic health problems at the feet of what Americans do and do not eat. *The Paleo Diet* was written by Loren Cordain, PhD, and has become popular with dieters, athletes, and many Americans looking to solve autoimmune disorders and other chronic health issues.

While not the first to look at how cavemen ate, Cordain brought the concept to a large audience by writing his diet book supporting the idea of a Paleolithic diet. S. Boyd Eaton was among the earliest supporters of eating like our ancient ancestors and the first to offer a scientific principle based on what he termed Paleolithic nutrition. He published his theory in a 1985 *New England Journal of Medicine* article in which he outlined the evolution of human genes and how he thought they interacted with their nutritional environment. He suggested that early man became used to the nutrients in his foods, while modern man finds the convenience foods of today incompatible with his genetic makeup. Eaton and later Cordain publically blame sugar and carbohydrate-filled foods for the current epidemic of obesity and diabetes in the United States.

Cordain took the idea of eating like our ancestors a step further and published his diet book in 2001 to moderate success. However, upon release of his revised edition in 2010, the word paleo had entered the national conversation, thanks to social media and the Internet where bloggers and others shared their own personal successes with Paleo-style eating plans. An Internet search can deliver testimonials from thousands of people who have written about their stories of weight loss and improved health once they ate like cavemen and removed most carbohydrates from their daily menu.

In fact, the Internet continues to provide a forum for others with similar eating plans including Robb Wolf, Sarah Fragoso, Dr. Kurt Harris, and Chris Masterjohn. Wolf, author of *The Paleo Solution*, is a biochemist and offers information as well as podcasts about his unique paleo-eating plan. Fragoso was introduced to paleo-style eating by Wolf and she also blogs and creates podcasts about her diet, which she calls everyday paleo. Dr. Kurt Harris calls himself an archevore and describes his diet as being based on essential principals. He is in private practice as a board-certified radiologist but blogs about nutrition with a focus on evolutionary biology. Masterjohn was influenced by Weston A. Price, and with a PhD in nutritional science, he has created a Web site that encourages a diet of quality animal foods based on his research that cholesterol is not the cause of heart disease in America.

In his book, Cordain made clear there are differences between his paleo diet and other similar eating plans as well as low-carbohydrate fad diets. For example, Cordain's paleo diet contains almost no carbohydrates when compared to the typical U.S. diet and includes more protein and more vegetables than the popular high-protein, low-carbohydrate diets like the Atkins plan. Cordain based his eating plan on studies he conducted as a researcher and professor of exercise physiology at Colorado State University.

SPECIFICS OF THE PALEO DIET

Cordain laid out seven fundamental characteristics of his paleo program that he said sets it apart from any other diet. They include a higher protein intake; a higher fiber intake from a bigger selection of fruits and vegetables; a smaller amount of carbohydrate foods, especially grains, and the drop in the glycemic index of foods eaten due to this lack of carbs; an increase in consumption of monounsaturated and polyunsaturated fats but not vegetable oils, and an improved balance of Omega-3 and Omega-6 fat levels; higher potassium and lower sodium levels; an increase in vitamins, minerals, antioxidants, and plant phytochemicals; and a change to the alkaline-acid load to the kidneys. Cordain reasoned that plant foods provide an alkaline balance rather than an acidic balance in the body. He suggested any increase in acidity is caused by other foods, especially processed foods or refined carbohydrate foods. An increase in acidity has been shown to increase bone and muscle loss along with high blood pressure. High acidity is also considered a factor in a number of kidney diseases including kidney stones.

So what exactly are paleo dieters eating? Most fruits are allowed along with nuts and seeds like almonds, chestnuts, pecans, and walnuts. Cordain is very specific about which oils he recommends and has narrowed the acceptable choices to olive oil, walnut oil, flaxseed oil, and avocado oil. He strongly recommends against eating any canola oil and suggests the only oil for cooking should be olive. Other paleo-style diets allow coconut oil or palm oils, even though they are high in saturated fats.

Forbidden foods include all dairy products; all sugars, especially sucrose, fructose, and molasses; all grains from cereals, breads, pastas and other wheat products as well as oats, rice, and even increasingly popular ancient grains like quinoa and amaranth; all legumes such as beans, lentils, coffee, soybeans, and peanuts; all starchy foods including potatoes and sweet potatoes. The diet also recommends that people avoid fatty, salty, processed meats such as bacon, sausage, hotdogs, and lunch meats; although in the updated version of Cordain's book he reassures those faithful to the basic principles of his paleo diet that they can eat those meats occasionally with no ill effects on their health. However, he strongly recommends that paleo followers seek out meats from animals that were not produced in a feedlot because they were raised on a grain-based diet. Instead, he recommends eating meat from wild animals or grass-fed animals.

A daily menu for the paleo diet is supposed to resemble what ancient people ate; only the choices are more contemporary. For example, foods like grass-fed meats, eggs, fish or other seafood, fresh vegetables and fruits along with olive, walnut, flaxseed, and avocado oils are all mainstays of the paleo menu. Cordain created three levels in his diet plan: Level I for those who want to move slowly into the diet and ease the feelings of deprivation that often go along with starting any diet; Level II for those willing to make a few more changes to their food choices; and Level III for those who can want to make long-term behavioral changes quickly and who want to see immediate weight loss or health benefits.

Breakfast in Level I might include a bowl of diced fruits and vegetables like apples, carrots, and raisins, plus poached eggs, or some leftover protein-like chicken breast. Lunch would be a vegetable-laden salad, maybe with tuna or some other seafood, and a sample dinner might be veal or halibut, a green or spinach salad with some other steamed or fresh vegetable or fruit plus nuts and berries for dessert.

Level II might start with something like an omelet with avocado or a breakfast steak and some fresh fruit slices, lunch would be a spinach salad with crabmeat or leftover chicken and vegetables from the previous dinner. Dinner might include fish, chicken, or beef, with squash or vegetable soup, and some fresh fruit for dessert.

A Level III sample menu would include melon and berries plus a broiled pork chop or beefsteak for breakfast, and lunch might include baked cod, salmon steak or some other fish, and a vegetable salad. Dinner would have a serving of fish and perhaps also some game meat like venison, buffalo, or pheasant along with a green salad, steamed asparagus, or other nonstarchy vegetables and baked apples or other fresh fruits like dates or figs. For those who still feel hungry after eating a paleo meal, Cordain recommends eating additional lean protein, chicken or turkey breasts, fish, lean beef, shrimp or crab, and more crisp vegetables or fresh fruit.

Critics of the diet point to the possible effects on the heart from the high amounts of meat and fats and suggest the increased intake of protein might also create kidney problems. Scientists question whether Paleolithic peoples would have exhibited many of our modern health problems if they had longer life spans. According to fossil remains, it is clear that most people of that time period did not live long enough to reach middle age, which is when chronic diseases like diabetes, heart disease, cancer, and osteoporosis frequently develop in adults.

The lack of whole food groups is also a concern for nutritionists when it comes to high-protein diets, and that is a worry voiced by critics of the paleo diet. Health experts agree that growing obesity rates and rising numbers of diabetics can be linked to our dependence on processed foods filled with fats and sugar, as well as an overall lack of exercise. They admit any diet that focuses on whole foods and increases daily fruit and vegetable intake can't be totally negative. However, the cost of eating a steady diet of specialty meats, fresh fruits, and vegetables can be extremely expensive for the average family.

See also: Atkins Nutritional Approach; Carbohydrates; Eat Right 4 Your Type.

FURTHER READING

Audette, Ray. *Neanderthin: Eat Like a Caveman to Achieve a Lean, Strong, Healthy Body.* New York: St. Martin's, 1999.

Challem, Jack. "Is the Paleo Diet for You? The Healthiest Diet for Today and Tomorrow May Very Well Be the Eating Habits of the Past." *Better Nutrition* 75, no. 4 (April 2013): 48(3).

Cordain, Loren. *The Paleo Diet: Lose Weight and Get Healthy by Eating the Food You Were Designed to Eat.* Hoboken, NJ: John Wiley & Sons, 2001.

Cordain, Loren, and Joe Friel. *The Paleo Diet for Athletes: A Nutritional Formula for Peak Athletic Performance.* Emmaus, PA: Rodale Books, 2005.

Sanfilippo, Diane. *Practical Paleo: A Customized Approach to Health and a Whole-Foods Lifestyle.* Las Vegas: Victory Belt Publishing, Inc., 2012.

Schmid, Ronald F. *Traditional Foods Are Your Best Medicine: Improving Health and Longevity with Native Nutrition.* Rochester, VT: Healing Arts Press, 1997.

Zuk, Marlene. "Pondering Paleo: Channeling Your Inner Caveperson." *Nutrition Action Healthletter* 40, no. 3 (April 2013): 9(3).

Phenylpropanolamine (PPA)

Phenylpropanolamine (PPA) is an amphetamine-like substance used at one time as an over-the-counter appetite suppressant or as a nasal decongestant. It disrupts hunger signals to the brain and dries out the mouth, making food taste bland and unappetizing, and it also clears nasal congestion by narrowing or constricting the blood vessels. It had been the main ingredient in several weight-loss products sold over the counter, including Dexatrim and Accutrim. In November 2000 the U.S. Food and Drug Administration (FDA) issued a public health warning cautioning consumers against taking such products. The FDA also asked manufacturers of products containing PPA to voluntarily replace it with alternative active ingredients.

The FDA determined that PPA was not safe for over-the-counter use based on the results of the Hemorrhagic Stroke Project, a study conducted between 1994 and 1999 by the Yale University School of Medicine that showed an increased risk of stroke in people taking drugs containing PPA. This action was aimed at diet products and also at over-the-counter allergy and cold medications. As part of the USA Patriot Act, which went into effect in 2005, the government passed the Combat Methamphetamine Epidemic Act, which required all retail sellers of ephedrine, pseudoephedrine, or phenylpropanolamine to become certified and submit monthly reports on sales of any products containing those drugs to the U.S. Drug Enforcement Administration. To further restrict unlawful use of these products, the Combat Methamphetamine Enhancement Act of 2010 was passed to include those who sell phenylpropanolamine, ephedrine, or pseudoephedrine containing products by mail.

In response to these various restrictions, many cold and cough recipes switched from PPA to pseudoephedrine, an ingredient already used in products like Sudafed. However, pharmacologists say there is no FDA-approved alternative to PPA for over-the-counter diet pills, only herbal ingredients that are considered dietary supplements and are not subject to FDA regulations under the Dietary Supplement Health and Education Act of 1994. Dexatrim manufacturers withdrew their PPA-containing product and introduced Dexatrim Natural, an herbal alternative containing ephedra. However, researchers continue to study the possibility that the human body may convert ephedra to PPA. In a November 2000 study published in the *New England Journal of Medicine*, researchers linked dietary supplements containing ephedra to serious side effects, including heart attacks, strokes, and seizures.

See also: Dexatrim; Dietary Supplement Health and Education Act (DSHEA); Ephedra/Ephedrine; Food and Drug Administration (FDA).

FURTHER READING

Brink, Susan. "Diet Drugs: What a Pill." *U.S. News & World Report*, November 20, 2000, 74.

"By the Way, Doctor—What's the Story with PPA?" *Harvard Women's Health Watch* 8, no. 9 (May 2001): 7–8.

"Combat Methamphetamine Epidemic Act of 2005." U.S. Department of Justice Drug Enforcement Administration Office of Diversion Control. http://www.deadiversion .usdoj.gov/meth/.

Haller, C. A., and N. L. Benowitz. "Adverse Cardiovascular and Central Nervous System Events Associated with Dietary Supplements Containing Ephedra Alkaloids." *New England Journal of Medicine* 343, no. 25 (December 21, 2000): 1833–38.

"Selling Ephedrine, Pseudoephedrine, or Phenylpropanolamine by Mail." *American Journal of Health-System Pharmacy* 67, no. 22 (November 15, 2010): 1900.

Phytochemicals

Phytochemicals are disease-fighting substances found in plant foods. These substances and antioxidants help reduce the risk of cancer, heart disease, and Alzheimer's disease. More and more research suggests that phytochemicals play an important role in overall health and may even slow down the aging process. Scientists have been able to identify several hundred types of individual phytochemicals over the past two decades and continue to study their link to human health. As the research continues health professionals suggest the best choice is to eat a colorful diet filled with fresh or steamed vegetables and fresh fruits.

Anthocyanins are antioxidants that help control high blood pressure and protect against diabetes-related circulatory problems. The best naturally occurring sources of this phytochemical are found in black or blue fruits such as blackberries, elderberries, black currants, and purple grapes. Red fruits and vegetables are also good sources of anthocyanins. Health professionals suggest the best choice is to eat red raspberries, sweet cherries, strawberries, cranberries, beets, red apples, red cabbage, red onion, and kidney beans.

Phenolics and anthocyanins also help reduce the risk of heart disease, cancer, and Alzheimer's, and may even slow down the aging process. The best naturally occurring sources of phenolics are prunes, eggplant, raisins, and plums.

Indoles help protect against breast cancer and prostate cancer. Indoles are found in broccoli, cauliflower, cabbage, and brussels sprouts. Lutein is an antioxidant that has been connected with better eye health. Lutein helps reduce the risk of forming cataracts and macular degeneration, both of which can cause vision loss in older people. Lutein is found in green leafy vegetables.

Beta-carotene is another antioxidant linked to a reduced risk of cancer and heart disease as well as giving an overall boost to the immune system. Beta-carotene is found in orange vegetables, such as carrots.

Bioflavonoids work together with vitamin C to improve overall health and heart health, to reduce the risk of cancer, to strengthen bones and teeth, and to promote more rapid wound healing. Orange- and yellow-colored fruits and vegetables supply both bioflavonoids and vitamin C.

Allicin may help lower cholesterol and blood pressure as well as work as an anti-infective for the body. It's found in garlic and onions.

Lycopene helps reduce the risk of several types of cancer. It's found in watermelons, pink grapefruits, and fresh tomatoes and tomato-based products, such as spaghetti sauce and tomato juice.

See also: Diabetes.

FURTHER READING

Fukushima, Rhoda. "The Top Ten." *St. Paul Pioneer Press*, April 7, 2002, F1.

Napier, Kristine. *Eat to Heal: The Phytochemical Diet and Nutrition Plan.* New York: Warner, 1998.

Stampfer, Meir J. "The Benefits and Risks of Vitamins and Minerals." *Harvard Special Health Report*, March 2006, 37.

Stieg, Bill, and Lisa Jones. "Guy-Friendly Food." *Men's Health*, June 2002, 44.

"Stronger than C." *Vegetarian Times*, May 2002, 13.

"10 Foods That Pack a Wallop: Eat, Drink and Be Healthy! Scientists Are Rapidly Identifying the Natural Chemicals That Give Preventive Punch to a Rainbow of Ordinary Edibles." *Time*, January 21, 2002, 76.

Prediabetes

Prediabetes is a condition affecting an estimated 79 million American adults aged 20 years or older according to 2010 statistics released by the Centers for Disease Control and Prevention. Prediabetes diagnosis means blood glucose levels are higher than normal but not yet diabetic. Even though cases of diabetes and prediabetes have nearly doubled in the United States since 1988, research from the Johns Hopkins Bloomberg School of Public Health has determined that obesity is apparently to blame for the surge, which means many of these cases can be prevented through lifestyle changes. One hopeful note from the study found that although cases of prediabetes and diabetes continue to increase, the number of undiagnosed cases is dropping, a statistics researchers say means screening and diagnoses are improving.

Lifestyle changes, primarily focusing on diet and physical activity, have been found not only to prevent the onset of diabetes but also to reduce the risk of heart disease and stroke significantly. Government health agencies and the American Diabetes Association are calling on physicians to begin screening overweight people age 45 and older for prediabetes, particularly if they have a family history of diabetes, low HDL cholesterol and high triglycerides, high blood pressure, a history of gestational diabetes or if a woman has given birth to a baby weighing more than 9 pounds, or belong to a minority group. African Americans, Native Americans, Hispanic Americans/Latinos, and Asian American/Pacific Islanders continue to be at increased risk for Type 2 diabetes.

A clinical trial run by the Health and Human Service involving more than 3,000 people found that diet and exercise resulting in a 5 to 7 percent weight loss lowered incidence of Type 2 diabetes by 48 percent. The press release stated that participants lost weight by cutting fat and calories in their diet and by exercising (most chose walking) at least 30 minutes a day, 5 days a week.

See also: Diabetes; Exercise; Insulin; Obesity.

FURTHER READING

American Diabetes Association press release. *HHS, ADA Warn Americans of 'Pre-Diabetes,' Encourage People to Take Healthy Steps to Reduce Risks*. Washington, DC, 27 March, 2002.

Centers for Disease Control and Prevention. *National Diabetes Fact Sheet: National Estimates and General Information on Diabetes and Prediabetes in the United States, 2011.*

Atlanta: U.S. Department of Health and Human Services, Centers for Disease Control and Prevention, 2011.

Rabin, Roni Caryn. "Diabetes on the Rise among Teenagers." *The New York Times*, May 21, 2012. http://well.blogs.nytimes.com/2012/05/21/diabetes-on-the-rise-among-teenagers/.

Selvin, E., C. M. Parrinello, D. B. Sacks, and J. Coresh. "Trends in Prevalence and Control of Diabetes in the United States, 1988–1994 and 1999–2010." *Annals of Internal Medicine* 160, no. 8 (April 15, 2014): 517–25. doi:10.7326/M13–2411.

President's Council on Physical Fitness, Sports, and Nutrition

The President's Council on Physical Fitness, Sports, and Nutrition (PCPFSN) was founded on July 16, 1956, by President Dwight D. Eisenhower after a study showed American children were less physically fit than children in other countries. Originally named the President's Council on Youth Fitness, the agency name was changed to the President's Council on Physical Fitness in 1960 by President John F. Kennedy to reflect an expanded mandate to serve Americans of all ages. And in 1968 President Lyndon B. Johnson added the word *sports* to the council title in a move to emphasize the importance of participation in sports. Johnson also began the tradition of presenting Presidential Physical Fitness Awards in 1966; the Presidential Sports Award program was created in 1972. Finally, in 2010 President Barack Obama announced the addition of nutrition to the name of the agency and an increase in Council members to support its expanded mission. That same year, the First Lady Michelle Obama announced the creation of her Let's Move program as a way to help reduce the incidence of childhood obesity in the United States.

The PCPFSN now includes 25 council members, up from 20 members, and each appointed by the President. Assisted by the U.S. Public Health Service, the PCPFSN provides guidance to the President and to the Secretary of Health and Human Services on how to encourage more Americans to be physically active and eat well. In its efforts to educate Americans about the benefits of physical fitness, the Council develops and distributes publications and pamphlets, and works with individual citizens, civic groups, private enterprise, community organizations, and others to promote fitness and good nutrition for all Americans. The PCPFSN encourages and supports the development of community recreation and sports programs and works with business, industry, government, and labor organizations to set up workplace physical fitness programs. The Council also works with agencies to encourage research in sports medicine, physical fitness, and sports performance.

In 2012, the White House announced a replacement for the Youth Fitness test, first initiated in 1966. The replacement, called the Presidential Youth Fitness Program, is a way to recognize athletic performance and assess student health and overall fitness. This updated program rates students by how well they meet their own goals rather than how they compare to classmates. The new program includes three key components that include resources for teachers, parents, and students; research-based assessment tools; and recognition for participating in the program. That same year the President's Council joined in a partnership with the Entertainment Software Association (ESA) to promote a healthy lifestyle through the use of active video games.

See also: Let's Move; Obama, Michelle.

FURTHER READING

"General Mills Collaborates with ADA, President's Council." *Pediatrics Week*, June 18, 2011, 75.
"Our History." *The President's Council on Fitness, Sports & Nutrition.* http://www.fitness.gov/about-pcfsn/our-history/.
"President's Council on Fitness, Sports & Nutrition Announces New Fitness Program Aimed at Helping Kids Stay Active." *President's Council on Fitness, Sports & Nutrition*, September 10, 2012. http://fitness.gov/news-highlights/press-releases/pr-10-sep-2012.html.

Pritikin, Nathan

Nathan Pritikin (b. August 29, 1915, in Chicago; d. February 21, 1985, in Albany, New York) was a self-taught nutritionist and an inventor who championed the concept that a low-fat, high-fiber diet of natural foods like fruits, vegetables, and whole grains, combined with regular aerobic exercise, could prevent and treat heart disease and other diseases of affluent society. He wrote six books, including the first, *Live Longer Now* (1974) and his best-selling *Pritikin Program for Diet and Exercise* (1979). Other titles included *The Pritikin Permanent Weight-Loss Manual* (1982), *The Pritikin Promise: 28 Days to a Longer, Healthier Life* (1983), *The Official Pritikin Guide to Restaurant Eating*, coauthored with wife Ilene (1985), and *Diet for Runners* (1985). Newer titles authored by Nathan Pritikin's son Robert Pritikin include *The New Pritikin Instinct* (1998) and *The Pritikin Principle: The Calorie Density Solution* (2000). In late 1984, Nathan Pritikin was hospitalized due to complications related to cancer treatment, and fully aware that he was deteriorating rapidly, took his own life in early 1985.

Although Pritikin received little formal education (he dropped out of the University of Chicago to work on the Nordon bombsight), he began his lifelong study of human anatomy and physiology as a youth. During World War II,

Pritikin began to develop his theory concerning the causes and cures of heart disease. Scientific thinking at that time held that heart disease was caused, in large part, by stress. Yet in looking over statistics on the civilian populations of Europe, he noticed that death rates due to heart attack had fallen during the stress-filled war years. In a 1991 interview in *Vegetarian Times*, Pritikin's son Robert said that his father had also noticed that while stress was high, rationing during the war meant people were eating very little meat and few dairy products. After the war, when rationing ended but stress subsided, Pritikin noted that the rates of heart disease went right back up.

Pritikin's years of research were put to the test in 1956 when he had his own cholesterol checked. It was over 300. He then underwent a stress electrocardiogram, which showed coronary insufficiency. A second cardiologist and second testing confirmed that Pritikin's arteries were clogging up. He was diagnosed with substantial coronary heart disease. He was 41 years old. A prestigious team of cardiologists gave him the standard prescription of the day: stop all exercise, stop climbing stairs, take it easy, and take naps in the afternoon. But Pritikin's readings of population studies had convinced him that dangerous arterial plaque would form at any cholesterol level over 160. If he could get his cholesterol level down with dietary measures, he figured he might have a chance of surviving. By April 1958, he had become a vegetarian. He had also started running three to four miles daily. By May, his cholesterol had fallen to 162. By January 1960, his cholesterol had dropped to 120, and a new electrocardiogram showed his coronary insufficiency had disappeared.

Encouraged by the results of his diet and exercise program, Pritikin launched several research projects over the next 25 years that validated the efficacy of his program. But the medical establishment was at first slow to accept Pritikin's theory that heart disease could be cured through dietary changes and exercise. Groups like the American Heart Association and the American Medical Association initially dismissed his claims and criticized the diet, saying it did not show lasting benefits and it was too restrictive as a life-long program. Pritikin ignored the criticism. His studies on heart disease, diabetes, hypertension, and nutrition were published in several key medical journals, including the *New England Journal of Medicine*, the *Journal of the American Medical Association*, and *Circulation*. Pritikin's theories and practices are similar to the low-fat, high-fiber diet recommended by Dr. Dean Ornish, a physician whose medical studies have also shown significant reduction in heart disease when patients are treated through diet, exercise, and stress reduction. Dr. John McDougall is another physician who developed an eating program sharing the common theme of low-fat and high-fiber foods. Like Pritikin and Ornish, McDougall also established his own health facility, the St. Helena Health Center.

The Pritikin diet calls for a menu rich in natural foods: fruits, vegetables, whole grains, all varieties of legumes (such as pinto beans, black beans, and lentils), moderate amounts of nonfat dairy products like nonfat milk and nonfat yogurt, and small amounts of poultry, lean meat, and seafood. Limited, too, are salt, sugar, and other refined carbohydrates like white flour. On a typical day an individual following the Pritikin diet would eat three meals and three snacks consisting of many different foods, such as hot oatmeal with banana and strawberries for breakfast; fresh fruit and yogurt for a midmorning snack; pasta with marinara sauce, fruit, and steamed vegetables for lunch; soups such as minestrone, lentil, or gazpacho for an afternoon snack; for dinner, broiled seafood, a large green salad, steamed asparagus, and a baked potato; and for dessert or an evening snack, popcorn or frozen yogurt.

Pritikin went public with his program through lectures, his presentations to medical communities, and the establishment of his Pritikin Longevity Center in 1975 in Santa Barbara, California, an in-residence program of nutrition, exercise, and lifestyle education that has attracted people from all over the world. The Pritikin Longevity Center in Florida continues to operate as both a lifestyle-training program and a research center, with a laboratory that works to investigate the relationship between diet, exercise, and disease prevention.

Pritikin also established the Pritikin Research Foundation, a nonprofit organization that both conducts and funds research examining the relationship between diet and disease. Robert Pritikin, Nathan's son, was named director of the Pritikin Program in 1985. In 1984, shortly before Nathan Pritikin's death, the National Heart, Lung, and Blood Institute announced that lowering blood cholesterol reduced the risks of heart attacks and coronary disease, vindicating Pritikin's earlier dietary recommendations.

Years before Pritikin first learned of his heart disease, he had been diagnosed with leukemia, an illness that would eventually lead to his death. Pritikin suspected that radiation he had been exposed to during World War II had contributed to his contracting leukemia. For decades, the leukemia was in remission. In 1984 the cancer reappeared. Pritikin suffered complications caused by his cancer treatments and grew increasingly weak. Even though his health was failing, Pritikin continued to work on new technology designed to remove fats from the blood without the use of drugs. Pritikin held more than two dozen patents in physics, chemistry, and electrical engineering, and marketed his inventions to companies including Honeywell, General Electric, Bendix, and Corning. Following his death, Pritikin's autopsy showed a heart and arteries that were in extraordinarily healthy condition, "like that of a 16-year-old," noted the supervising pathologist. Nathan Pritikin was buried in Santa Monica, California.

See also: Life Choice Diet; McDougall Program; Ornish, Dean; Pritikin Program for Diet and Exercise.

FURTHER READING

Almanac of Famous People. 6th ed. Farmington Hills, MI: Gale Research, 1998.

Barnard, Neal D. "The Pritikin Legacy." *Vegetarian Times*, May 1991, 64–73.

Hoover, Eleanor. "When His Health Deserted Him, Diet and Fitness Guru Nathan Pritikin Turned to Suicide." *People Weekly*, March 11, 1985, 57–59.

Pritikin, Nathan. *The Pritikin Program for Diet and Exercise*. New York: Grosset and Dunlap, 1979.

Scribner Encyclopedia of American Lives. Vol. 1: *1981–85*. Farmington Hills, MI: Gale Group, 1998.

Shute, Nancy. "A Childhood without Twinkies: Young Pritikin Modifies His Father's Draconian Fat-Free Message." *U.S. News & World Report*, January 12, 1998, 62.

Pritikin Program for Diet and Exercise

The Pritikin Program for Diet and Exercise by Nathan Pritikin, a self-taught nutritionist and inventor, is a program Pritikin developed in 1979 while he was treating his own heart disease. This diet and exercise plan in 2010 was named the first residential education program in the United States to be covered by Medicare and Medicaid Services. The four-week program is based on a low-fat, high-fiber diet and exercise plan available through the Pritikin Longevity Center, also spelled out in Pritikin's many best-selling books, including *The Pritikin Program for Diet and Exercise* (1979), and in his son Robert Pritikin's books. Pritikin called his diet "a declaration of war against the American dependence on processed foods, fats, sugars, proteins, salt, caffeine, alcohol, and nonfoods." It focuses on complex carbohydrates, fresh fruits, and vegetables eaten raw or cooked. The Pritikin Diet advocates a fat level that averages no more than 10 percent of total calories daily. The average American diet may run from 30 to 40 percent fat while the U.S. Department of Agriculture (USDA) Dietary Guidelines for Americans recommend eating no more than 30 percent or less of daily calories from fat.

Unlike many fad diets, the Pritikin Program does not limit specific food groups but instead divides foods into those to use versus those to limit or avoid altogether. In his book *The Pritikin Permanent Weight-Loss Manual,* dieters who want more structure are advised to find daily menu plans outlining four different calorie-intake levels. Most breakfast menus contain some grain foods to help dieters meet important nutritional requirements and also because whole grains are filling and provide a substantial start for the day. Breakfast grains include hot cereals of cracked wheat, rolled oats, or cornmeal, plus recommended cold cereals like shredded wheat or grape-nuts.

The Pritikin diet strongly encourages snacking between meals, saying the body functions best when food is eaten more frequently during the day. People who attend the Pritikin Longevity Center eat seven to eight meals a day with few restrictions on quantity of food eaten. Good snack choices include low-fat, high-fiber soups like minestrone and other bean-based varieties, whole fruits, vegetables, and salads. Lunch and dinner often include pasta dishes, seafood rich in omega-3 fatty acids, Asian rice and vegetable entrées, Mexican dishes like burritos and enchiladas, and a wide variety of salads and soups. Pritikin called fresh fruit the best dessert but his book also features other dessert recipes. He cautioned that many of his recipes did contain generous amounts of fruit juice sweeteners and should be restricted or reserved for only occasional use. Each of Pritikin's books also contains daily menu ideas as well as many recipes.

A typical breakfast on the Pritikin Program menu includes hot oatmeal, sliced bananas and blueberries, nonfat milk, half a grapefruit, and a cup of green tea. Lunch might include a large green salad with nonfat dressing, a veggie or garden burger on whole wheat bread topped with onion and tomato, an ear of corn, fresh fruit, and herbal tea or mineral water. A typical dinner would be poached salmon, roasted new potatoes, steamed asparagus, a green salad with balsamic vinegar or nonfat dressing, fruit salad, and a glass of wine or herbal tea. Snacks throughout the day would include fat-free plain yogurt mixed with fresh fruit, fresh vegetables like carrots and cherry tomatoes, popcorn, salsa with baked tortilla chips, or baked potatoes with fat-free sour cream.

The Pritikin program also emphasizes foods, like fruits and vegetables, that are low in calorie density; in other words, nutrient-rich foods that fill you up with the least amount of calories. These foods include most fruits; vegetables; nonfat dairy products; many unrefined carbohydrates, such as pasta, hot cereals like oatmeal, brown rice, yams, and corn; beans, peas, and lentils; and lean animal protein like seafood, chicken breast, and turkey breast.

Pritikin cautioned against high-protein diets such as the Scarsdale Medical Diet and Dr. Atkins's Diet Revolution. He said high-protein, low-carbohydrate diets had immediate as well as long-term adverse effects, including nausea; constipation; vitamin and mineral depletion; mineral imbalances; accumulation of toxic substances such as ketones, uric acid, and ammonia; elevated blood cholesterol that narrows arteries; increased kidney malfunction; and possible increased risk of colon disease. In his book *The Pritikin Program for Diet and Exercise*, he wrote, "There is nothing good that can be said for high-protein diets. I am against them because of their inherent dangers, because they discourage people from adopting healthy and satisfying eating habits and because they are of dubious effectiveness even in the short term."

In announcing the Medicare eligibility, Paul Lehr, President of the Pritikin Longevity Center & Spa suggested that the Pritikin model of diet and exercise successfully addresses the health crisis in the United States by offering preventive solutions rather than relying on disease management measures such as surgery and medication. The late Pritikin did encourage people to exercise daily, and said a good exercise program would improve well-being, build resistance to heart disease, and help any weight-loss effort. Pritikin was himself an avid jogger, and followed a regular exercise routine until the last year of his life.

See also: Atkins Nutritional Approach; Dietary Guidelines for Americans; Ketones/Ketosis; Scarsdale Diet.

FURTHER READING

American National Biography. New York: Oxford University Press, 1999.

Barnard, Neal D. "The Pritikin Legacy." *Vegetarian Times*, May 1991, 64–73.

Gever, John. "Ornish, Pritikin Cleared for Medicare Payment." *MedPage Today*, August 13, 2010. http://www.medpagetoday.com/Cardiology/Prevention/21675.

Pritikin, Nathan. *The Pritikin Permanent Weight-Loss Manual*. New York: Grosset and Dunlap, 1981.

Pritikin, Nathan. *The Pritikin Program for Diet and Exercise*. New York: Grosset and Dunlap, 1979.

"The Pritikin Program Approved by Medicare in Landmark Decision." *Medical Devices & Surgical Technology Week*, September 5, 2010, 155.

Protein Power

The Protein Power plan is a high-protein, low-carbohydrate plan developed by Dr. Michael Eades and Mary Dan Eades. The concept behind the Protein Power plan is that reducing intake of carbohydrates will reduce the amount of insulin released into the body. Protein Power also suggests avoiding "bad fats," which include fried foods, hydrogenated fats, and trans fats or trans fatty acids, such as margarine.

The Protein Power Web site offers minimum requirements for protein, depending on your level of activity and "lean body mass." For example, a sedentary person needs only 0.5 grams of protein per pound of lean body mass compared to a very active person (one who exercises an hour or more at least five times a week) who needs 0.8 grams of protein per pound of lean body mass.

In calculating carbohydrates, the Eades use the "effective carbohydrate content." This is the total carbohydrates in a food, minus the dietary fiber. In other words, high-fiber carbohydrate foods have a lower carbohydrate rating than a simple sugar might, even if the total carbohydrates listed on the Nutrition Facts label are the same.

Low-carbohydrate, high-protein diets have become increasingly popular in recent years. Diets from Scarsdale and Atkins to Paleo and the Dukan diet all point to carbohydrates as the cause for weight gain. An article in the *Journal of the American Dietetic Association* suggested that carbohydrates became the dieters' taboo "because the low-fat diets of the 1980s and 1990s failed consumers who mistakenly believed that consumption of low-fat products was license to eat voraciously while paying no mind to the amount of sugar and energy being consumed. Many people find irresistible the basis of low-carbohydrate diets: eating as much protein as desired—including steaks, eggs, and other fatty foods that they had previously been told by media reports and medical practitioners to shun—and still losing weight, so long as intake of carbohydrates is strictly limited."

Yet many critics of these restrictive carbohydrate plans say severely limiting carbohydrates is not good either. All high-protein, low-carbohydrate plans put the dieter at risk of loss of vitamin B, calcium, and potassium, resulting from lack of carbohydrates in the diet, and risk of coronary heart disease from eating more high-protein foods that are also high in fat.

While a low-carbohydrate diet will help a dieter lose weight initially, critics say the dieter will feel lethargic. Because there are so few carbohydrates to burn as energy, the body begins to burn lean muscle mass for energy. The Eades respond on the Web site, noting, "In the first seven to ten days, some people may feel tired. This is because it may take a week or two for your body to manufacture the necessary enzymes to effectively handle your new nutritional structure. Your body will make the enzymes it needs, but there is a short lag in the time it takes to do so. During this period, you may feel slightly fatigued, but that should quickly pass. Be sure that you are taking your potassium supplement. You should try to pamper yourself in the first couple of weeks on the plan. Get some extra rest. Take it easy on any hard-core exercise."

Nonetheless, most nutritionists and physicians would recommend a carbohydrate-moderating diet, not a severe reduction.

See also: Ketones/Ketosis; Trans Fatty Acids.

FURTHER READING

Eades, Michael R., and Mary Dan Eades. *Protein Power: The High Protein/Low Carbohydrate Way to Lose Weight, Feel Fit and Boost Your Health—In Just Weeks.* New York: Bantam Books, 1997.

Eades, Michael R., and Mary Dan Eades. *The Protein Power Lifeplan.* New York: Warner Books, 2001.

Gotthardt, Melissa Meyers. "The New LowCarb Diet Craze." *Cosmopolitan,* February 2000, 148.

"Protein Power!" *Flex,* May 2013, 28.

Stein, Joel. "The Low-Carb Diet Craze." *Time,* November 1, 1999, 71–79.

Stein, Karen. "High Protein, Low-Carbohydrate Diets: Do They Work?" *Journal of the American Dietetic Association,* 100, no. 7 (July 2000): 760.

Turner, Richard, and Joan Raymond. "The Trendy Diet That Sizzles: A Counterintuitive Program Reaches Critical Mass." *Newsweek International,* September 13, 1999, 62.

Wilgoren, Jodi. "Low-Carb Diet: Lose the Bun, Not the Burger." *New York Times,* January 11, 2000, D7.

www.eatprotein.com.

Qsymia

Qsymia, a combination of phentermine and topiramate, two U.S. Food and Drug Administration (FDA)-approved drugs, is one of two prescription weight-loss medications that was approved by the FDA in 2012. Prior to that, the FDA had not approved a prescription weight-loss medication in 13 years. The other drug approved in 2013 is called Belviq.

The drug is approved for use in adults with a body mass index (BMI) of 30 or greater (obese) or adults with a BMI of 27 or greater (overweight) who have at least one weight-related condition such as high blood pressure, Type 2 diabetes, or high cholesterol. Qsymia is designed to be used as part of a reduced-calorie diet and exercise program.

Among its side effects, one highly stressed effect is that the drug should not be used by pregnant women and any adult woman taking the medication should be very careful not to become pregnant. A fetus exposed to one of the key ingredients topiramate, an anticonvulsant, in the first trimester of pregnancy has an increased risk of oral clefts (cleft lip with or without cleft palate). The other drug in the combination, phentermine, is an appetite suppressant.

In two FDA clinical trials for Qsymia, results showed that after one year of treatment at two doses of Qsymia, the patients had an average weight loss of 6.7 percent (at the lower dose) and 8.9 percent (at the higher dose) over those who were treated with placebo. Approximately 62 percent and 69 percent of patients lost at least 5 percent of their body weight with the recommended dose and highest dose of Qsymia, respectively, compared with about 20 percent of patients treated with placebo.

The drug maker, Vivus Inc., is required to conduct 10 postmarketing requirements, including a long-term study to measure whether using Qsymia increases the risk for heart attack and stroke. Other weight-loss drugs were taken off the market in 1997 because of the increased risk to the cardiovascular system.

See also: Belviq.

FURTHER READING

Boyles, Salynn. "Combo Drug Qsymia Tops for Weight Loss." *MedPage Today*, October 29, 2013. http://www.medpagetoday.com/endocrinology/obesity/42563.

DeNoon, Daniel J. "Weight Loss Pill Qsymia Now for Sale." webmd.com, September 18, 2012. http://www.webmd.com/diet/news/20120918/weight-loss-pill-qsymia-now-for-sale.

Grohol, J. "Qsymia and Belviq Drugs for Obesity, Weight Loss." Psych Central, 2012. http://psychcentral.com/lib/qsymia-and-belviq-drugs-for-obesity-weight-loss/00013443. Accessed April 13, 2014.

Press Release FDA Approves Weight-Management Drug Qsymia. U.S. Food and Drug Administration, July 17, 2012. http://www.fda.gov/NewsEvents/Newsroom/PressAnnouncements/ucm312468.htm.

Raw Foods

Fresh food means different things to different people. To a person following the Paleo diet, it might look like grass-fed beef or apples just picked from the tree. To someone following the Master Cleanse, it might mean fresh squeezed lemons and little else. To someone following a raw foods diet, it includes only nutrient-rich plant foods that have not been processed by heat in any way.

With a striking resemblance to the Garden of Eden, a raw foods diet includes fruits, vegetables, nuts, along with seeds, legumes, and grains that are sprouted instead of cooked. Although some raw foodists do eat some unpasteurized dairy products or raw fish and meat, most follow a vegan eating plan.

The theory behind raw foods is that when foods are heated, the important vitamins, minerals, and enzymes are destroyed. In a raw foods diet, there are no calorie restrictions; dieters eat as much as they want of the fresh fruits and vegetables. Those who do not cook their food report feeling more energy and mental clarity, and are free of toxins. Celebrities who have joined the raw food ranks at one time or another include Sting, Madonna, Demi Moore, and actor Woody Harrelson.

While health care professionals agree that eliminating processed and fast foods from the standard American diet would bring improved health, many are convinced a raw food lifestyle can also create health problems. Due to all the restrictions and the need to avoid cooked grains, beans, or legumes, those following a raw food diet do have difficulty staying on it for the long term. Also, followers need to be very careful to meet their needs for vitamins and other essential nutrients that often come from a large variety of foods. Researchers have discovered that cooking can unleash more essential nutrients from many vegetables, something that allows the body to absorb them more completely.

Food safety experts also suggest that food poisoning can come from eating raw or improperly cooked foods, if those foods have been exposed to *Salmonella* or *E. coli* and are not properly washed before they are eaten.

Those who support a raw diet suggest the pros outweigh the cons especially when it comes to the quality of the food eaten on a raw diet. Processed foods like pasta, pizza, hot dogs, or bread often contain hydrogenated, saturated, or other cooked fats, all things that require extra energy to digest. And anyone who suffers from food allergies would automatically avoid much of the wheat, dairy, soy, and corn that can trigger a reaction when raw foods are eaten. Supporters say another plus comes from the support a raw foods lifestyle provides to sustainable farming. With that comes a reduction in the carbon footprint needed to provide food. Plus, raw food can be grown and purchased in its natural state and requires no extra packaging, one more aspect that decreases unnecessary waste.

People who have turned to a raw foods diet to lose weight have had some success since the diet by virtue of what is eaten is low in fat, low in sodium, and filled with fiber, vitamins, minerals, and antioxidants. Medical professionals caution that it is important to consult a doctor before making a change to a raw food diet for any reason. In fact, there is little research available that shows that eating only raw, uncooked food is the key to staying healthy. However, there is plenty of science that shows eating fruits, vegetables, seeds, nuts, and other fresh foods is a cornerstone to good health. Anyone thinking of beginning a raw food diet should consult with a health care professional to make sure it is the best choice.

See also: Gluten-Free; Master Cleanse Diet; Paleo Diet.

FURTHER READING

"Going Raw: Pros and Cons." *Environmental Nutrition* 36, no. 3 (March 2013): 3.

Ladermann, Dan, and Cherie Sorie. "The Raw Truth about Raw Meals." *USA Today (Magazine)* 141, no. 2816 (May 2013): 60.

MacDonald, Marianne. "Will Eating a Raw Diet Give Me More Energy?" *Prevention* 65, no. 10 (October 2013): 62.

Sharma, Himanshu. "Raw Food Diet: Easy Way to Lose Weight." Onlymyhealth.com, October 4, 2013. http://www.onlymyhealth.com/lose-weight-with-raw-food-diet-1380890028.

Registered Dietitian (RD)

Only registered dietitians—those who have completed an academic program accredited by the American Dietetic Association, and gained related experience—can use the letters "RD" after their name. Registered dietitians must keep up with continuing professional education to maintain their certification.

In some states, dietitians are licensed by the state, and only state-licensed dietetics professionals are permitted to provide nutrition counseling. Not all states require licensing, however. Some states have less restrictive certification or registration regulations. According to the American Dietetic Association, "Consumers in these states [without licensing requirements] who are seeking nutrition therapy assistance need to be more cautious and aware of the qualifications of the provider they choose."

Who should work with a registered dietitian? Health care professionals suggest many Americans would benefit from consulting with an RD as a way to improve their diet, especially those with diabetes. For diabetics, the need to manage blood glucose levels is of paramount importance. An RD can work with an individual to find the best way to safely adjust unhealthy eating habits and replace them with positive choices based on the latest nutrition information. Anyone who consults an RD can expect for the dietitian to take into account their medical history, body measurements, present health, economic concerns, and food allergies or preferences to craft a plan to improve their health through their food choices.

See also: Diabetes.

FURTHER READING

Neithercott, Tracey. "Eating Expertise: What to Expect When Working with a Registered Dietitian." *Diabetes Forecast* 66, no. 12 (December 2013): 58(4).
Strom, Stephanie. "Dietitians Pay Off for Supermarkets." *The New York Times*, August 25, 2012, B1.

Relaxacisor

The Relaxacisor was a handheld device designed to help people firm and tone their muscles by delivering a mild electric shock through contact pads. The shocks caused muscle spasms, which were supposed to be firm and tone and tighten problem areas in a woman's figure. The Relaxacisor was billed as an easy solution to being "out-of-shape"; Relaxacisor, Inc., sold more than 400,000 of the machines from 1949 until 1970 when the FDA banned them as ineffective and dangerous. According to Stephen Barrett and William Jarvis, authors of *The Health Robbers*, it took years of investigation and a five-month court battle to eventually produce the federal ban on the devices.

In his final decision, federal Judge William P. Gray said the Relaxacisor could cause miscarriages and could aggravate many preexisting medical conditions, including hernia, ulcers, varicose veins, and epilepsy. Following the decision, many of those who had purchased the devices requested refunds while the firm filed an appeal. The appeal was dismissed and the FDA promptly sent posters to all U.S. post offices warning against use of the devices. The government also warned that the sale of secondhand Relaxacisors was illegal. Owners were encouraged to either destroy them or make them inoperable to avoid the possibility of harm to "unsuspecting users."

The standard model had three control knobs and six pads to exercise six muscles at a time. The deluxe model was twice as large. A 1956 magazine advertisement for the device promoted it as passive exercise. "It's a modern mode of NO-EFFORT exercise that you can concentrate on the areas that need it most. Relaxacisor, for example, can exercise just the muscles of your tummy while the rest of you RESTS!" Magazine advertisements in the 1950s and 1960s pictured shapely models reclining with a book or magazine. The pads were visible, attached to hips, thighs, buttocks, and stomachs, and each woman appeared completely relaxed.

Known as electrical muscle stimulators (EMSs), these devices have limited usefulness in physical therapy for people with spinal cord injuries who can no longer voluntarily control their muscles, according to doctors. They are also still used to reduce muscle shrinkage in bed-ridden patients.

See also: Exercise.

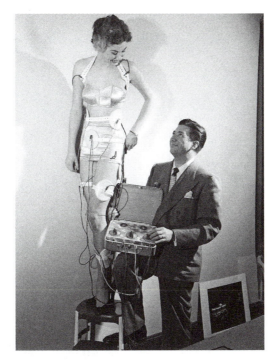

The Relaxacisor and other electric fat-reduction
machines delivered a mild electric shock to help
tone muscles. It was banned in 1970 for being both
dangerous and ineffective. (Bettmann/CORBIS)

FURTHER READING

Barrett, Stephen, and William T. Jarvis. *The Health Robbers: A Close Look at Quackery in America*. Buffalo, NY: Prometheus Books, 1993.

"Eminently Suitable Affair: Relaxacisor." *Vogue*, March 1, 1968, 88.

Gilbert, Susan. *Medical Fakes and Frauds*. New York: Chelsea House Publishers, 1989.

Simon, Stephanie. "A Gaggle of Quackery Going Mainstream." *Los Angeles Times*, February 4, 2002, A12.

Resting Metabolic Rate

Resting metabolic rate is the rate at which your body consumes calories during
rest. Your body burns up calories simply to support its basic functions. To create
a baseline for the appropriate overall calorie intake, it might be helpful to know

your resting metabolic rate. Once you determine it, you can multiply it by another factor, depending on your activity level, to calculate an approximate daily calorie need.

Men and women use different formulas to calculate their resting metabolic rate.

For women, start with 655, then add your weight × 4.3, add your height in inches × 4.3, and subtract your age in years × 4.7.

Here's an example for a 20-year-old female, 5'4" or 64 inches tall, weighing 130 pounds.

655 + (130 × 4.3 = 559)

+ (64 × 4.3 = 275) − (20 × 4.7 = 94)

or

655 + 559 + 275 − 94 = 1,395

That means this young woman's resting metabolic rate is about 1,395 calories per day.

For men, the formula is this:

66 + (weight × 6.2) + (height in inches × 12.7) − (age in years × 6.8)

Our example here is a 22-year-old male, 5'10" or 70 inches tall, weighing 190 pounds.

66 + (190 × 6.2 = 1,178)

+ (70 × 12.7 = 889) − (22 × 6.8 = 150)

or

66 + 1,178 + 889 − 150 = 1,983

Knowing your resting metabolic rate is just a starting point in determining the amount of calories to consume. Your active metabolic rate, or the amount of calories you burn while moving around and doing other physical activities, will obviously be higher. About 65 to 80 percent of the calories your body burns up are consumed while your body is at rest. One rule of thumb is that sedentary people should multiply their resting metabolic rate by 1.2; moderately active people can multiply it by 1.4; and serious athletes can multiply it by 1.8. Studies released by Duke University Medical Center looked at the difference between using aerobic activity and resistance training to lose weight. Researchers determined that a combination of both would be helpful; however, the aerobic exercise was the more effective of the two in reducing fatty tissue.

See also: Aerobic Activity; Calories.

FURTHER READING

"Aerobic Exercise Beats Resistance Training for Weight and Fat Loss: Physical Activity, Such as Walking, Running and Swimming, Seems Best for Losing Both Weight and Body Fat." *Duke Medicine Health News* 19, no. 3 (March 2013): 7.

Reynolds, Gretchen. "Dieting vs. Exercise for Weight Loss." *The New York Times*, August 1, 2012. http://well.blogs.nytimes.com/2012/08/01/dieting-vs-exercise-for-weight-loss/.

Rotation Diet

The Rotation diet, written in 1986 and revised and updated in 2012, is Dr. Martin Katahn's answer to helping people lose up to a pound per day, and most importantly, never gain it back. Katahn was director of the Vanderbilt University Weight Management Program near Nashville at the time he wrote his best seller. When first released, the Rotation diet was so popular that it grew into a city-wide fad, with more than 75,000 Nashville residents dieting collectively to shed 1 million pounds in 12 weeks. As the Rotation diet gained popularity, people began joining the "Melt-a-Million" at their local Kroger grocery stores. The supermarket chain served as diet headquarters, giving away thousands of sample rotation menus and running weekend public weigh-ins. Nashville restaurants, fearing huge business losses, even added Rotation diet specials to their menus. Nashville was "rotating."

The basic rotation plan calls for dieters to eat less fat and more fish, and walk or incorporate other exercise into their daily routine. What makes it different is the rotation aspect, which requires both men and women to vary the number of calories they consume during a three-week period. After the three weeks, dieters are encouraged to take a diet vacation and return to normal eating habits for anywhere from a week to a month. Katahn then suggests that those who need to lose more weight can follow another three-week rotation, completing the cycle as many times as it takes to reach a target weight.

The rotation theory is based on Katahn's belief that the majority of diets routinely fail because people tire of eating the same, boring foods and because metabolism gradually slows during any diet that strictly limits calories. Katahn's other theory, that hormone and enzyme levels increase after dieting and send signals to the body to regain and store any lost weight, has been bolstered by recent research on ghrelin, an appetite-stimulating hormone. Research published in a May 2002 issue of the *New England Journal of Medicine* showed that ghrelin is present in the stomach and increases following weight loss.

Katahn insists that his program will deliver permanent weight loss, because dieters who follow the plan keep their metabolism at a consistent level and avoid regaining weight when they return to eating what they consider normal amounts of food. But he warns users that the Rotation diet is forever, and was quoted in a 1986 *People* interview as saying, "If you go back to eating the way you did before, you're going to gain your weight back." Katahn also cites research conducted using participants in the Vanderbilt Weight Management Program. He said Vanderbilt studies show that there was no reduction in metabolic rate for participants who followed the Rotation diet. Instead, he says their metabolic rate increased, meaning dieters were able to eat normally after the diet without any weight gain.

Critics of the diet caution that losing 3 to 4 pounds a week is excessive and they questioned the safety of eating only 600 calories per day. The daily calorie count for women using this plan rotates between 600, 900, and 1,200, and men eat 1,200, 1,500, or 1,800 calories daily. By following Katahn's suggested menus, the first three days for women are at the lowest calorie level, 600. Female dieters then increase their calories to 900 per day for four days. The entire second week for women calls for a daily level of 1,200 calories and the third week rotates back to the 600 and 900 limits. Men follow the same schedule, substituting slightly higher calorie allowances. During the maintenance period, dieters are encouraged to gradually increase their intake of calories until they reach a point where they can eat and not regain any weight.

The menu for men and women on the Rotation diet is basically the same, but men eat an additional two servings of grain, 50 percent larger portions of meat, fish, or fowl, and three extra-safe fruits. A typical 600-calorie breakfast is half a grapefruit, one slice of whole wheat bread with an ounce of cheese, and a no-calorie beverage, usually water. In fact, Katahn recommends that dieters drink 8-ounce glasses of water per day and he discourages the consumption of artificially sweetened drinks. The Rotation diet allows up to two cups of coffee or tea per day and suggests a beverage of low-salt bouillon for a change of pace.

A Rotation diet lunch might include a protein food such as salmon, tuna, or cottage cheese along with unlimited free vegetables, salad, crackers, or a slice of bread. Dinner ideas range from baked chicken and salad to poached fish served with a variety of steamed vegetables and fruit desserts. To soothe hunger pangs, especially during low-calorie days, dieters are allowed to eat unlimited amounts of free vegetables and fruits.

Katahn classifies free vegetables as anything that has so few calories, it can be eaten in unlimited quantities: spinach, watercress, cucumber, celery, endive, lettuce, parsley, and asparagus are all free vegetables and allowed as snacks. Safe fruits—fruits that are low in calories and high in fiber—include apples, berries, grapefruit, melon, oranges, peaches, pineapple, and tangerines. *The Rotation Diet* book includes recipes for dishes like almond chicken, royal Indian salmon, baked or broiled rainbow trout, gingered beets, and braised carrots and celery.

The Rotation diet program, sponsored by the Nashville Kroger stores, eventually generated millions of dollars in free TV, radio, and newspaper publicity, as other supermarket chains jumped on the diet bandwagon. Stores, from BI-LO to Farm Fresh Supermarkets, Publix, and Wegman's, offered in-store programs and promotional efforts. Every chain reportedly contacted the state health department before endorsing or recommending the diet and hired professional nutritionists, home economists, or dietitians to answer any diet-related questions, according to a 1986 article in *Supermarket News*. Despite the success of the Rotation diet, some Nashville supermarkets did not offer the diet in their stores, stopping short of promoting this specific diet. Instead, they urged customers to follow a healthy eating plan based on the Dietary Guidelines for Americans, devised by the U.S. Department of Health and Human Services and the U.S. Department of Agriculture.

The author's theory came from his own personal experience of losing 70 pounds in 1963 following a heart attack at the age of 35. Katahn said in a 1986 *People* interview that it took him 18 months to lower his weight to 154 from 230 pounds by following his own rotation principle, and by adding a daily physical exercise program. *The Rotation Diet* recommends up to 45 minutes of daily exercise, from walking to jogging, tennis, or swimming.

Katahn wrote some 14 diet manuals, including *The T-Factor 2000 Diet*, a revised edition of his original 1989 *T-Factor Diet; The Tri-Color Diet: A Miracle Breakthrough in Diet and Nutrition for a Longer, Healthier Life* (1996); *The Cancer Prevention Good Health Diet* (2000); and *How to Quit Smoking without Gaining Weight* (1994). *The T-Factor Diet*, another best seller, resembles Katahn's rotation plan and was among the early diet books that promoted reducing dietary fat as a practical way to lose weight.

Both the Rotation and T-Factor diets contain the same elements and similar menu suggestions, but the T-Factor system only counts daily fat intake, not total calories. In his T-Factor plan, Katahn argues that the source of calories eaten is more important than the total number of calories ingested. By understanding the "T-factor," or thermogenic effect, in which carbohydrate calories are burned faster than fat calories, Katahn believes dieters can successfully lose weight. In his T-Factor books Katahn explains how to choose foods that naturally maximize the T-Factor level and activate the body's hidden fat-burning potential. The plan also provides two daily diet menus—one for people who want moderate weight loss and another for those who want quick results. Critics raised concerns about the rapid weight loss and called the fat and fiber counter in the book difficult to use, with foods listed according to type instead of alphabetically by name.

Katahn retired from his position at Vanderbilt University in 1991 and is now professor of psychology emeritus there in Nashville.

See also: Dietary Guidelines for Americans; Ghrelin; T-Factor Diet.

FURTHER READING

"Campus Life: Vanderbilt; 400 Students Join 3-Week Program on Eating Smart." *The New York Times*, March 25, 1990. http://www.nytimes.com/1990/03/25/style/campus-life-vanderbilt-400-students-join-3-week-program-on-eating-smart.html.

Chu, Dan. "Nashville Hopes to Shrink Its Population by a Million—A Million Pounds, That Is." *People Weekly*, March 10, 1986, 52–55.

Davis, Tim, and Rachel Kaplan. "Rotation Diet: A Heavy-Weight Promotion; Stores Get Publicity and Traffic Increases." *Supermarket News*, August 18, 1986, 1–3.

Katahn, Martin. *The Rotation Diet*. New York: W. W. Norton & Company, 1986.

Katahn, Martin. *The T-Factor 2000 Diet*. New York: W. W. Norton & Company, 1999.

Stoddard, Maynard Good. "The Diet That Consumed Nashville." *Saturday Evening Post*, July–August 1986, 26–29.

Toufexis, Anastasia. "Hey, Are You Rotating?" *Time*, April 14, 1986, 108.

Zilberter, Tanya. "To Count or Not to Count? The T-Factor and Rotation Diets." www.chasefreedom.com. Accessed June 10, 2003.

Scarsdale Diet

The Complete Scarsdale Medical Diet (1987), by Herman Tarnower, MD, and Samm Sinclair Baker, became an instant best seller, and dieters were losing up to 20 pounds per week with this high-protein, low-carbohydrate, and low-calorie regime.

The Scarsdale diet was designed to be followed precisely and it contained no "bewildering array of choices." Instead, users merely followed an exact list of menus for 14 days and then were advised to stop. Dr. Tarnower explained in the book that it worked well because people had such specific directions, plus the short duration made the rigid regime less daunting. As the doctor noted, "You won't develop any vitamin or mineral deficiency in two weeks, even on a starvation diet." But he cautioned dieters that it was important to stop the diet at the two-week mark. At that point, users would follow the Scarsdale maintenance diet for one or two weeks. His suggested timetable for success was two weeks on the diet, two weeks off, and then two weeks back on.

In the book Tarnower discussed the mind of an obese person who is desperately trying to lose weight and failing. He wrote, "The more you worry about food, the more you even think about it while you're on a diet, the more difficult and tiresome the whole process can become." The Scarsdale diet also maintained that quantities of foods were less important than the chemical reactions between them. Yet, the meals were very low calorie, designed to average 1,000 calories or less per day with triple the amount of protein recommended by the U.S. Department of Agriculture's (USDA) Dietary Guidelines for Americans.

Breakfast each day was the same and included half a grapefruit or fruits in season; one slice of protein bread, toasted with no spread, and coffee or tea with no sugar, cream, or milk. Lunch included assorted cold cuts, such as chicken, turkey, beef, or tongue, plus tomatoes and coffee, tea, or diet soda. Because all food choices were allowed in any amount desired, Tuesday's dinner, for example, called for "plenty of steak," tomatoes, lettuce, celery, olives, cucumbers, or Brussels sprouts. Sunday's dinner was the same minus the tomatoes, lettuce, and olives. Thursday's dinner included two eggs, cottage cheese, cabbage, and a slice of dry protein toast. Protein bread was any bread with high protein content, such as gluten or whole wheat bread. The diet suggested the bread be chewed in little bites so that it would be more satisfying, and no margarine, spreads, or jams were allowed.

Substitutions were taboo except for one "official" lunch substitution: 1/2 cup low-fat cottage cheese mixed with 1 tablespoon of low-fat sour cream, sliced fruit, and 6 halves of walnuts or pecans sprinkled over the fruit. That could be eaten any day in place of an afternoon meal. All foods were prepared without butter; all salads without dressings except lemon and vinegar. No alcohol was allowed and the only approved between-meal snacks were raw carrots and celery.

Critics of high-protein reducing plans like the Scarsdale or Atkins diets strongly disagree with this style of high-protein, low-calorie, and low-carbohydrate diets. Scientists with the USDA and the American Dietetic Association say carbohydrates are essential for providing energy for the body and without them the body will burn its own fat, reacting to what it perceives as starvation. Problems develop because the body does not burn this fat completely, causing substances called ketones to form. They are eventually released into the bloodstream, which increases the levels of uric acid in the blood. Doctors say abnormally high ketone levels in the blood cause ketosis, which can trigger kidney disease, gallstones, gout, or cardiac complications in some people. However, abnormally high ketone levels in the body make dieting easier because they decrease appetite by causing nausea, weakness, dehydration, headaches, and constipation or diarrhea.

Tarnower maintained that his carefully designed combination of foods increased the fat-burning process and provided rapid weight loss. In answer to concerns about the lack of carbohydrates, he suggested that dieters who produced ketones were "enjoying fast fat metabolism," a desired state. And he wrote that ketones were a good thing because they acted to curb the appetite, making the dieting process "less burdensome and cutting down any need for appetite-depressing drugs." The book told readers that ketones are washed out through the urine, which is a helpful, cleansing part of the increased fat-burning process.

Researchers suggest that a gradual loss of 1 pound per week is a healthy goal in contrast to the Scarsdale diet average of 1 pound per day. The position of the ADA on weight management recommends a gradual, incremental weight loss, a far cry from the quick, dramatic losses experienced by Scarsdale dieters. Instead, the ADA suggests that prospective dieters reduce their focus on actual weight loss and food, and instead establish a more constructive focus in life. And the American Heart Association continues to caution dieters about the problems associated with protein-rich regimens like the Scarsdale diet. They recommend following the USDA Food Guide Pyramid, a model that includes moderate amounts of lean protein foods as well as fresh fruits and vegetables and complex carbohydrates. They caution against foods full of saturated fat and cholesterol that can increase the risk of heart disease.

See also: Dietary Guidelines for Americans; Food Guide Pyramid; Ketones/Ketosis; Tarnower, Herman.

FURTHER READING

"Dieting with a French Accent." *Staying Healthy from the Faculty of Harvard Medical School.* Boston, MA: Harvard Health Publications Group, 2006.
Dullea, Georgia. "The Sensational Scarsdale Diet." *New York Times,* July 7, 1978, 10.
"1978: Gunning for Calories." *Men's Fitness* 19, no. 10 (October 2003): 18.
Tarnower, Herman, and Samm Sinclair Baker. *The Complete Scarsdale Medical Diet.* New York: Rawson, Wade Publishers, Inc., 1978

Sears, Barry

Barry Sears (b. June 6, 1947, Long Beach, California) is a biochemist and the author of *Enter the Zone: A Dietary Road Map*. Since its publication, the *New York Times'* best seller has sold millions of copies and been translated into more than 20 different languages. Sears continues to write diet books and continues his research to support his beliefs about the cause behind the country's obesity crisis. Sears focuses on what he calls the high levels of omega-6 fatty acids in U.S. diets and the lack of omega-3 fats. His studies have linked eicosanoids, specialized hormones, with the development of many serious diseases. According to Sears, this imbalance in the omega fats creates inflammation and increases the risk of cancer, heart disease, diabetes, and obesity for many Americans.

Sears first published his theories in his diet book, which recommends a daily intake of 40 percent carbohydrates, 30 percent fat, and 30 percent protein. Sears maintains that his own studies show that food has a potent, drug-like effect on the hormonal system and eating the right combination of foods leads to a "zone" metabolic state in which the body works at peak performance while decreasing hunger, increasing energy, and losing weight.

His interest in dietary theory followed his father's death from heart disease at age 53. In fact, Sears's grandfather, father, and three uncles all died of heart attacks before the age of 54. In his book, Sears describes how this personal tragedy changed the focus of his research as he sought to understand the role of fat in heart disease. That research became his first best seller, written in 1995 in collaboration with professional health writer Bill Lawren. Sears followed with the sequel, *Mastering the Zone* (1997), which spent 11 weeks on the best-seller list. Other titles include *The Anti-Aging Zone* (1999); *The Soy Zone* (2000); *Zone Perfect Meals in Minutes* (1997); *Zone Food Blocks: The Quick & Easy, Mix & Match Counter for Staying in the Zone* (1998); and *A Week in the Zone* (2000). Other titles also include *The Anti-Inflammation Zone* (2005) and *Toxic Fat* (2008).

Following an undergraduate degree from Occidental College, Sears earned a doctorate in biochemistry in 1971 from Indiana University. A lanky six-foot-five, he described himself in a 1997 *Time* magazine article as a "pointy-headed scientist." His book jackets list him as a "former MIT researcher," where he was a technical staff member at the Francis Bitter Magnet Laboratory at MIT, a facility that studies condensed matter physics, not nutrition. As a practicing biochemist, Sears also holds 12 patents for biomolecular inventions from the 1970s and 1980s. Those inventions involve systems for delivering cancer and heart-disease drugs into the bloodstream on a fat-molecule carrier.

Over the years, critics of the Zone diet have included the American Cancer Society (ACS), which recommends that people adopt a diet high in fruits and vegetables, but low in meat and fat. And ACS studies show that high-fat, high-protein foods may be associated with up to one-third of the 500,000 cancer deaths in the United States each year from colorectal, stomach, lung, mouth, throat, larynx, esophagus, prostate, and possibly breast cancer. But Sears writes in his book that he believes the opposite—that a high-carbohydrate diet brings with it cardiovascular risks and medically approved low-cholesterol, low-fat diets actually cause heart disease.

Criticism of the Zone and Sears from the medical community seems to have enhanced Sears's image as a crusader fighting the national nutrition and medical establishment. Many celebrities and professional athletes have followed his diet, including Madonna, Janet Jackson, Arnold Schwarzenegger, former president Bill Clinton, and 1992 Olympic gold medal swimmer Jenny Thompson.

See also: Carbohydrates; Eicosanoids; The Zone.

FURTHER READING

"Don't Look for Magic Bullets." *Consumers' Research Magazine*, July 2000, 24.

"Dr. Sears Blames Obesity Crisis on Omega 3–6 Imbalance." *Nutraceuticals World* 14, no. 5 (June 2011): 14.

Norris, Eileen. "High-Protein Diets: Where's the Beef?" *Harvard Health Letter* 22, no. 3 (January 1997): 1–3.

Ratnesar, Romesh. "Against the Grain: The Low-Carb Zone Diet Rises from Fad to Fixture." *Time*, December 15, 1997, 86.

Seigel, Jessica. "Zoned Out: The Medical Miracles Promised by Barry Sears, Diet Guru of the Moment, Are Sometimes Hard to Swallow." *Los Angeles Magazine*, February 1997, 34–42.

Shamblin, Gwen

Tennessee dietitian Gwen Shamblin founded the Weigh Down Workshop, Inc., in 1986 using the principles she developed as part of her own successful weight loss. "I was a thin eater growing up," she confessed in her 1997 best seller, *The Weigh Down Diet*. But with college came the familiar freshman weight gain and the beginning of her self-described battle with food.

A registered dietitian, Shamblin graduated from the University of Tennessee with a master's degree in food and nutrition. Following graduation she was employed by health departments in Tennessee and Mississippi but later began a weight control consulting practice in 1980 in Memphis. During that time she started counseling people toward the spiritual dimension of weight loss and away from a focus on food. After several years she launched the Weigh Down Workshop, which tailored her weight-loss program for church-sponsored classes. It's centered on a 10-week program that starts by teaching participants what hunger is. The idea is to help dieters understand the difference between being physically hungry and being spiritually hungry. By beginning the diet with a fast, participants can feel hunger pangs—something to which they are probably unaccustomed. Critics of the diet plan say that it does not provide enough nutritional guidance, especially not for people with poor eating habits.

Shamblin's program for children, named "the Last Exodus," is aimed at dieters as young as eight years old. Shamblin took a controversial stand in 2004 when she contributed to the defense fund for parents, members of a chapter of Shamblin's Remnant Fellowship, who were charged in the death of their son. Shamblin founded Remnant in 2002 based in Nashville. Shamblin also created controversy in 2000 when she publically rejected the doctrine of the Trinity.

According to Shamblin, most overeaters eat to fill the void in their lives and some develop an unhealthy passion for food. She suggests participants fill that emptiness with a passionate relationship with God. Critics charge she combines the superficial nutritional advice of diet personalities like Susan Powter with the evangelistic fervor of televangelists such as Jimmy Swaggart. In recent years Shamblin's theological beliefs have also created some controversy when various church leaders questioned her views on the Trinity. Their concerns were based on comments Shamblin posted on her Weigh Down Web site.

See also: Christian Diets; Weigh Down Diet.

FURTHER READING

Ellin, Abby. "Seeing Overeating as a Sin, and God as the Diet Coach." *The New York Times*, May 29, 2004, A13.

Mulrine, Anna. "A Godly Approach to Weight Loss." *U.S. News & World Report*, May 5, 1997, 12.

Shamblin, Gwen. *The Weigh Down Diet*. New York: Doubleday, 1997.

Smith, Pam. *The Diet Trap*. Washington, DC: LifeLine Press, 2000.

"The Weigh Down Diet." *Publishers Weekly* 244, no. 8 (February 24, 1997): 8.

Winner, Lauren F. "The Weigh & the Truth." *Christianity Today*, September 4, 2000, 50.

Simmons, Richard

Richard Simmons (b. July 12, 1948, New Orleans) reached the status of popular-culture icon in the 1980s with his zeal for dancing off the pounds. In his autobiographies and numerous press interviews, Simmons details the humiliation of being an overweight child and his conflicted relationship with his father. By second grade, he was seriously overweight and a doctor put him on a diet. He cheated, he wrote in his autobiography, *Still Hungry—After All These Years*, adding, "My best shot lasted three days."

He documented the years of dieting struggles and trying to find a gym where he was comfortable, particularly one that involved a regimen based on dance. He recalls waiting in line to join one such club. "I heard one of the trainers refusing to sell a membership to an overweight woman in front of me, saying she was

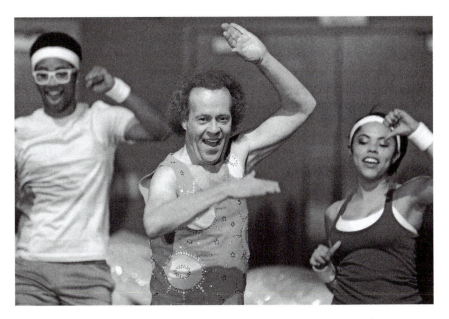

Richard Simmons danced his way into becoming a popular culture icon in the 1980s. His aerobic workouts and energetic chatter have endeared him to many. (AP Photo/ Dominic Chan/Canadian Press)

an insurance risk. Well, as you can imagine, I was horrified! I left the line *and* the gym, and I found the woman outside and said, 'Here's my card. I'm going to open a gym, and you can come to *my* gym any time you want!'" Shortly after, he created Slimmons, his own gym with an attached salad bar called Ruffage—so people could get exercise and eat healthy foods. In his book, he recalls that because he couldn't afford a piano player, he brought in his own records. Simmons still teaches one exercise class per week at the studio. The club became popular in Beverly Hills and, soon afterward, Simmons was playing the role of an aerobics exercise instructor on the soap opera *General Hospital*. After four years on *General Hospital*, he became host of his own show, *The Richard Simmons Show*. In his autobiography, he recalls that he had his mother on as a regular guest to do some of the cooking segments.

By 1986, Simmons was running infomercials on television, and his diet Deal-A-Meal and more recent FoodMover plans and exercise videos, including *Sweatin' to the Oldies*, were well known. Simmons, with his Afro hairstyle and his uniform of short shorts and tank top, is part funny-man, part motivational speaker, and part exercise guru. Today, the Richard Simmons Web site lists the more than 30 videos he has developed. These include the *Sweatin' to the Oldies* series, "Dance Your Pants Off," "Groovin' in the House," "Blast Off the Pounds," and "Sit Tight"—a special workout program for people in wheel chairs or anyone else who needs to remain sitting during an exercise session. He also personally participates in a seven-night special session on Carnival Cruise Lines called "Cruise to Lose." He also markets his FoodMover program, a combination of a cookbook, video, calorie charts, and an instructional booklet. Plus, the Web site offers his newest Slim Away Every Day program—a 30-day plan to help dieters get into good habits.

The combination of eating less—a minimum of 1,200 calories—and exercise has earned Simmons's programs favorable comments from most dietitians. Some criticize the recent addition of nutritional supplements into Simmons's lineup, however.

One of the characteristics that has most endeared Simmons to his followers is his genuine concern for them. In his autobiography, he wrote, "One thing I've always done throughout my career has been my daily telephone calls—talking to people about their weight issues and offering them all the encouragement I can, and helping them to get started on a program of healthy eating and exercising." Since the mid-1970s, Simmons has been making 40 to 50 calls per day, even while traveling. On busy days, he wrote, he can make as many as 100 calls. And most days are busy days. The Web site notes that Simmons makes about 300 appearances a year.

FURTHER READING

Dalka-Prysby, Sandra, and Richard Simmons. *Slow but Sure: How I Lost 170 Pounds with the Help of God, Family, Family Circle Magazine and Richard Simmons*. New York: Signet, 2001.

"Dancing Raising Turn to Aerobics." May 2000. www.preparedfoods.com/archives/2000/2000_05/0005marketwatch.htm. Accessed June 12, 2003.

Emmons, Steve. "Clown Prince of Weight Loss Takes Big Interest in Fans." *Los Angeles Times*, July 14, 1991, E2.

Simmons, Richard. *The Richard Simmons Farewell to Fat Cookbook*. New York: Good Times Publishing, 1996.

Simmons, Richard. *Richard Simmons' Never-Say-Diet Cookbook*. New York: Warner Books, 1985.

Simmons, Richard. *Still Hungry—After All These Years: My Story*. New York: GT Publishing, 1999.

Stewart, Susan. "Richard Simmons Holds Nothing Back." *Knight-Ridder/Tribune News Service*, January 21, 1994.

Wedlan, Candace A. "Exercising Discipline." *Los Angeles Times*, May 1, 1996, E3.

Weinraub, Judith. "Richard Dishes Up Dessert." *Washington Post*, January 14, 1998, E1.

www.richardsimmons.com.

Slim Chance Awards

Since 1989, more than 100 questionable or downright dangerous items have been given the Slim Chance award—an annual event to shine some light on what the sponsor, Healthy Weight Network, calls quackery and fraud in the weight-loss industry. While some of these diets and ideas are discussed in greater detail in other parts of this volume, this section will highlight the award recipients for this dubious distinction.

In 2013 winners, there were four Slim Chance awards presented.

Worst Weight Loss Plan: The Special K Challenge™. Kellogg claims that by replacing two meals and snacks a day with Special K products, including cereals, protein shakes, and protein meal bars, a weight loss of up to six pounds in 14 days will occur. Why the idea is deemed bad: "First, a focus on quick weight loss just sets people up for the yo-yo diet cycle of losing and regaining that makes people fatter, not thinner," said Marsha Hudnall, MS, RDN, CD, president and co-owner of Green Mountain at Fox Run, which sponsored the January 2014 ceremony. "It may also foster chronic inflammation, which leads to all sorts of health problems, including weight gain for many."

Most Overrated: Non-Invasive Body Contouring Procedures. These procedures are marketed to treat problem area. The network selected this award because, "These kind of 'miracle' procedures feed body dissatisfaction and encourage unhealthy behaviors," said Ashley Solomon, PsyD. "When people are only focused on reducing fat, losing inches or weighing less, they set themselves up for disappointment."

Most Outrageous: Cotton Ball Diet. The press release announcing the awards said, "The Cotton Ball Diet started popping up on YouTube earlier in 2013, unveiling a disturbing fad diet most popular among young women. Dieters dip cotton balls in juice and ingest them. The objective is to feel full without actually consuming real food. Risks include a blockage in the digestive system, which could result in surgery."

Worst Gimmick: The Tongue Patch Diet. The press release states, "In this reversible procedure a plastic mesh patch is fitted to the patient's tongue. The purpose is to make chewing extremely painful, thus limiting the dieter to only liquid. Users have reported up to 20 lbs. of weight loss in a month." But critics say that nothing about this enhances good nutrition.

In 2012, Dr. Memet Oz (known to TV viewers as simply, Dr. Oz) received the group's Worst Claim award for his endorsement of raspberry ketones. Although Dr. Oz did say on his show that good diet and exercise are essential to healthy weight loss, his enthusiastic endorsement of raspberry ketone as "the number one miracle in a bottle to burn your fat" has been used by many marketers of products.

Other 2012 awards went to QuickTrim as the Worst Product, which had been touted by the Kardashian sisters, because its ingredients include stimulant laxatives and unspecified amounts of caffeine; the Ab Circle Pro as the Worst Gimmick, an exercising disk with knee rests and handlebars that allegedly would "melt inches and pounds," if users kneeled on it and rotated their bodies side-to-side; acai berry scammers who received the Most Outrageous award for their deceptive advertising.

The Healthy Weight Network has called out fad and famous diets, supplements, patches, wraps, pills, creams, and more. The network is run by Francie M. Berg, MS, LN, a licensed nutritionist and adjunct professor at the University of North Dakota School of Medicine. She is the founder, editor, and publisher of *Healthy Weight Journal* and author of 12 books.

See also: Ephedra/Ephedrine; Grapefruit Diet, Weight-Loss Earrings.

FURTHER READING

Press release of Worst Weight Loss Schemes of 2013 Selected by Healthy Weight Week Expert Judges: Slim Chance Awards Call Out Most Questionable Weight Loss Products, Plans, Claims & Gimmicks, January 2, 2014. http://www.healthyweightnetwork.com/fraud.htm.
www.healthyweightnetwork.com.

Slim-Fast

Slim-Fast has been synonymous with easy weight loss to millions of dieting Americans. Considered a dominant player in the growing $1.3 billion diet products market, Slim-Fast had net sales of $611 million in 1999, according to industry figures, with sales growth of more than 20 percent. However, in the four years leading up to 2014, those sales have disappeared, dropping some 40 percent to just under $200 million.

In its early days, the company's advertising efforts have continuously put Slim-Fast in the public eye, thanks to commercials featuring celebrities like baseball manager Tommy LaSorda, television entertainer Kathy Lee Gifford, and actresses Elizabeth Ashley and Shari Belafonte. In 1992, Slim-Fast scored a national marketing coup, thanks to residents of the small town of Pound, Wisconsin, who took part in a Slim-Fast weight reduction plan for four months and lost a combined 2,800 pounds.

A Slim-Fast diet averages about 1,200 calories a day, some 500 calories less than the typical American woman eats and at least 1,000 calories less than the typical American male consumes. One of the most common meal replacement diets available, the plan requires a shake for breakfast and lunch along with a sensible dinner. Dieters following the Slim-Fast plan are also allowed two additional pieces of fruit as well as a Slim-Fast Bar for snacks during the day. In an effort to revive sales, the brand introduced a new line of shakes in 2011, calling them the richest, creamiest, and best-tasting shakes. In an attempt to reach new customers they also changed from cans to bottles. The size and shape of the bottle was designed by the company to satisfy hunger for up to four hours and included 10 grams of protein, 5 grams of fiber, and two-dozen vitamins and minerals.

A sensible meal, according to the Slim-Fast program, looks something like this: 4–6 ounces of poultry, fish, or lean meat; half a baked potato; three steamed vegetables; and fruit for dessert. Basically, the plan controls calorie intake and reducing calories means losing weight. Nutrition experts say the program is not a good choice for long-term dieting, but Slim-Fast can be an acceptable supplement if dieters remember to eat fruits, vegetables, and whole grains as part of their one daily meal. But critics say dieters must also remember that the shakes and bars are processed foods and while they contain added vitamins and minerals, they still lack important fiber, antioxidants, and the other health benefits associated with eating fresh foods.

While Americans can buy the familiar diet drink everywhere, Slim-Fast has struggled to keep pace with competitors in the digital age. Despite the trend toward diet smartphone apps, Slim-Fast has failed to provide its own diet app. According to *Consumer Reports* magazine, Slim-Fast also ranked last in a survey of satisfaction among dieters and was beaten by the Paleo diet and Atkins diet.

Slim-Fast was first introduced in 1977, the same year some 58 dieters died as the result of following very low-calorie liquid protein diet products. Although Slim-Fast was not involved in the deaths, it was pulled from shelves that same year as sales all but disappeared. It was reintroduced again in the early 1980s by originator S. Daniel Abraham. At the same time that Slim-Fast was returning to store shelves, concerns were being raised about PPA, phenylpropanolamine, an ingredient now banned by the Food and Drug Administration (FDA) after studies linked it to an increased risk of stroke. The FDA action was aimed at diet pills containing PPA, like Dexatrim and Metabolife, and also at over-the-counter cold and allergy remedies. Partly due to consumer concerns over PPA, sales of the reintroduced Slim-Fast showed dramatic improvement from $149 million in 1983 to $197 million in 1984.

Slim-Fast faced a minor public relations problem in 1999 when it was discovered that some of the ready-to-drink diet shakes were filled with diluted cleaning solution. The statement released by the company said only a few cans were involved but as a safety precaution about 192,000 cans of Ultra Slim-Fast shakes were pulled off the shelves. The recalled cans were from Arizona, California, Colorado, Michigan, New York, Ohio, Oregon, Utah, Virginia, and Wisconsin. In 2000, Unilever PLC acquired Slim-Fast Foods Company for $2.3 billion in cash. Industry analysts say the move reflects Unilever's commitment to developing its burgeoning functional foods business.

See also: Calories; Liquid Protein Diets; Paleo Diet; Phenylpropanolamine (PPA).

FURTHER READING

Berman, Phyllis, and Amy Feldman. "An Extraordinary Peddler." *Forbes*, December 9, 1991, 136–39.

Boyle, Matthew. "Unilever's Slim-Fast Goes from Juggernaut to Afterthought." *Bloomberg .com*, January 15, 2013. http://www.bloomberg.com/news/2013–01–14/unilever-s-slim-fast-goes-from-juggernaut-to-afterthought.html.

Eder, Rob. "Unilever Purchases Slim Fast Foods." *Drug Store News* 22, no. 7 (May 22, 2000): 31.

Harrison, Joan. "Unilever Joins Other Food Giants Scrambling to Get Healthy." *Mergers & Acquisitions*, June 2000, 19.

Johnsen, Michael. "Slim Fast Gets a New Look, Focuses on Snack Replacement." *Drug Store News* 24, no. 3 (March 4, 2002): 35.

"Slim-Fast Introduces Its Best Tasting Shakes Ever in New On-the-Go Bottles in Time for Diet Season." *Food Weekly News*, October 27, 2011, 124.

"Slim Fast Recalls a Batch of Shakes." *New York Times*, April 18, 1999, 27.

Somers, Suzanne

Suzanne Somers (b. October 16, 1946, in San Bruno, California), the actress best known for playing the "ditzy blonde" character of Chrissy on the 1970s comedy series *Three's Company*, has developed a successful career writing diet books following years as a model, actress, and owner and spokesperson for ThighMaster exercise equipment. Her eating plan, called "Somersizing," requires dieters to follow a two-part system of weight loss and maintenance where proteins and fats are eaten together but never with carbohydrates. Although Somers brings no nutrition credentials to bear on her books, she credits endocrinologist Dr. Diana Schwarzbein with helping her develop the low-carbohydrate, controlled-sugar intake program. Schwarzbein, who first self-published her own book for her diabetic patients, has written the foreword for Somers's best-selling title *Suzanne Somers' Eat Great, Lose Weight*. Other best-selling books by the actress include *Get Skinny on Fabulous Food; 365 Ways to Change Your Life;* and *Eat, Cheat and Melt the Fat Away*.

Somers got her first taste of acting while appearing in a high school musical. In the spring of 1977 she won the part of Chrissy in *Three's Company* and became a television star. Somers left the show in 1982. She first hit the lecture circuit after her 1988 best-selling autobiography *Keeping Secrets*, detailing her childhood plagued by her alcoholic father's all-night rages. She published a book of interviews with people from abusive families titled *Wednesday's Children* (1992), and founded the Suzanne Somers Institute for the Effects of Addiction on Families to set up outpatient centers to treat addicts and family members of addicts.

The actress then moved into the fitness business when she and her husband Alan Hamel invested in the company that made ThighMaster Exercise equipment. Somers was pictured on the box and also starred in infomercials touting its benefits. ThighMaster quickly became part of American pop culture, mentioned on television shows like *Saturday Night Live*. Somers wrote in her second autobiography, *After the Fall: How I Picked Myself Up, Dusted Myself Off, and Started All Over Again* (1998), that in a move to revitalize her entertainment career she appeared in Las Vegas, and in 1991 costarred in a new sitcom, *Step by Step*. She also produced and starred in a television movie based on her autobiography.

Somers wrote in her first diet best seller, *Suzanne Somers' Eat Great, Lose Weight*, that she reached a nutritional turning point at age 40 when her struggle to stay slim intensified. That was when she developed her eating plan based on the concept of food combining. In her book, she emphasizes the importance of eliminating sugar and foods high in starch, then combining foods to aid in weight loss and digestion. Those who follow the "Somersize" plan stop eating what she calls Funky Foods, all sugars from white and brown sugar to corn syrup, molasses, and honey along with maple syrup, beets, and carrots. Starches to avoid are anything made with white or semolina flour, pasta or couscous, white rice, corn, popcorn, sweet and white potatoes, pumpkin, winter squashes, and bananas. She also cautions again eating nuts, olives, liver, avocados, coconuts, low-fat or whole milk, and any tofu or soy milk. Her plan also eliminates caffeine and alcohol, except in cooking, which burns off the alcohol but leaves the flavor behind.

The rest of the food choices are separated into "Somersized food groups" for mixing and matching. Somers maintains that when proteins and carbohydrates are eaten together, their enzymes create a halt in the digestion process and cause weight gain. She says her book is different from similar high-protein diet programs, such as the Zone, Sugar Busters!, and the Atkins diet, because those plans encourage dieters to eat animal proteins and fats, as long as very few carbohydrates are eaten. Somers's plan does allow such carbohydrates as whole grain bread, cereal, and pasta but never at the same meal as proteins and fats. In *Eat, Cheat, and Melt the Fat Away* she praises Atkins for having "the courage to take on the medical establishment and, in doing so, has paved the way for a new way of thinking."

Critics of Somers's plan, however, don't see many differences between it and the other high-protein diet programs. The American Institute for Cancer Research (AICR) cautions that the high amounts of cholesterol and saturated fat prescribed in these protein-packed eating plans increases the risk of heart disease and possibly some cancers. There is also recent evidence that a diet featuring excessive protein may leach valuable calcium from the bones. A 1997 AICR report, *Food, Nutrition and the Prevention of Cancer: A Global Perspective*, identified numerous studies possibly linking a high-fat intake with increased risk of several cancers and other chronic diseases.

See also: Atkins Nutritional Approach; Beverly Hills Diet.

FURTHER READING

Breu, Giovanna. "Let the Patient Beware: Cancer Expert Barrie Cassileth Warns that Alternative Treatments May Pose Serious Dangers." *People Weekly*, April 30, 2001, 77.

Eberle, Girard. "Go Ahead, Order the Combo Plate: The Rules of Food Combining Are an Unforgiving Master, But Is that Tangerine after Lunch Really Evil Incarnate?" *Women's Sports and Fitness* 19, no. 5 (June 1997): 78–80.

Newsmakers 2000. Issue 1. Detroit: Gale Group, 2000.

Pierce, Ellise. "On Tour with Suzanne Somers." *People Weekly*, March 3, 1997, 42.

Quinn, Judy. "Science of Sugar Brings Sweet Diet Book Sales." *Publishers Weekly* 246, no. 31 (August 2, 1999): 21.

Schneider, Karen S., and Elizabeth Leonard. "A Matter of Choice: Coping with Breast Cancer and the Controversy over her Unorthodox Treatment Plan, Suzanne Somers Faces the Future with Serene Self-Assurance." *People Weekly*, April 30, 2001, 72–78.

Somers, Suzanne. *After the Fall: How I Picked Myself Up, Dusted Myself Off, and Started All over Again.* New York: Crown, 1998.

Somers, Suzanne. *Suzanne Somers' Eat, Cheat and Melt the Fat Away.* New York: Random House, 2001.

Wolfson, Nancy. "The Suzanne Somers Diet." *Good Housekeeping*, July 2000, 110–12.

South Beach Diet

For dieters who are not suffering from kidney disease and are not uncomfortable with potential bouts of low blood sugar, excessive fluid loss, cramping, dehydration, dizziness, or hypoglycemia, the South Beach diet is a popular choice that many Americans have turned to for quick weight loss. Cardiologist Dr. Arthur Agatston published his diet after seeing a need for a simple weight-loss program for his obese patients. He named it the South Beach diet. The diet was published in 2003 as a way for Agatston to help his patients who were struggling with what he called the standard American Heart Association type low-fat eating plan. Agatston put together his three-phase, low-carbohydrate plan that emphasized foods with a low glycemic index number while also minimizing consumption of saturated fat. The restriction on saturated fat is what Agatston suggests separates the South Beach plan from other carbohydrate-restrictive plans like the Atkins and Zone diets.

While the glycemic index and its role in weight gain and loss has been debated for years, it was Agatston, whose book remained on the *New York Times* best-seller list for over a year, who focused media attention on the concept. Agatston appeared on a number of television shows including *Good Morning America, Dateline,* and *Fox and Friends.* The glycemic index compares foods on a scale of 1 to 100 based on how much each food increases glucose or sugar in the blood when eaten. Foods with a low glycemic index have been shown to raise blood sugar less than those foods with a high glycemic index. And low GI foods satisfy hunger longer and minimize cravings for food. When people eat foods that contain a lot of glucose or sugar their insulin levels go up rapidly, which causes the body to secrete more insulin. Increased insulin has been shown to eventually lead to diabetes or a condition known as insulin resistance.

The overriding principle of the South Beach diet is the importance of eating good carbohydrates such as fruits, vegetables, and whole grains while at the same time dieters must give up bad carbohydrates, generally recognized as processed foods with no fiber and lots of sugar. The diet also suggests that to compensate for the lack of carbohydrates, dieters should eat ample proteins and fats as long as they are the unsaturated and polyunsaturated fats like olive oil and nuts.

The three phases are designed to first do away with any cravings for high glycemic index foods like pasta, sugar, bread, and potatoes. This is also where high carbohydrate foods including many fruits, cereal, alcohol, and some vegetables are restricted and replaced by protein-rich foods. Phase one should not be extended past the suggested two weeks in order to prevent problems including loss of bone and muscle mass as well as increased strain on the kidneys that could lead to kidney stones or other kidney damage. Plus, any ketosis-induced dehydration that occurs during phase one could contribute to the loss of other important minerals, vitamins, and upset electrolytes.

Ketosis occurs when there are not enough carbohydrates for the body to convert into blood sugar. The human body typically runs on glucose or blood sugar supplied by eating carbohydrates. That lack of carbohydrates forces the body to use blood sugar stored in the liver and muscles. On a low- or no-carbohydrate diet, there is an immediate and rapid weight loss because human muscle includes lots of water and the body burns muscle for energy. If the carbohydrate restriction continues, the body eventually begins to burn fat for fuel. Unfortunately, along with the quick weight loss, ketosis comes with irritability, headaches, stress on the kidneys, and more serious heart palpitations.

Phase two eases restrictions on some carbohydrate foods including whole wheat pastas, breads, and many fruits. At this point weight loss can average one to two pounds each week, down from the rapid weight and water loss in the first phase. This second phase focuses on a menu of low glycemic index foods. A sample menu for phase two of the diet would include a breakfast of yogurt, coffee, tomato juice, and a bowl of oatmeal. A morning snack might include strawberries or some other low glycemic fruit plus coffee. Lunch would be a salad with tuna. An afternoon snack might include a hard-boiled egg and some celery or cucumber sticks, while dinner would be lean meat such as a London broil or chicken, roasted asparagus, and salad.

Phase three is designed to maintain the overall weight loss as a lifetime eating plan. Techniques include focusing on low glycemic index foods with an occasional allowance of a high glycemic treat. If weight gain occurs, the diet suggests that phase one or two be reintroduced until goal weight is achieved.

Critics of the diet say the restrictive nature of the eating plan and potential for nutritional deficiencies make it difficult for many people to follow. Without an emphasis on exercise critics also suggest that the loss of muscle and bone mass during phase one can create long-term health problems for those who attempt to follow the diet. However, nutritionists find the focus on replacing saturated fats with unsaturated fats, a healthy part of the South Beach diet along with its eventual focus on unprocessed and complex carbohydrate foods.

Agatston has written several other South Beach books including his latest *The South Beach Diet: Gluten Solution* (2013). Although the first phase of the South Beach diet was grain-free as a way to decrease cravings for high glycemic foods, Agatston claimed he discovered that dieters were finding that joint pain, fatigue, and rashes were clearing up as well. Agatston wrote his book based on his assumption that Americans have been overloaded by gluten, which can now be found in almost all processed foods including toothpaste, tomato sauce, soy sauce, and lipstick. The author also added a walking plan to his diet plan to answer criticism of his lack of exercise. The walking plan is included in the *South Beach Diet Supercharged* (2008).

See also: Atkins Nutritional Approach; Gluten-Free; The Zone.

FURTHER READING

Agatston, Arthur. *The South Beach Diet: The Delicious, Doctor-Designed Foolproof Plan for Fast and Healthy Weight Loss*. New York: Rodale Press, 2003.

Bachman, John, and Donna Scaglione. "South Beach Diet Guru: Hidden Gluten Can Wreck Your Health." *Newsmax*, April 26, 2013. http://www.newsmaxhealth .com/Headline/South-Beach-Diet-hidden-gluten-gluten-free-diet-DrArthur-Agatston/2013/04/26/id/501479.

Sass, Cynthia. "The Worst Diet for Your Heart." *Prevention* 60, no. 4 (April 2008): 78.

Scales, Mary Josephine. *Diets in a Nutshell: A Definitive Guide on Diets from A to Z*. Clifton, VA: Apex Publishers, 2005.

Starch Blockers

Starch blockers are a so-called miracle weight-loss cure that claims to block the absorption of starches or carbohydrates. The theory behind starch blockers, an extract made from a protein in various beans, is simple. Essentially an enzyme in the beans prevents the breakdown of starch molecules. This, according to their manufacturers, allows dieters to lose weight even as they fill up on pizza, pasta, and bread. Starch blockers were marketed heavily in the 1970s but were finally forced off drugstore shelves by the Food and Drug Administration (FDA) in 1983, when the FDA ordered more than 200 manufacturers and distributors to stop selling the pills, pending further investigation into their long-term effects. Thanks to the Internet, many products not available in U.S. retail outlets are available online. That is true with items banned by the FDA such as starch blockers. Bottles with various brand names can be purchased for prices that range from $14 dollars to $30 dollars per bottle.

The FDA made its ruling after receiving more than 100 reports of problems associated with starch blockers, side effects ranging from abdominal pain and diarrhea to vomiting and other extreme reactions. Problems developed with the pills when undigested starch ended up being dumped into the colon. And while dieters suffered no permanent damage, they did not enjoy permanent weight loss either.

Following the FDA ruling, there was a flurry of legal wrangling between the government and starch blocker manufacturers as they sued to get the ban overturned. At one point, the FDA seized a shipment of starch blocker pills valued at $480,000, as some distributors attempted to defy the government ban on their sale.

The manufacturers argued that the pills were food supplements and did not need to be proven safe and effective under the law. However, the FDA pushed to classify the pills as a drug, meaning the product was intended to affect the function of the body and anything labeled a drug falls under government purview. At that time there were only two categories of products—food or drugs. Now, following the passage of the Dietary Supplement Health and Education Act of 1994, manufacturers have another category for products, that of dietary supplement.

In recent studies, researchers at the Mayo Clinic have suggested higher doses of the bean extract and wheat germ extract used in many starch blocker formulas may be more effective in slowing carbohydrate digestion.

Critics of the pills include health organizations, such as the American Medical Association (AMA). Physicians with the AMA's Department of Foods and Nutrition, quoted in *Newsweek*, stated that there are no clinical studies that prove starch blockers actually help people lose weight. In fact, researchers suspect that starch blockers do not work for two possible reasons. Either the protein-digesting enzyme breaks down the bean extract before it can act to block the starch, or there are more enzymes secreted than needed and they lead to carbohydrate absorption in spite of the starch blocker. Either way, scientists, nutritionists, and health-care professionals say pills like starch blockers or fat blockers continue to cast doubt over the credibility of the dietary supplements industry.

See also: Dietary Supplement Health and Education Act (DSHEA); Fat Blockers.

FURTHER READING

Barrett, Stephen. "Be Wary of Calorie-Blockers." www.quackwatch.com. Accessed June 10, 2003.

Biddle, Wayne, and Margot Slade. "FDA Outlaws 'Starch Blockers.'" *New York Times*, July 4, 1982, E9.

"Fragakis, Allison Sarubin, RD." *Prevention,* November 2011. http://www.prevention
    .com/weight-loss/diets/low-carb-diets-and-diet-pills.
Seligmann, Jean. "Starch Blockers: How Safe?" *Newsweek,* July 12, 1982, 83.

Stevia

The American battle of the bulge has resulted in the creation of substitutes for sugar known as artificial sweeteners, which are used to replace sugar and to reduce calories in a variety of foods. The sweeteners themselves are divided into two groups, nutritive sweeteners, which add calories to food, and nonnutritive sweeteners, which add very few or no calories to food.

Nutritive sweeteners include natural sugars like sucrose, fructose, and galactose, as well as a group of carbohydrate compounds called polyols. The polyols are also known as sugar replacers, sugar-free sweeteners, or novel sugars, and while they develop naturally from plants, they are produced commercially.

One controversial example of a polyol is the herbal sugar substitute made from the leaves of the stevia shrub found in South America, called stevia. It has been used for many years in food and beverages in the United States as well as countries like South Korea, China, Japan, and Brazil. However, stevia has never been accepted by the U.S. government as an artificial sweetener and remains categorized as a dietary supplement, which leaves it unregulated.

Stevia was first introduced in the United States as a dietary supplement when the Food and Drug Administration (FDA) delayed approval of it, calling it neither sweetener nor food additive. In fact, in 1991 the FDA issued a statement labeling stevia as an unsafe food additive and denied its import into the United States. Finally, with the passage of the 1994 Dietary Supplement Health and Education Act stevia was admitted as a dietary supplement, a classification not under the FDA's regulatory authority. Passage of that legislation redefined foods, foods supplements, and dietary supplements and removed all supplements from the FDA's control. Stevia can now be sold in the United States, just not as a food or food additive.

The stevia bush or plant can be found in an area that stretches from Paraguay through Mexico and Central America into the southern region of the United States. The bush grows to a height of some 40 inches and is commonly known as candy leaf, sweet honey leaf, sugarleaf, or stevia, the name widely used in the United States.

The leaves of the plant are long with lightly serrated edges and are the only part of the plant used for making the sweetener, which is about 300 times as sweet as common table sugar. Records show Dr. Moises Santiago Bertoni of the College of Agriculture in Asuncion, Paraguay, studied the plant as early as 1887. Dr. Bertoni used the dried leaves and suggested the plant be named Stevia rebaudiana to honor Paraguayan chemist Ovidio Rebaudi who was the first scientist to actually examine the chemical components of the stevia leaves.

The early concerns at the FDA were based on studies that suggested stevia caused reproductive problems in animals. However, other studies later suggested stevia was safe. While research continues countries including Canada, Australia, and the European Union, like the United States, have all been slow to grant approval for the use of stevia. Canada finally approved Stevia's use as a food additive and dietary supplement in 2012. That same year, the FDA released a statement saying the use of whole-leaf stevia and crude stevia extracts are not permitted in the United States because these particular substances have not been accepted as a food additive. The American Dietetic Association has followed the lead of the FDA and does not endorse stevia as a sugar substitute for Americans with diabetes. Concerns about stevia cited on the FDA Web site include its possible effects on the human reproductive, cardiovascular, and renal systems.

Reported side effects from heavy stevia use include hypoglycemia or low blood sugar and hypotension or low blood pressure. While studies have hinted at health problems for animals that were fed high concentrations of stevia over long periods of time, there are no significant reports of problems with human consumption.

While stevia as a nutritive sweetener has had its share of controversy, accepted nonnutritive sweeteners have also raised health concerns over the years. Nonnutritive sweeteners are synthetic compounds including saccharin, aspartame, acesulfame potassium, also known as acesulfame-K, and sucralose and neotame. These sweeteners are between 200 and 13,000 times as sweet as sucrose or table sugar, which is the government's standard means of comparison. The federal government classifies what it accepts as artificial sweeteners in just two categories, either food additives or GRAS, generally regarded as safe.

The term "food additives" stems from the Federal Food, Drug and Cosmetic (FD&C) Act of 1938. Legislation was created when a company mistakenly added an antifreeze ingredient to a liquid medicine and tragically killed more than 100 men, women, and children. The law passed the next year provided a legal definition of a food additive to prevent other tragedies and to give the government oversight of ingredients added to processed foods and medicines. The GRAS designation was developed in 1958 when the FD&C was modified with the Food Additives Amendment. That amendment set up the GRAS status and designated those items that experience or common use in foods had shown were safe for public consumption. Only a few of the sweeteners have GRAS status, most are still considered food additives.

Will the FDA accept stevia as an artificial sweetener in the future? It depends on which side you ask. Stevia supporters suggest the artificial sweetener manufacturers are behind the FDA's position to prevent competition. The FDA and other official organizations remain cautious and want stevia to stay classified as a dietary supplement. Under that designation the FDA cannot regulate its content or purity, leaving consumers to decide on their own. The best advice is to use all substances in moderation, a rule of thumb that remains true in the case of stevia.

See also: Artificial Sweeteners.

FURTHER READING

"Background on Carbohydrates and Sugars." *Food Insight.* International Food Information Council Foundation, September 26, 2009. http://www.foodinsight.org/Resources/ Detail.aspx?topic=Background_on_Carbohydrates_Sugars.

Elkins, Rita. *Stevia: Nature's Sweetener.* Chapmanville, WV: Woodland Press, 2007.

"Is Stevia an FDA Approved Sweetener?" U.S. Department of Health and Human Services, U.S. Food and Drug Administration, April 4, 2012. http://www.fda.gov/ AboutFDA/Transparency/Basics/ucm214864.htm.

"Nutritive and Nonnutritive Sweeteners." Food and Nutrition Information Center. United States Department of Agriculture (USDA), January 19, 2014. http://fnic.nal .usda.gov/food-composition/nutritive-and-nonnutritive-sweetener-resources.

Stevia.Net. "A Tale of Incredible Sweetness and Intrigue." February 29, 2008. http://www .stevia.net.

Subway Diet

Every day millions of Americans eat at fast-food restaurants. In recent years as more and more people consider healthy food choices, those chain restaurants have tried to improve the public perception of their food. Calorie counts, fats grams, and protein amounts are available online and in the actual restaurants for consumers hoping to make healthy choices among the fast food options. One chain in particular, Subway, has promoted itself as "healthy" fast food for over a decade, thanks to the weight-loss plan created by Jared Fogle, an obese college student who lost 245 pounds eating a daily diet of Subway sandwiches and little else.

Fogle had tried several other diets, everything from frozen low-calorie meals to diet shakes to drop weight from his 425 pound high and finally settled on the Subway Seven under 6 Grams of Fat menu at a restaurant near his apartment during the spring of 1998. By 1999 he had lost over 100 pounds and had started walking for exercise. The weight continued to come off and when Fogle ran into a friend who marveled at his dramatic weight loss, the friend wrote about Fogle's diet in the college newspaper. Although this was pre-social media, Fogle's story was picked up and shared by a number of different news organizations including the Associated Press. Finally, after the information appeared in major health magazines in 2000 the agency handling advertising for Subway contacted Fogle and asked him to appear in commercials for the restaurant chain.

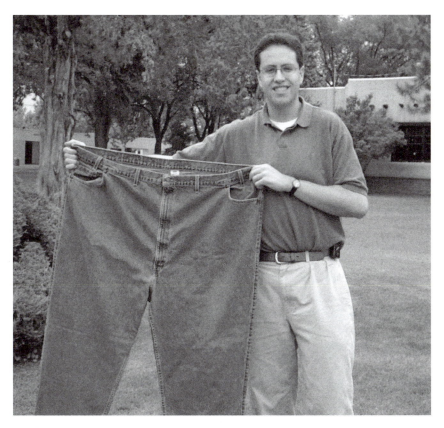

Jared Fogle attributes his success in losing 245 pounds in a year to eating Subway
sandwiches. In this 2001 photo, he holds up the pair of jeans he used to wear.
(AP Photo/Ivan Chavez)

With the commercials highlighting his success, others were inspired to also
follow their own versions of Fogle's diet. Subway officials did not specifically
endorse what became known as the "Jared Diet" according to Subway news
releases at the time, but they did promote their lower-fat food choices and
encouraged Americans to exercise. As Fogle toured the country and spoke to
audiences about the importance of diet and exercise, he also created a foundation, called the Jared Foundation, to bring awareness to the problem of childhood obesity.

While Fogle was able to lose and maintain a substantial weight loss with a very
limited choice of foods, nutritionists caution that a more balanced diet and daily
exercise are important for overall health and weight loss. Still Fogle's biggest ac-
complishment was that he was able to demonstrate healthy choices were available from fast-food restaurants. His daily intake amounted to about 1,000 calories.

Fogle admitted he rarely ate breakfast and the Subway sandwich was his first food of the day. He did snack on fruit and took a daily multivitamin but overall his routine included a six-inch sub for lunch and dinner from the seven choices of ham, roasted chicken breast, club, sweet onion chicken teriyaki, turkey breast, turkey breast, and ham or the vegetarian sandwich. He usually added a bag of baked chips or pretzels and a diet soft drink. He alternated between wheat and white bread and added lots of vegetables to his sandwiches including lettuce, green, or other peppers and pickles while he avoided cheese or condiments that contained fat.

It was clear that Fogle used the restaurant because it was convenient. That convenience extended to automatic portion control. Fogle was able to pay attention to fat and calories, thanks to the nutritional information provided by the company, and he was able to include vegetables without having to buy or prepare them. Once he began his career as a public speaker, he routinely recommended to his audiences that dieters consult with a doctor or a dietitian before starting any diet. He said he discussed his Subway plan with a dietitian, and his father, who was a physician, monitored his health. While he was successful with his plan, both Fogle and a Subway dietitian publically acknowledged the lack of some nutritional elements in his specific eating regimen. In fact, federal guidelines in the Dietary Guidelines for Americans suggest Americans consume a wide variety of foods from all of the recognized food groups including fruits, vegetables, calcium-rich foods, whole grains, and lean proteins.

While Fogle's "Subway diet" lacked nutritional balance, the Center for Science in the Public Interest (CSPI) did commend the restaurant chain in 2002 for helping to lead the way to healthier fast food and advocating for health and nutrition. Over a decade later, researchers have examined fast-food habits in adolescents and have discovered that current food choices at Subway were not much healthier than the choices made at McDonalds. The study, published in the *Journal of Adolescent Health*, found that the youngsters, ages 12 to 21, ate too many calories at both restaurants. The Institute of Medicine recommends youngsters not eat more than 2,400 calories in one day and the McDonalds meals averaged 1,038 calories, while the subway meals were an average of 955. While researchers did call the nutrient profile at Subway slightly healthier, the food still contained three times the recommended amount of salt. The scientists also recommended that customers at McDonalds would do well to eliminate sugary drinks and French fries from their meals. Those eating at Subway were advised to consume fewer calories by eating the smaller sized subs, ordering less processed meats, and adding more vegetables to the sandwiches.

See also: Dietary Guidelines for Americans.

FURTHER READING

Connolly, Ceci. "The Subway Guy, Still on a Roll; Jared Fogle Eats More Now, but Manages to Save Room for Success." *The Washington Post*, October 12, 2003, D1.

Fogle, Jared, and Bruno, Anthony. *Jared, the Subway Guy: Winning through Losing: 13 Lessons for Turning Your Life Around.* New York: St. Martin's Press, 2006.

"For Adolescents, Subway Food May Not Be Much Healthier than McDonald's, UCLA Study Finds." *Obesity, Fitness & Wellness Week,* May 25, 2013, 547.

"Jared Fogle-The Man the Myth and the Legend." *Folio SLCC'S Art & Literary Magazine,* November 12, 2013. http://www.folioslcc.org/2013/11/jared-fogle-man-myth-and-legend.html.

The Jared Foundation, Inc. http://www.jaredfoundation.org.

Oberliesen, Elise. "Jared Fogle-A Look at the Man behind the Sub Sandwich." *American Fitness* 29, no. 2 (2011): 41.

Sugar Busters!

Sugar Busters makes this attention-grabbing point: "Sugar is toxic." Not in the sense that sugar can kill you instantly. But the four authors, three of whom are MDs, argue that significant amounts of refined sugar can cause digestive and metabolic problems, as well as being a major factor in weight gain. That is because sugar stimulates production of the hormone insulin. Insulin regulates blood-sugar levels but overproduction of insulin causes the body to store excess sugar as fat and stimulates the liver to make cholesterol.

Sugar Busters! is the name of the *New York Times* number-one best seller, authored by H. Leighton Steward, Morrison C. Bethea, MD, Sam S. Andrews, MD, and Luis A. Balart, MD. Sugar Busters menu options are available at some restaurants. The underlying principle is that sugar contributes to weight gain and overall poor health. The authors point out that refined sugar became a part of the diet only around the 1700s and in the past century our consumption of it has grown exponentially. In 1980, Americans consumed 124.6 pounds of sugar per year and in 1994, that figure was up to 149.2 pounds.

Consumption figures for sugar were downgraded in 2012 based on new estimates of how much sweetened food is eaten versus how much is thrown away by consumers. The number for 2012 was just over 76 pounds, a dramatic difference from the 152 estimated for 2000. "Sugar just may be the number-one culprit in lowering quality of life and causing premature death," the authors state. However, their sugar busting doesn't stop at the sugar jar on the kitchen counter. Since carbohydrates are turned into sugars in the body, some carbohydrates are to be avoided on this diet plan. In particular, Sugar Busters requires you to avoid potatoes, corn, white rice, bread from refined flour, beets, carrots, refined sugar, corn syrup, molasses, honey, sugared colas, and beer.

Instead, the Sugar Busters menu encourages eating high-protein foods, such as meats, nuts, and some vegetables. Because these high-protein foods supply very little glucose to the body, the liver biosynthesizes glucose in a process called gluconeogenesis. Glucagon is a hormone that stimulates the mobilization of previously stored fat cells.

The fundamental point of Sugar Busters is that sugary foods, including many carbohydrates, promote production of insulin, which causes the body to store excess sugar as fat, while protein foods prompt the body to use up previously stored fat cells.

The book contains a 14-day menu and various recipes, developed at New Orleans restaurants, following the principles of the plan. The menu typically calls for a whole grain cereal or hot oatmeal for breakfast. Lunch is often a sandwich on whole grain bread with meat, lettuce, tomato, and mayonnaise. Dinners are grilled or baked meat, such as pork tenderloin, salmon or other fish, chicken, veal, steak, or lamp chops. These are generally accompanied by a whole wheat pasta, brown rice, salads, and fresh steamed vegetables. Suggested drinks are limited to milk, water, tea, coffee, and diet drinks. Desserts are on the menu about every other night, and are typically a dozen almonds or other nuts, two thin slices of cheese, sugar-free ice cream or frozen yogurt, or a Sugar Busters chocolate mousse recipe.

Throughout the book, the foods that raise the most concern are sugary or high-carbohydrate foods. The authors dispute the "myths" surrounding traditional weight-loss regimens, discounting the dangers of fats and foods high in cholesterol, contending that calorie counting isn't necessary, and even downplaying the role that exercise plays in weight control. While they acknowledge that most Americans eat a diet too high in saturated fats, they make the point of distinguishing among different types of fat. While they agree that very high cholesterol levels are "significantly related" to coronary artery disease, they don't believe that total cholesterol alone is a reliable indicator for the risk of heart disease. About calories, they write, "Our view is that calories per se are not as important as the types of food we eat . . . . What we do know is that normal, even significant, amounts of the proper types of food can be consumed for indefinite periods without causing weight gain." And exercise, while good for the body, isn't necessary for weight loss.

The book and the Web site (www.sugarbusters.com) contain plenty of success stories, from overweight noninsulin-dependent diabetics who lost weight and were able to control their diabetes with diet alone, to people who were unable to control their weight through any other diet plan. In fact, short of serious athletes or exercise "fanatics," who need higher levels of sugary foods for immediate energy, the authors say this food-choice lifestyle will work for anyone.

However, the Sugar Busters plan has its critics. The Physicians Committee for Responsible Medicine gives the book only two stars out of a possible five, rating it "not satisfactory." The group states that Sugar Busters "menus are low in fiber and high in fat and cholesterol with cheese, eggs, butter, yogurt, and cream not restricted in the meal plans. These foods squeeze out others that are higher in fiber and lower in fat."

Some dietitians and endocrinologists have suggested that the reason people lose weight on the Sugar Busters plan is that they limit overall calories, not insulin production. They argue that the body does not distinguish between carbohydrates from milk and carbohydrates from chocolate bars. And the downside of the plan is that the high-in-fat, low-in-fiber menu options limit variety, the basis of a healthy diet.

See also: Calories; Carbohydrates; Cholesterol (Dietary).

FURTHER READING

Gorman, Christine. "Sugar Busters! What You Should Know about the New Diets That Blame Insulin, Not Calories, for Your Extra Girth." *Time,* July 6, 1998, 1.
Grieger, Lynn. "Sugar Busters—Truth or Bust?" *Nutrition Guide,* May 27, 1999.
Kenney, Jay. "Do Potatoes Inhibit Weight Loss?" *Communicating Food for Health,* January 1999, 1–5.
Steward, H. Leighton, Morrison C. Bethea, Sam S. Andrews, and Luis A. Balart. *Sugar Busters!* New York: Ballantine Publishing Group, 1998.
Strom, Stephanie. "U.S. Cuts Estimate of Sugar Intake of Typical American." *The New York Times,* October 27, 2012, B1.
"Sugar Myths—A Trick or Treat." American Dietetic Association Web site. http://www .eatright.org. Accessed June 12, 2003.
Taubes, Gary. "What If It's All Been a Big Fat Lie?" *The New York Times,* July 7, 2002. http://www.nytimes.com/2002/07/07/magazine/07FAT.html?pagewanted=1.

Supersize

The *Oxford Dictionary* defines it as a verb. It means to create something or produce something in a larger size. Supersize has become synonymous with American fast food, specifically with McDonalds, but it actually first appeared in 1967 in a movie theater chain that wanted to boost sales of popcorn and soda. It was a way to increase profits; the company could charge quite a bit more than the cost of the extra popcorn. Sales were immediately successful.

David Wallerstein, a manager for the movie chain eventually was headhunted by McDonalds where he once again applied the concept that bigger was better for profits. Wallerstein had realized customers would not buy more than one of an item, fearing it would make them seem gluttonous but if given the chance to order a larger size, they would see it as a good value since it cost less than buying two portions. At the same time, the fast-food industry also realized that people had a hard time resisting sugar and fat.

The 2004 documentary *Super Size Me* by Morgan Spurlock was a hit at the Sundance Film festival. In it, Sherlock spent just 30 days eating only McDonalds food and had his meals supersized every time an employee offered that option. During the month, his weight ballooned, his cholesterol levels rose dramatically, and his general health deteriorated. McDonalds' officials called the movie a supersized distortion of the quality, choice, and variety available at McDonalds. However, soon after they also removed the supersized value meals from the menu. Officials announced that the phasing out of supersizing had nothing to do with the release of the movie. A company spokesman said they were simply cleaning up a cluttered menu. While a supersizing choice on fast-food restaurant menus no longer exists,

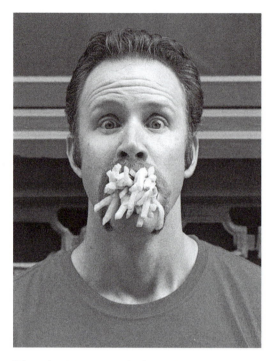

Filmmaker Morgan Spurlock's 2004 documentary
Super Size Me was a hit at the Sundance Film Festi-
val. He spent 30 days eating only supersized fast food.
(AP Photo/Julie Soefer)

portion sizes have risen dramatically and America is forever linked with the concept of supersizing.

What has also been linked with supersizing are the figures for overweight and
obese Americans, numbers that have more than tripled since 1980 according to
the Centers for Disease Control and Prevention (CDC).

See also: Cholesterol (Dietary); Nutrition Facts Label.

FURTHER READING

Gorin, Amy. "Fast Food Alert! The Return of Supersizing." *Prevention* 60, no. 2 (February
    2008): 82.
Orr, Gillian. "Supersized: Why Our Portion Sizes Are Ballooning." *The Independent*, June
    15, 2012. http://www.independent.co.uk/life-style/food-and-drink/features/supersized-
    why-our-portion-sizes-are-ballooning-7852014.html.
Tavernise, Sabrina. "New F.D.A. Nutrition Labels Would Make 'Serving Sizes' Reflect
    Actual Servings." *The New York Times*, February 27, 2014, A14.

Target Heart Rate

Fitness experts refer to a target heart rate—an optimum number of beats per minute—during aerobic exercises. There are several ways to figure out your target heart rate—and online calculators that can help determine it—but they're based on figuring out your maximum heart rate and working at between 50 and 85 percent of that. The prevalent formula for figuring out your maximum heart rate is subtracting your age from 220. So a 20-year old would have a maximum heart rate of 200 (220–20) and a target heart rate of between 100 and 170. A 40-year-old would have a maximum heart rate of 180 (220–40) and a target heart rate of between 90 and 153. The more sedentary person should start at the lower end of the scale, while an extremely fit person can push toward the higher end.

Are there differences in what target rates should be for men or women? Research from the Ohio State University Medical Center found there is a need for a gender-specific formula. In that study, women multiplied their age by 88 percent then subtracted that number from 206 instead of 220. While the studies continue, health professionals do agree it is important to exercise no matter how high you get your heart rate up.

How do you know your heart rate? The least expensive way is to measure it yourself or have a friend do it for you. Place your index and middle finger over the pulse—the inside of your wrist. Count the number of beats in a 10-second interval and multiply by six to get your heart rate per minute. Take the pulse as soon as you finish exercising or even in the middle of a workout. Your heart rate begins to slow down quickly as soon as you stop exerting yourself.

To get the maximum benefit from your exercise routines, the American College of Sports Medicine recommends exercising at an intensity of 60 to 85 percent of your target heart rate for 20 to 60 minutes, three to five days a week. This doesn't mean taking a brisk hour-long walk every day. Exercise intervals can be as short as 10 minutes to get the benefit. Just do them three times a day or more.

See also: Exercise.

FURTHER READING

Noonan, Peggy J. "Target Heart Rate Formula Made Especially for Women." *USA Today*, September 9, 2011. http://usatoday30.usatoday.com/news/health/story/health/story/2011–09–21/Target-heart-rate-formula-made-especially-for-women/50501680/1.

Reynolds, Gretchen. "Finding the Right Heart Rate." *The New York Times*, February 11, 2014, D4.

Stockton, William. "Fitness; Target Heart Rate: Is It Important, or Overrated?" *The New York Times*, April 4, 1988. http://www.nytimes.com/1988/04/04/sports/fitness-target-heart-rate-is-it-important-or-overrated.html.

Tarnower, Herman

Herman Tarnower (b. March 18, 1910, in New York; murdered March 10, 1980) was a physician and cardiologist who achieved worldwide fame on the basis of his book *The Complete Scarsdale Medical Diet* (1978). By the time of Tarnower's death in 1980, more than 2 million copies of his book had been sold. The Scarsdale diet and the 1973 Dr. Atkins's Diet Revolution were forerunners of the high-protein, low-carbohydrate regimens popular in newer diets like the Zone and Protein Power. Tarnower said in his book that his diet's success came from a metabolic change brought on when dieters restricted carbohydrates and filled up on protein.

An internist and cardiologist for over 40 years, Tarnower never followed the diet himself but he did counsel heart patients about losing weight. The actual Scarsdale diet began as a list he created of good and bad foods for his patients. Over the years the list was passed by word of mouth until friends from the publishing business suggested that Tarnower write a book selling his diet to a larger audience. He worked with Samm Sinclair Baker, author of the popular *Dr. Stillman's 14-Day Shape-Up Program*. The Scarsdale book included recipes, successful case histories, and Tarnower's thoughts on weight, eating, and health.

Tarnower, the son of Jewish immigrants Dora and Harry Tarnower, received his MD degree in 1933 from Syracuse University in New York and completed his internship and residency in internal medicine at Bellevue Hospital in New York. He traveled abroad in 1936 and 1937 on a New York Academy of Medicine fellowship and following World War II was selected as one of only two doctors to head a study of the possible aftereffects of radiation suffered by Japanese civilians in Nagasaki and Hiroshima. He was a founder and senior staff member of the Scarsdale Medical Group and was a clinical professor of medicine from 1975 until his death at the New York Medical College in New York City. Tarnower died at the hands of Jean S. Harris, a longtime companion whom he credited with helping him write the Scarsdale diet book. During her trial, she maintained the shooting was accidental; she was convicted of second-degree murder and was incarcerated before being pardoned in 1992.

See also: Atkins Nutritional Approach; Scarsdale Diet; The Zone.

FURTHER READING

American College of Physicians. *Biographical Directory of the American College of Physicians.* New York: R. R. Bowker Co., 1979.

Feron, James. "Scarsdale Diet Doctor Is Slain; Headmistress Is Charged." *New York Times,* 12 March 1980, A1.

Trilling, Diana. *Mrs. Harris: The Death of the Scarsdale Diet Doctor.* New York: Harcourt Brace Jovanovich, 1981.

Television

Why is there an entry on television in this encyclopedia? For the simple reason that watching television might be related to childhood obesity and overall poor quality diets. A study published in the June 2002 issue of *Pediatrics,* the *Journal of the American Academy of Pediatrics,* found that young children who had televisions in their bedrooms were more likely to be overweight than those who did not. About 40 percent of the children in the study had a television in their room, and these children spent 4.6 hours more per week watching TV/video than children without a TV in their bedroom. A 2014 study by the Yale University Prevention Research Center confirmed that placing a TV in a child's bedroom is still linked to weight gain. However, results also suggested that active video games may help youngsters lose unwanted pounds. Calling technology a "double-edged sword," researchers found not all video games contributed to obesity in kids.

Still, television viewing remains a problem and watching television may be linked with an overall decline in the quality of the diet. A press release issued by the North American Association for the Study of Obesity noted, "Children who watched television during dinner and snacked while watching television— practices that are greatly influenced by their parents—consumed less milk, fruits and vegetables than those who turned off the television at dinnertime and didn't snack while watching television."

Other studies have shown that, in older children, body mass index tends to increase along with the number of hours spent watching television.

The number of hours Americans watch television has been creeping upward. According to Census Bureau numbers, in 1993, the average American over 18 years of age spent 1,535 hours per year watching television. By 1998, the figure had increased to 1,573. The average increased to more than 1,700 hours per person per year in 2010.

The authors of the *Pediatrics* study concluded, "This study extends the association between TV viewing and risk of being overweight to younger, preschool-aged children. A TV in the child's bedroom is an even stronger marker of increased risk of being overweight. Because most children watch TV by age 2, educational efforts about limiting child TV/video viewing and keeping the TV out of the child's bedroom need to begin before then." Researchers suggested that taking the TV out of a child's bedroom is an important way to reduce that child's risk for weight gain.

See also: Childhood Obesity; Obesity.

FURTHER READING

"Bassett Study Reports Early Childhood Obesity Not Recognized by Most Parents." Bassett Healthcare Research Institute press release, May 22, 2000.

Costley, Kevin C., and Timothy Leggett. "Childhood Obesity: A Heavy Problem." U.S. Department of Education, 2010. www.eric.ed.gov/ERICWebPortal/contentdelivery/servlet/ERICServlet?accno=ED508702.

Dennison, Barbara A., Tara A. Erb, and Paul L. Jenkins. "Television Viewing and Television in Bedroom Associated with Overweight Risk among Low-Income Preschool Children." *Pediatrics* 109, no. 6 (June 2002): 1028–35.

Reinberg, Steven. "TV in Child's Bedroom Tied to Weight Gain; But 'Active' Video Games Might Help Youngsters Stay Slim, Researchers Stay." *Consumer Health News*, March 3, 2014. http://consumer.healthday.com/fitness-information-14/misc-health-news-265/childhood-obesity-technology-offers-pluses-minuses-685426.html

"Watching TV May Be Related to Poor Quality Diet and Increased Risk of Child Obesity." North American Association for the Study of Obesity press release, October 10, 2001.

T-Factor Diet

The T-Factor diet, written in 1989 by Dr. Martin Katahn, calls itself a scientific breakthrough and promises dieters they can lose weight safely and quickly without cutting back or counting calories. The thermogenic effect, or "T-factor," according to Katahn, is the way the body generates heat by burning carbohydrates, fats, and proteins at different rates. The author points to studies that suggest that fat in the diet turns into body fat more easily than do carbohydrates. By getting dieters to eat a much higher proportion of carbohydrates to fats, Katahn maintains that, over time, without extra fat coming in, excess pounds will simply melt away. In other words, eat less fat, store less fat, and lose weight. Since the 1990s the discussion of whether fats or carbohydrates cause weight gain has raged with some nutritionists suggesting that fewer carbohydrates and more lean protein are the better choices to avoid weight gain. In other words, they content carbohydrates could be acting as a fat storing device, and what affects weight gain is both the quality and quantity of the carbs eaten.

However, in his book, *The T-Factor 2000 Diet*, Katahn tells dieters that the source of calories eaten is more important than the total number of calories taken in. He instructs dieters to choose foods that naturally maximize the T-factor level and activate what he calls the body's hidden fat-burning potential. This simply means dieters must choose low-fat foods instead of fat-laden favorites; choose a baked potato instead of french fries.

The diet itself earns high marks for being well balanced, with plenty of fruits, vegetables, and whole grains. Yet critics point to the plan's strictness, saying it is too difficult to follow, since it recommends that only 15 to 20 percent of daily calories come from fat. Other low-fat, high-fiber diets, like the eating plans by Dr. Dean Ornish, Dr. John McDougall, and Nathan Pritkin, have been criticized for being too difficult to follow because they are also very low in fat. Americans traditionally consume closer to 40 percent of their calories as fat and nutritionists note that many people have difficulty dropping that to the newest American Heart Association recommendation of a 30 percent level.

The T-factor formula for weight loss is 20 to 40 grams of fat per day for women and 30 to 60 grams of fat per day for men. People wishing to lose weight quickly should cut their fat intake to the bottom limit of the recommended range—20 grams of fat for women and 30 grams of fat for men. Katahn also tells dieters to compensate for the reduction of fat in their diet with "whatever increase in carbohydrate foods feels good and satisfies your appetite." The book offers lists of fruits, vegetables, and grain foods that have little or no fat and can be eaten in unlimited amounts, as well as a fat substitution guide that suggests that dieters substitute foods like ground turkey for ground beef, bouillon for fatty sauces, skim milk for whole milk or cream, and water chestnuts for nuts in some dishes.

Sample menus in the book are basic and easy to follow. Breakfast for a typical day includes a banana or fresh fruit, dry cereal, one cup of skim milk, and coffee or tea, for a fat total of 3 grams. Lunch weighs in at 4 grams, with half a cup of cottage cheese, assorted raw vegetables, 5 whole-wheat crackers, and fresh fruit. Dinner includes up to 10 grams of fat with a small serving of baked chicken, brown or wild rice, a tossed salad with fat-free dressing, and fruit. Snacks are plain, nonfat yogurt, fresh fruit, or low-fat crackers. This particular example adds up to a daily total of 20 grams of fat.

The T-Factor Diet was published a few years after Katahn's best seller *The Rotation Diet* in 1986. That diet, which measures calories, instructed women to complete a dieting cycle by eating 600, 900, and then 1,200 calories per day in rotation. But Katahn writes in his diet book that the T-factor plan is an improvement over his earlier effort. "When I created the Rotation Diet, I was unaware of the direct relationship between the fat content of your body and the fat content of your diet." He adds that the rotation plan, "unfortunately failed many people in maintenance," and also did not adequately stress the importance of continuing to control fat intake when dieters reached goal weight.

The T-Factor diet, like the Rotation Diet, was heavily promoted in Katahn's hometown of Nashville, although the T-factor program fell short of the earlier rotation craze. In 1986, the author had the entire city "rotating," as some 75,000 residents collectively dieted to shed 1 million pounds in 12 weeks as part of a "Melt-a-Million" program sponsored by the Nashville Kroger grocery stores.

Katahn also includes what he calls "an advance over the Rotation Diet," a concept called the Quick Melt, where dieters can get the quick weight loss they desire by following the T-Factor diet and then cutting calories. In this way, he writes, "By cutting calories, not just substituting carbohydrates for fat, you create a deficit that pulls even more fat from your fat cells." The menus he provides have a daily calorie count for women of 1,100 to 1,300 and 1,600 to 1,800 calories for men. However, the rotation theory is absent from the Quick Melt and dieters are not instructed to vary calorie intake to prevent their metabolism from slowing down, as they were in the rotation plan. Instead, they are cautioned to add calories back slowly and to increase exercise after such a restricted diet to prevent any rapid weight gain.

However, unlike the Rotation diet, the T-factor book does devote a chapter to the importance of exercise in weight loss and in maintaining that loss. The author divides activities into "carb burners" and "fat burners." The carbohydrate-burning activities are what he calls start-stop choices like tennis, football, or calisthenics classes. The steady-state activities, or fat burners, require continuous whole-body movement like jogging and swimming and, according to Katahn, these aerobic activities burn fat more efficiently. The author lost 75 pounds on his diet and during that time became a strong supporter of daily exercise as a way to achieve fitness and a healthy weight.

See also: McDougall Program; Ornish, Dean; Pritikin, Nathan; Rotation Diet.

FURTHER READING

Katahn, Martin. *The Rotation Diet.* New York: W. W. Norton & Company, 1986.
Katahn, Martin. *The T-Factor Diet.* New York: W. W. Norton & Company, 1989.
Katahn, Martin. *The T-Factor 2000 Diet.* New York: W. W. Norton & Company, 1999.
Taubes, Gary. "What Really Makes Us Fat." *The New York Times,* June 30, 2012, SR5.
Toufexis, Anastasia. "Hey, Are You Rotating?" *Time,* April 14, 1986, 108.

TOPS, Take Off Pounds Sensibly

TOPS, Take Off Pounds Sensibly, founded in 1948 by Milwaukee housewife Esther Manz, was the first of the weight-watching organizations to successfully advocate the use of praise for weight loss. According to the organization's official Web site, TOPS was born around a kitchen table when Manz and three other women gathered to support each other in an effort to lose weight for health reasons. There are at least 10,500 chapters, located in the United States and in Canada, but many members now enroll online and participate from their home rather than attending chapter meetings. Manz saw obesity as a disease and believed sufferers should not face their problem alone. She conceived of the idea of a mutually helpful group, much like the support meetings of Alcoholics Anonymous. Years later, Overeaters Anonymous began, another nonprofit organization that offers group support and recommends seeing a doctor or health professional for an eating plan. According to its Web page, TOPS does endorse a standard exchange diet like the one offered by Weight Watchers, Inc.

TOPS differs from the Weight Watchers program, founded in 1963, in several significant ways. With its brand name diet foods and other products, Weight Watchers, Inc., is a profitable business. However, TOPS remains a nonprofit and noncommercial group. Leaders are volunteers and each chapter is designed to offer individuals support, encouragement, and educational opportunities that focus on healthy eating and lifestyles. There is now a small fee for joining and for Internet access to various resources available through the group's Web site.

Members who reach their goal weight become honored KOPS, Keep Off Pounds Sensibly. Any TOPS money left over from member dues is used for research into the causes of obesity. The group has contributed over $4 million to obesity research, much of it to the TOPS Center for Metabolic Research at the Medical College of Wisconsin, which includes the Esther Manz Laboratory and the Ronald K. Kalkhoff Library. The late Dr. Kalkhoff was TOPS's original medical advisor. Manz, the organization's founder, died at age 88 in 1996.

See also: Overeaters Anonymous; Weight Watchers.

FURTHER READING

Mitchell, Nia S., L. Mirim Dickinson, Allison Kempe, and Adam G. Tsai. "Determining the Effectiveness of Take Off Pounds Sensibly (TOPS), a Nationally Available Nonprofit Weight Loss Program." *Obesity* 19, no. 3 (March 2011): 568–73. doi:10.1038/oby.2010.202.
"TOPS Club, Inc. (Take Off Pounds Sensibly). Healthfinder.gov." http://healthfinder.gov/FindServices/Organizations/Organization.aspx?code=HR0678.

Trans Fatty Acids

Trans fatty acids, just about everywhere in the typical American diet, may finally be going away, much to the relief of public health advocates. Trans fats are created through the hydrogenation process that turns liquid oils into stick margarines or shortening and they are used in foods like crackers, cookies, and doughnuts, as well as frozen pizzas, microwave popcorn, and ready-made frosting. They make pie crusts flakier and french fries crispier. Trans fats are important to food manufacturers because they increase the shelf life and flavor stability of products. Unfortunately, research has shown that gram for gram, trans fats may be even more damaging than saturated fat. In other words, french fries cooked in partially hydrogenated vegetable shortening have as much artery-clogging potential as potatoes fried in lard or beef tallow.

Finally, after decades of research has linked trans fats to an increase of heart disease, the Food and Drug Administration (FDA) has removed them from its "generally recognized as safe" (GRAS) list of approved food additives. That change means manufacturers must now prove the trans fats in their foods are safe to eat, a difficult challenge since studies for decades have clearly shown they are not safe. The Institute of Medicine announced there is no safe level for consumption of trans fats, a fact the FDA added to its ruling.

Although nutritionists are still studying how a diet high in trans fats compares to one heavy in saturated fats, there is growing evidence that those trans fats may be raising concentrations of the so-called bad form of cholesterol, or LDL, in the body while lowering levels of HDL, the good cholesterol, setting the stage for heart disease. In 1993 investigators from Harvard reported the results of a study using female nurses. Even after accounting for other heart disease risk factors, women who consumed the most trans fatty acids had one and a half times more heart attacks than those who consumed the least trans fat. A 1994 Harvard study of men also found that those who ate large amounts of trans fats had more than twice the number of heart attacks as men who ate small amounts.

Unfortunately, until 2006 trans fats had been nearly invisible to consumers because food labels listed the amount of saturated fat per serving, but not the trans fat. After continuing debate and delay over a proposed law that would require food manufacturers to list the percentage of trans fat in their foods, the FDA added trans fats to label requirements for fat. Groups like the Center for Science in the Public Interest (CSPI) petitioned the FDA for the label change so consumers could see how much artery-clogging fat was in different products. Even though the measure has stalled for years, the FDA declared in 2006 that consumers would now see on the Nutrition Facts label how much of all three—saturated fat, trans fat, and cholesterol—are in the foods they choose to buy and eat.

The strongest opposition to the rule came from groups like the National Frozen Pizza Institute (NFPI). In a statement the NFPI called the rule premature, since no consensus exists on the effects of trans fatty acids on heart health.

Consumers trying to avoid trans fats in foods can follow several suggestions: read ingredients lists and stay away from products with the words "partially hydrogenated oil" (if this is one of the first ingredients listed, the product likely has lots of trans fat); when buying margarines and spreads, the softer the spread the lower in trans fats; use olive or canola oil instead of butter, margarine, or shortening whenever possible; avoid deep-fried foods; buy and eat low-fat foods, since the lower the fat per serving, the lower the trans fat will be; shop in natural-food stores whenever possible, since the majority of their product lines are trans-free; read labels and look for hidden trans fats in all kinds of foods, including whole wheat breads and peanut butters, prepared mixes for muffins, cakes, and cookies, and boxes of macaroni and cheese.

The wide variety of names and types of fats continues to confuse American consumers. Basically, different categories of fats get their names from their patterns of hydrogen atoms. All fatty acids, which make up fats, contain chains of carbon atoms, with hydrogen atoms attached to some or all of the carbon atoms. Fats with one double bond are called monounsaturated; those with more double bonds are called polyunsaturated. Both monounsaturated and polyunsaturated fats are considered good fats by nutritionists. Good fats, the heart-healthy kind, include olive oil, canola oil, walnut oil, peanut oil, nuts, and avocados plus omega-3 fatty acids from fatty fish. These fats provide the HDL or high-density lipoprotein cholesterol that protects artery walls by carrying away the LDL cholesterol back to the liver, where it is excreted into the intestines and out of the body.

Saturated fats, those found in animal fats, palm oil, and processed foods like margarine and pastries, don't have what scientists call double bonds. Saturated fats, for decades considered the bad fats, were thought to promote high blood-cholesterol levels by raising LDL cholesterol levels. These LDL or low-density lipoproteins damage artery linings and form deposits on artery walls, eventually slowing blood flow.

When early research linked saturated fats to a variety of health problems like heart disease, high blood pressure, and diabetes, consumers switched to unsaturated fat products, going from butter to margarine. At first, trans fatty acids, because they contain a type of unsaturated fatty acid, were not considered a health risk. But nutritionists now say studies show that when vegetable oils are changed into semisolid or solid substances, those newly created trans fats act like saturated fats, or worse, and increase the blood level of LDL.

With so many confusing categories of fats, consumers look to health organizations like the ADA and the FDA for recommendations on healthy eating. The 2014 Dietary Guidelines for Americans recognized a shift in established thinking concerning fats. As a result of additional research, organizations like the American Heart Association and the American Diabetes Association are giving saturated fats another look as studies question whether saturated fat is the problem consumers were told it was concerning heart disease.

See also: Cholesterol (Dietary); Dietary Fat; Dietary Guidelines for Americans.

FURTHER READING

Dausch, Judith G. "Trans-Fatty Acids: A Regulatory Update." *Journal of the American Dietetic Association* 102, no. 1 (January 2002): 18–20.

Gorman, Jessica. "New Studies Add to These Fats' Image Problem." *Science News,* November 10, 2001, 300–302.

"Headless FDA Begins 2002 with Broad Agenda." *Food Chemical News* 43, no. 47 (January 7, 2002): 3.

McCord, Holly, and Gloria McVeigh. "How to Shop Trans-Free." *Prevention,* April 2000, 70.

O'Connor, Anahad. "Study Questions Fat and Heart Disease Link." *The New York Times,* March 17, 2014. http://well.blogs.nytimes.com/2014/03/17/study-questions-fat-and-heart-disease-link/.

Palmer, Sharon. "FDA Bans Trans Fat." *Environmental Nutrition* 37, no. 2 (February 2014): 2.

Tavernise, Sabrina. "F.D.A. Ruling Would All but Eliminate Trans Fats." *The New York Times,* November 7, 2013, A1.

"Trans Fat Now Listed with Saturated Fat and Cholesterol." *U.S. Food and Drug Administration*, December 17, 2013. http://www.fda.gov/food/ingredientspackaginglabeling/labelingnutrition/ucm274590.htm.

Wootan, Margo, Bonnie Liebman, and Wendie Rosofsky. "Trans: The Phantom Fat." *Nutrition Action Healthletter* 23, no. 7 (September 1996): 1–6.

Vegetarian Diet

A vegetarian diet is a plant-based diet that does not include meats. The number of vegetarians in the United States varies widely, depending on which organization is doing the survey. According to a 2012 Gallup survey, some 5 percent of American adults call themselves vegetarian and that figure has not changed significantly since a 2000 poll. Another 2 percent of youth (aged 6 to 17) also considered themselves vegetarian.

This variety in polling numbers does not indicate a sudden drop in those eating a vegetarian diet, but rather reflects the differing audiences (all Americans as opposed to American adults). It also reflects the variety in vegetarian diets themselves. For example, lacto-ovo vegetarian, a popular type, describes a diet that includes milk, cheese, yogurt, and eggs. This is easiest in terms of menu planning and you will also find food choices in most restaurants and fast-food restaurants. Those who eat dairy but not eggs are called lacto-vegetarians. Those who eat eggs but no dairy, by contrast, are called ovo-vegetarians. And those who choose to eat no animal products at all are called vegans. Vegan diets are based on vegetables, fruits, grains, legumes, nuts, and seeds, and exclude all meat, fish, poultry, dairy, and eggs. Many vegans are also philosophically opposed to animal products, such as wool, leather, honey, and cosmetics and soaps from animal products. A raw foodist eats uncooked nuts, fruits, vegetables, and sprouted seeds. Fruitarians are people who eat only raw fruits, nuts, and berries. A pollo-vegetarian eats a diet similar to lacto-ovo but incorporates poultry. A pesca-vegetarian eats fish and seafood along with the lacto-ovo diet.

Many nutritionists and doctors acknowledge the health benefits of a plant-based diet when compared to a meat-based diet high in cholesterol and saturated fat. Research shows that, on the whole, vegetarians eat a more healthy diet than nonvegetarians and consume about two to three times as much fiber as their meat-eating counterparts. And a diet high in fiber can actually lower the chances of developing certain cancers, particularly colon cancer, according to the National Cancer Institute.

In fact, the National Cancer Institute, the American Dietetic Association (ADA), the American Heart Association, and the U.S. Department of Health and Human Services now support a well-planned vegetarian diet and its associated health benefits. The ADA stated in a 1997 position paper, "Appropriately planned vegetarian diets are healthful, are nutritionally adequate, and provide health benefits in the prevention and treatment of certain diseases." The paper also stated that vegetarian diets have been used successfully to reverse severe coronary artery disease as well as offer protective benefits from hypertension and some cancers.

But health concerns are not the only reason that young adults give for changing their diets. Some make the choice out of concern for animal rights. When faced with the statistic that some 90 percent of animals raised as food live in confinement, many teens give up meat to protest those conditions. Others turn to vegetarianism to support the environment. Meat production uses vast amounts of water, land, grain, and energy while creating problems with animal waste and subsequent pollution. It takes more than three times as much fossil fuel to feed a meat eater as it does to feed a person who eats no meat or dairy products, according to EarthSave, an organization founded in 1988 to educate people about the environmental benefits of a plant-based diet. Whatever the reason you choose to become a vegetarian, your choice brings with it questions from parents about your health and nutrition. By becoming an educated vegetarian, you can achieve good nutrition as well as support a more humane and ecological world and do your part to reduce global hunger.

A vegetarian diet does not have to be bland, brown, and boring. The plant kingdom is a multicolored world of crunchy, chewy, creamy, and meaty textures. From portobello mushrooms to polenta, from summer corn to seitan, there are wonderful tastes to try. In fact, you are already familiar with many basic and classic meatless dishes: eggplant parmesan, spaghetti with marinara sauce, pasta with pesto sauce, bean burritos, stuffed peppers, split pea soup, vegetable lasagna, and baked potatoes with broccoli and cheese sauce. Gourmet cuisine is also part of the vegetarian experience, with foods like roasted pepper and tomato soup; fassolada, a Greek bean soup; and mango raita, a fruity yogurt sauce. Or maybe you would prefer your fresh mango in a couscous salad or fajita wraps with salsa verde and chocolate rum cake. Many Italian dishes are vegetarian naturals and pasta in its myriad forms makes numerous meatless meals. Mexican cooking is often meatless as well, using tortillas, beans, and cheese. Other ethnic cuisines have made a culinary art out of vegetables, like the Greek spinach dish, spanakopita. Asian stir-fries are another example of delicious meatless cooking, as are Indian curries and Ethiopian dishes of assorted vegetables and beans. Overall, a vegetarian diet is an indulgence in good food and in good health.

Well-known vegetarians include Leonardo da Vinci, Albert Einstein, Benjamin Franklin, Charles Darwin, Thomas Edison, Leo Tolstoy, Henry David Thoreau, Mahatma Gandhi, and Clara Barton; all abstained from eating meat. Today's famous vegetarians include Chelsea Clinton, Brad Pitt, Madonna, and Beatle Paul McCartney.

The 1970s saw a resurgence in vegetarianism with the 1971 publication of Frances Moore Lappé's *Diet for a Small Planet*. Lappé criticized the inefficiency of a diet based on animal foods, calling beef cattle "a protein factory in reserve" because cattle consume much more protein than they ever provide as meat. She raised the discussion to a global level by addressing the environmental effects of food production, like the destruction of rain forests and the politics of world hunger. She called for a large-scale move to a plant-based diet. Lappé wrote, "What we eat is within our control, yet the act ties us to the economic, political and ecological order of the whole planet. Even an apparently small change, consciously choosing a diet that is good for both our bodies and for the earth, can lead to a series of choices that transform our whole lives."

Public attention also turned to issues of animal cruelty. People for the Ethical Treatment of Animals (PETA) and others brought the stories and photographs of slaughterhouse conditions to the forefront. Formed in 1980, PETA encourages vegetarianism for humane reasons and works through a combination of advocacy, public relations, and advertising to expose the American people in sensational and graphic terms to what the organization calls the inhumanity of animal agriculture.

As is true of a diet that includes meat, variety is fundamental. A look at the U.S. Department of Agriculture's (USDA) MyPlate lists meat, fish, and poultry as the primary sources of protein. In 1998, a vegetarian alternative to the earlier USDA Food Guide Pyramid was unveiled at the International Conference on Vegetarian Diets. That alternative pyramid promotes protein from soy, legumes, dairy, nuts, and seeds, and emphasizes a wide base of foods to be eaten at every meal, including fruits and vegetables, whole grains, and legumes. The middle band of the pyramid, to be eaten daily, includes nuts and seeds, egg whites, dairy and soy milk, and plant oils. The pyramid top shows optional foods or foods that should be eaten in small quantities, and includes eggs and sweets.

A vegetarian diet is not, by definition, either a healthy or a low-calorie eating plan. Nutritionists say the biggest mistake new converts make is to fill up on fattening foods such as cheese, french fries, pizza, avocados, and nuts. They say the best diet is rich in fiber and complex carbohydrates and low in fat—consider apples, oranges, bananas, bagels, popcorn, pretzels, bean tacos or burritos, salads, frozen juice bars, smoothies, or rice cakes. Other good meal choices include non-cream soups and salads.

Misuse of vegetarian eating has also been associated with eating disorders like anorexia and bulimia. Teens who choose to be vegetarian should be doing it correctly and with the right motivation rather than trying to camouflage an eating disorder. A report in the *Archives of Pediatrics & Adolescent Medicine* in August 1997 looked at how some teens hid eating disorders behind the healthy façade of vegetarianism. The study reported that although vegetarian teens ate more fruits and vegetables than their meat-eating peers did, they were also twice as likely to diet frequently. The meatless teens were also four times as likely to diet intensively and eight times as likely to abuse laxatives. According to the study, this was the first population-based look at eating disorders and their connections to vegetarianism. The authors suggested that due to the increased social acceptance of vegetarian diets, teens who adopt a meatless diet should be evaluated carefully by their parents and health care professionals. Excessive dieting, binge eating, intentional vomiting, and laxative abuse are more obvious red-flag behaviors associated with anorexia and bulimia, and teens may try to hide them by changing to a vegetarian diet. This is not to say that every teen who decides to go vegetarian is going to develop an eating disorder, but when it is pursued to extremes there is potential for serious problems.

See also: Anorexia Nervosa; MyPlate.

FURTHER READING

Atlas, Nava. *Vegetariana: A Rich Harvest of Wit, Lore and Recipes*. New York: Little Brown, 1984.

Bode, Janet. *Food Fight: A Guide to Eating Disorders for Pre-Teens and Their Parents*. New York: Simon and Schuster, 1997.

David, Marc. *Nourishing Wisdom: A New Understanding of Eating*. New York: Random House, 1994.

Goodman, Brenda. "Vegetarian Diet May Help Lower Blood Pressure, Research Suggests; Japanese Review of 39 Studies Shows a Meatless Menu Might Boost Cardiovascular Health but the Findings Are Preliminary." *Consumer Health News*. February 24, 2014, NA.

Harel, Zeev. "Adolescents and Calcium: What They Do and Do Not Know and How Much They Consume." *Journal of the American Medical Association* 279, no. 21 (June 3, 1998): 1678.

"How Many Teens Are Vegetarian? How Many Kids Don't Eat Meat?" *Vegetarian Journal* xix, no. 6 (January/February 2001). www.vrg.org/journal/v2001jan/2001janteen.htm. Accessed June 12, 2003.

Krizmanic, Judy. *A Teen's Guide to Going Vegetarian*. New York: Viking and Puffin Books, 1994.

Krizmanic, Judy. *The Teen's Vegetarian Cookbook*. New York: Viking and Puffin Books, 1999.

Lappé, Frances Moore. *Diet for a Small Planet*. 20th Anniversary ed. New York: Ballantine Books, 1991.

Lemlin, Jeanne. *Quick Vegetarian Pleasures*. New York: HarperCollins, 1992.

Madison, Deborah. *The New Vegetarian Cooking for Everyone*, rev ed. Berkeley, CA: Ten Speed Press, 2014.

Maradino, Cristin. "The Pyramids Go Veg: New Food Guide." *Vegetarian Times*, January 1998, 18.

Messina, Virginia, and Mark Messina. *The Vegetarian Way: Total Health for You and Your Family*. New York: Crown, 1996.

Neumark-Sztainer, Dianne, Mary Story, Michael D. Resnick, and Robert W. Blum. "Adolescent Vegetarians: A Behavioral Profile of a School-Based Population in Minnesota." *Archives of Pediatrics and Adolescent Medicine* 151, no. 8 (August 1997): 833.

Newman, Judith. "Little Girls Who Won't Eat: The Alarming New Epidemic of Eating Disorders." *Redbook*, October 1997, 120.

Newport, Frank. "In U.S., 5 % Consider Themselves Vegetarians." *Gallup Well-Being*, July 26, 2012. http://www.gallup.com/poll/156215/consider-themselves-vegetarians.aspx.

O'Connor, Amy. "8 Nutritional Myths: Debunking Accepted 'Truths' About Your Diet."
    Vegetarian Times, July 1997, 78.
Parr, Jan. *The Young Vegetarian's Companion*. New York: Franklin Watts, 1996.
Pierson, Stephanie. *Vegetables Rock!* New York: Bantam Books, 1999.
Reilly, Lee. "Bites of Passage: What You Need to Know When Your Teen Goes Vegetar-
    ian." *Vegetarian Times*, November 1997, 78.
Richmond, Akasha. *The Art of Tofu*. Torrance, CA: Morinaga Publications, 1997.
Robbins, John. *Diet for a New America*. Walpole, NH: Stillpoint Publishing, 1987.
Spencer, Colin. *The Heretic's Feast: A History of Vegetarianism*. London: The Fourth Estate,
    1993.
Springer, Ilene. "Are You Ready to Go Vegetarian?" *Cosmopolitan*, October 1995, 130.
Stepaniak, Joanne. *The Vegan Sourcebook*. Los Angeles: Lowell House, 1998.
VanTine, Julia. "When Kids Say 'No More Meat!'" *Prevention*, November 1999, 52.
Vegetarian Times Vegetarian Beginner's Guide. New York: Macmillan, 1996.
Visser, Margaret. *Much Depends upon Dinner*. New York: Macmillan, 1988.

Vitamins

Vitamins are the natural components in food—different from proteins, carbohydrates, and fats—which help ensure normal metabolism. They are essential for
good health and growth and when they are deficient or absent dramatic problems can develop. Vitamins fall into two categories, essential and nonessential.
The essential vitamins are needed to sustain life and to maintain good health
but the body must get them from outside sources. Nonessential vitamins are vital
but the body can manufacture them on their own.

The word *vitamin* was derived from the term *vitamine*, Latin's *vita* for "life"
and *amine* for "organic compound." The term was coined by biochemist Casimir
Funk to describe an organic base, or amine, later found to be thiamine. In 1912,
biochemists Sir F. G. Hopkins and Funk formulated the vitamin hypothesis of
deficiency disease, meaning that certain diseases are caused by a dietary lack of
specific vitamins. Dramatic examples of these diseases include scurvy from lack
of vitamin C; pellagra from lack of niacin; and beriberi from lack of thiamine.

Vitamins are classified by their ability to be absorbed in fat or water. The water-
soluble vitamins are the eight B vitamins and vitamin C. They must be eaten
frequently because they cannot be stored, with the exception of some B vitamins. The fat-soluble vitamins—A, D, E, and K—are generally eaten along with
fat-containing foods and can be stored in the body's fat, so they do not need to
be eaten every day. Vitamin D is the only one manufactured by the body; all the
others must come from the diet.

A well-balanced diet should satisfy the Recommended Dietary Allowance
(RDA) of each vitamin. RDAs are guidelines first developed by the Food and
Nutrition Board and the National Academy of Sciences–National Research
Council based on the nutritional needs of an average healthy person. The U.S.

government eventually adopted the National Research Council's RDAs. They are expressed in milligrams or international units (IU) and these recommendations differ for adults and children as well as for people who must follow special diets or women who are pregnant or lactating.

The vitamins include vitamin A; the eight vitamin B complex group of B_1, or thiamine; B_2, or riboflavin; B_3, or niacin; B_5, or pantothenic acid; B_6, or pyridoxine; B_7, or biotin; B_9, or folic acid; and B_{12}, or cobalamin; vitamin C; vitamin D; vitamin E; and vitamin K.

Vitamin A is fat-soluble and comes from animal foods like liver, egg yolks, cream, or butter or from beta-carotene that occurs in leafy green vegetables and in yellow fruits and vegetables. Vitamin A is important to skeletal growth as well as the health of the skin and mucous membranes. A deficiency of this vitamin can cause slowed skeletal growth, skin abnormalities, and susceptibility to serious infection. In very severe cases it can cause death.

Thiamine, B_1, is part of the vitamin B complex and plays an important role in the metabolism of carbohydrates. It also helps maintain appetite, normal intestinal function, and the health of the cardiovascular and nervous systems. Yeast, legumes, whole grains, thiamine-enriched cereal products, and nuts are all good sources of thiamine.

Riboflavin, also known as B_2, is needed for the body to effectively metabolize carbohydrates, fats, and respiratory proteins. Good sources of riboflavin include liver, milk, meat, dark green vegetables, whole grain and enriched cereals, and mushrooms. Deficiency can cause skin lesions and sensitivity to light.

Niacin, B_3, aids in the release of energy from nutrients. A deficiency of niacin causes pellagra, whose symptoms include a sunburn-like eruption that breaks out when skin is exposed to sunlight. Other symptoms are a red and swollen tongue, diarrhea, mental confusion, and depression. Large doses of niacin have been used to reduce levels of cholesterol in the blood, but over long periods they can cause liver damage. Good sources of niacin are liver, poultry, meat, tuna and salmon, dried beans and peas, and nuts.

Pantothenic acid, B_5 vitamin, plays a role in the metabolism of many substances, including fatty acids, steroids, and carbohydrates. The adrenal gland is an important site of pantothenic acid activity. Pantothenic acid is abundant in many foods, including liver, kidney, eggs, and dairy products, and there is no known problem with deficiency since it is also manufactured by intestinal bacteria.

Pyridoxine, or vitamin B_6, is needed for the absorption and metabolism of amino acids, glucose, and fatty acids. It also plays a role in the formation of red blood cells. The best sources are liver and other organ meats, along with spinach, avocados, green beans, bananas, whole grain cereal, and seeds.

Biotin, a B vitamin, also plays a role in the metabolism of carbohydrates, fats, and amino acids. It is synthesized by intestinal bacteria and is widespread in foods, especially egg yolk, tomatoes, yeast, kidney, and liver. There is no known deficiency in humans.

Folic acid, or vitamin B_9, is rich in green leafy vegetables, fruits, dried beans, sunflower seeds, and wheat germ. It works to form body protein and hemoglobin, and deficiencies have been linked to neural tube defects, a type of birth defect that causes serious brain or neurological disorders such as spina bifida. Folic acid is lost in foods stored at room temperature and during cooking, so to increase access to this important vitamin the government has required enrichment of flours, cornmeal, rice, and pasta with folic acid since 1998. Unlike other water-soluble vitamins, folic acid is stored in the liver and does not need to be eaten daily.

Vitamin B_{12}, cobalamin, is the most complex of all known vitamins and is important in nervous system functioning. It comes only from animal sources—liver, kidneys, meat, fish, eggs, and milk—and vegans or vegetarians, who eat few or no dairy products, are advised to take a supplement to ensure that they have adequate amounts. This vitamin is also necessary for folic acid to fulfill its role, and both are involved in the synthesis of proteins.

Vitamin C is perhaps the best known of the vitamins and is important in the formation and maintenance of collagen, a protein that help form bones and teeth. Vitamin C also enhances the absorption of iron from foods. Deficiency of this vitamin causes scurvy, whose symptoms include hemorrhages, loosening of teeth, and bone problems, especially in children. The use of large doses of vitamin C in treating common colds is the subject of continuing research.

Vitamin D is needed for healthy bones and for the retention of calcium and phosphorus in the body. Called the sunshine vitamin, it can be manufactured in the body with as little as a half-hour of sunlight. Rickets, from vitamin D deficiency, is usually caused by a lack of exposure to sunlight rather than a dietary deficiency. Symptoms include bowlegs, knock knees, and other bone deformities, or, in adults, softening of the bones. However, because this is a fat-soluble vitamin, it is stored in the body. To prevent deficiencies, the government requires milk to be fortified with Vitamin D. On the other hand, excessive consumption can cause nausea, loss of appetite, and kidney damage. Good food sources of vitamin D include egg yolk, liver, tuna, and vitamin D–fortified milk or juice.

Vitamin E plays a role in forming red blood cells and muscle and other tissues. It is also a potent antioxidant, and studies show that it protects against arterial plaque buildup and cancer. It is found in vegetable oils, wheat germ, green leafy vegetables, and liver. Scientists believe it may have an anticoagulant effect on the blood, but that has not been substantiated although research is ongoing.

Vitamin K is necessary for the clotting of blood and its richest sources are alfalfa and fish livers. Other sources include leafy green vegetables, egg yolks, soybean oil, and liver. The bacterial synthesis of this vitamin usually provides enough for a healthy adult but those suffering from blood diseases can experience some deficiency.

See also: Malnutrition; Nutrition Facts Label.

FURTHER READING

"Should You Take Vitamins?" *Focus on Healthy Aging* 13, no. 3 (March 2014): 4.
"Vitamin Therapy: A Good Idea?" *Harvard Health Commentaries*, August 21, 2006, NA.
Zimmer, Carl. "Vitamins' Old, Old Edge." *The New York Times*, December 9, 2013, D1.

Walking

Never underestimate the power of a good pair of sneakers. Walking is something nearly everyone can do—and it's one of the easiest, most convenient, and least expensive ways to begin an exercise regimen. On the Physical Activity Pyramid (see Exercise), walking is listed as one of the "everyday activities." These first-level activities should total 30 minutes and should be repeated most days of the week. If you can't find one 30-minute interval, try finding two 15-minute opportunities to take a walk around the block, run an errand on foot instead of getting in the car, hop off the bus a stop or two before your usual one, or take the stairs instead of the elevator.

Set reasonable goals for yourself. Don't insist on walking 5 miles per day only to realize after two days that it's too much. Instead, say to yourself that you're going to "go for a walk" twice a day. As time goes on, either find a route that involves more hills or walk for longer stretches of time. Encourage a friend to walk with you. Time seems to go faster when you're enjoying conversation. And realize that even though it's "just" walking, it is exercising and it has cumulative benefits. Walking briskly can burn off about 100 calories per mile.

See also: Calories; Exercise.

FURTHER READING

"Heart Disease Risk Is Improved by Walking." *Focus on Healthy Aging* 17, no. 3 (March 2014): 2.
Reynolds, Gretchen. "Why a Brisk Walk Is Better." *The New York Times*, December 4, 2013. http://well.blogs.nytimes.com/2013/12/04/why-a-brisk-walk-is-better.
"Walking: A Step in the Right Direction toward Better Health." *UWIRE Text*, April 10, 2014, 1.

Weigh Down Diet

The Weigh Down Diet (1997) could literally be called an answer to author Gwen Shamblin's prayers. A registered dietitian with a master's degree in food and nutrition, Shamblin describes in the book how for many years she was "food focused," constantly struggling with her weight. Then she happened upon the simple concept that God can take away the desire to overeat and the Weigh Down Diet was born. The premise is simple; you don't have to starve yourself to lose weight. Overeating is a problem of the soul, and those who can put their spiritual life in order can, and will, lose weight.

The diet does not focus on the usual diet strategy of counting calories and makes very little mention of exercise. Still this 1997 best seller has grown into a multimillion-dollar, Nashville-based corporation called the Weigh Down Workshop, Inc. The diet is part of a 10-week program that starts by teaching participants what hunger is. Instructors do not prescribe a specific menu nor do they encourage participants to cut out bad foods or empty calories from their lives. Instead, dieters focus on when they are physically hungry as opposed to when they are spiritually hungry.

In her book, Shamblin gives a sample of her daily menu, but cautions participants to choose the foods they want in the amounts they select. Although fasting is not a goal in the diet, the program starts with an initial fast so dieters can feel hunger pangs, something they may not have felt in a long time. With Weigh Down, the use of fasting is seen as a way to gain more control over eating problems. Shamblin writes, "Fasting is all over the Old and the New Testaments as an offering to God. God would not be asking us to damage the body." But doctors say fasting poses health risks and is sometimes used by women to mask the signs of anorexia or bulimia. Although the book briefly cautions anorexics not to fast, Shamblin suggests that those with eating disorders work to "be obedient to hunger or emptiness by eating every time they sense emptiness." Critics question the program's use of fasting and lack of insight into its related risks.

While instructors spend the first few weeks teaching that participants should eat the way God intended, many skeptics point out that the diet offers no upfront nutritional information, leaving people with bad eating habits doomed to failure. Opponents of Weigh Down call this approach shortsighted, charging that it ignores documented scientific principles such as the U.S. Department of Agriculture's (USDA) Dietary Guidelines for Americans.

An even more controversial aspect of the Weigh Down Diet is the clear message that fat is sin and God wants people to be thin. However, Shamblin makes no apologies for this approach, saying that if you crave a food, you should eat it, and God will help you stop when you are satisfied. But critics worry about the people who do not lose or who gain their weight back. Those people, theologians fear, might believe they are letting God down, they may question their faith, or even give up on God.

Although Weigh Down teaches people to trade an obsessive focus on food for an all-out focus on God, there are other Christian dieting programs that offer more nutritional direction and regimentation. Consider the program 3D—Diet, Discipline, and Discipleship. 3D was founded in 1973 by Carol Showalter, a Presbyterian pastor's wife, who believes that Christians, meeting in small groups, can lose weight if they lead disciplined lives, a combination of disciplined eating and disciplined prayer. Another similar program, First Place, was founded in 1981 in Houston. Its national director, Carole Lewis, says this program supports a recognized food plan using food exchanges and the USDA Food Guide Pyramid.

Early Christian diet books have also enjoyed success long before the *Weigh Down Diet* was written. *Pray Your Weight Away* (1957), by Presbyterian minister Charlie Shedd, is believed to be the first overtly Christian diet book published for a mainstream audience. Shedd, pastor of the Memorial Drive Presbyterian Church of Houston, lost 100 pounds after which he wrote this best seller explaining how to wage war against gluttony and overeating through prayer. Fifteen years later he wrote a second book, titled *The Fat in Your Head* (1972), based on his experiences as a board member of a psychiatric hospital. Other popular Christian diet book titles include *Help Lord, The Devil Wants Me Fat!* (1978), by Dr. C. S. Lovett, and *I Prayed Myself Slim* (1960) by Deborah Pierce.

See also: Anorexia Nervosa; Bulimia Nervosa; Christian Diets; Dietary Guidelines for Americans.

FURTHER READING

Barber, Christine. "Gaining the Pounds? That's How Satan Likes It." *The Santa Fe New Mexican*, October 15, 2008, D.

Brown, Deneen. "Dieting Faithfully; Proponents of the Weigh Down Diet Turn to God for the Will to Resist Overeating." *Washington Post*, April 11, 2000, Z14.

Goodman, Ellen. "The Perils of Paunches and Pounds." *Washington Post*, December 12, 1977, A23.

Kennedy, John W., and Todd Starnes. "Gwen in the Balance." *Christianity Today*, October 23, 2000, 15.

Shamblin, Gwen. *The Weigh Down Diet*. New York: Doubleday, 1997.

Winner, Lauren F. "The Weigh & the Truth." *Christianity Today*, September 4, 2000, 50.

Weight Watchers

Weight Watchers is one of the best-known weight-loss support organizations in the world. Spokespeople for the organization have ranged from actress Lynn Redgrave, Sarah Ferguson, the Duchess of York, former NBA star Charles Barkley, Grammy winning singer Jennifer Hudson, and actress Jessica Simpson. Weight Watchers helps people lose weight at a moderate pace and keep it off with a program that offers a healthy food plan, exercise, and behavior modification in a group support environment.

The Weight Watchers concept was begun by Jean Nidetch in 1961—at the time, a 200-plus-pound New Yorker who met with friends to talk about effective

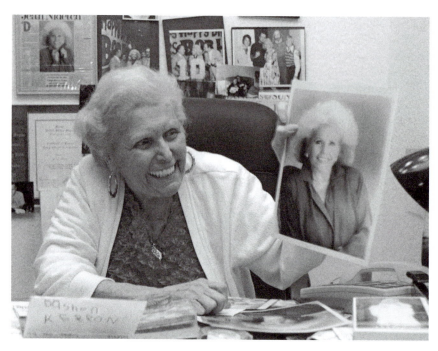

Jean Nidetch, shown in a 2011 photo, co-founded Weight Watchers in 1961. With the support and encouragement of other overweight friends, Nidetch lost 72 pounds and formally created the organization in 1963. (AP Photo/Alan Diaz)

weight loss and provide each other with moral support. With the support of other overweight friends, Nidetch lost 72 pounds and the organization was formally launched in 1963. Since then, the organization has enrolled millions of members worldwide. In 1978, H.J. Heinz purchased Weight Watchers, and 20 years later, it was purchased by Luxembourg's Artal Group. In November 2001, the company went public and listed on the New York Stock Exchange.

Weight Watchers offers the Points weight-loss system that includes the Daily Points Range and a new Simple Start plan for immediate results. The Daily Points Range is assigned based on the amount of weight to lose. Rather than measure portion size or count calories, points are easier to track, and accomplishes much the same. Stay within the Daily Points Range and you'll lose weight. For example, a scoop of ice cream is 4 points; a bottle of beer is 3 points, a slice of pizza is 9 points, and a cup of grapes is 1 point. Weight Watchers members are encouraged to eat the daily allowance of food points and are told not to go below the Daily Points Range in an effort to speed up weight loss. People can, however, "earn" extra points by stepping up their physical activity level. The point system was adapted in 2010 to take into account a more complex formula that recognizes each items mix of protein, fiber, carbohydrates, and fat. While some members embraced the new system, others, especially long-standing members, are more comfortable with the original point system.

An adult who wants to lose at least 5 pounds can join Weight Watchers. Weight Watchers stresses that it does not market to teens. All members who join start with a preliminary goal to lose 10 percent of their body weight. For example, a person who weighs 200 pounds and has perhaps been struggling and yo-yo dieting for years to try to reach 150 pounds may quickly find herself or himself disappointed. With the 10 percent goal, the person would reach the first goal at 180 pounds—a weight loss of 20 pounds. That builds up confidence in ability to lose weight. Then he or she can set the next goal.

Weight Watchers is not a quick-fix diet scheme. On its Web site, www.weight watchers.com, it states that the organization promotes a "healthy rate of weight loss—up to two pounds per week after the first three weeks."

Weight Watchers produces a bimonthly magazine and numerous cookbooks and inspirational books for those trying to lose weight and maintain that weight loss. Weekly meetings are key to the concept of Weight Watchers. The Weight Watchers Web site states,

"Preliminary scientific research shows that people who regularly attend Weight Watchers meetings lose more weight than people who try to lose weight on their own. Weight Watchers Leaders, who have all risen through the ranks as Weight Watchers meeting members and learned how to lose and successfully control their weight, lead meetings that follow a weekly curriculum. Their experience, techniques, and suggestions for solving problems can help you do what you're having trouble doing on your own: lose weight. Weight Watchers meeting members are also encouraged to share their weight-loss challenges and to celebrate their weight-loss victories at meetings . . . knowing that others are facing the same issues you're facing and hearing firsthand how they've solved or are working to solve similar problems can help keep you motivated and inspire you to stay the course."

For those who cannot join weekly meetings, Weight Watchers also offers online support through an Internet-based journal for tracking daily points, an online newsletter, and other support.

Weight Watchers generally receives good ratings from nutritionists because its emphasis is on moderate fat and balanced nutrients.

The Web site contains a FAQ section, success stories, and a search engine that allows a user to find the closest Weight Watchers meetings. Membership charges and special promotions are listed on the local group's contact information.

See also: Celebrity Endorsements; Hudson, Jennifer; Yo-Yo Dieting.

FURTHER READING

Ferguson, Sarah, Duchess of York. *Win the Weight Game: Successful Strategies for Living Well*. New York: Simon and Schuster, 2000.

Ferguson, Sarah, Duchess of York with Weight Watchers. *Energy Breakthrough: Jump-Start Your Weight Loss and Feel Great*. New York: Simon and Schuster, 2002.

Fletcher, Anne M. "Inside America's Hottest Diet Programs." *Prevention*, March 1990, 54.

Frascella, Larry. "An Exclusive Visit with Jean Nidetch." *Weight Watchers Magazine*, January 1988, 37.

Gootman, Elissa. "Weight Watchers Upends Its Points System." *The New York Times*, December 3, 2010, A1.

Heshka, Stanley, James W. Anderson, Richard L. Atkinson, Frank L. Greenway, James O. Hill, Stephen D. Phinney, Ronette L. Kolotkin, Karen Miller-Kovach, and F. Xavier Pi-Sunyer. "Weight Loss with Self-Help Compared with a Structured Commercial Program: A Randomized Trial." *Journal of the American Medical Association* 289 (April 9, 2003): 1792.

"Meet the Patrons of Prevention's Hall of Fame." *Prevention*, September 2000, 158.

Miller, Holly G. "Hips, Hips Away!" *Saturday Evening Post*, November 1988, 48.

Neal, Mollie. "Weight Watchers' Winning Marketing Strategy." *Direct Marketing*, August 1993, 24.

Nidetch, Jean. *Story of Weight Watchers*. New York: New American Library, 1979.

Olson, Elizabeth. "For Weight Watchers, Jennifer Hudson Wins a Losing Battle." *The New York Times*, April 6, 2010, B3.

Tisdale, Sallie. "A Weight That Women Carry: The Compulsion to Diet in a Starved Culture." *Harper's Magazine*, March 1993, 49.

Weight Watchers International, ed. *Weight Watchers New Complete Cook Book*. New York: John Wiley & Sons, 1998.

Weight Watchers International, ed. *Weight Watchers Stop Stuffing Yourself: 7 Steps to Conquering Overweight*. New York: John Wiley & Sons, 1999.

Weight-Loss Earrings

Spandex and tummy-control pantyhose are fashion staples for many who want to disguise some bulky spots—but weight-loss earrings are meant to be worn for others to see. Some use the concept of acupressure and aurilism, the mapping of key acupressure points on the ear. The magnetic earrings that are designed to put pressure on points of the ear that suppress appetite increase the metabolic rate and/or boost energy. Other available options are silicone toe rings that sellers say improve metabolism by enhancing foot massage.

While there are a number of magnetic weight-loss earrings advertised through eBay, Groupon, and Amazon, one brand of magnetic weight-loss earrings with its own Web site, called Aurislim, says that the product combines "traditional Chinese acupressure and three advanced scientific innovations: Magnetic Acupressure, Far Infrared Ultrasonic Auriculotherapy and Negative Ionization to achieve positive health benefits such as weight loss, faster metabolism, better rest and sleep, reduction of fats and cholesterol, healthy cardiovascular function and circulation, increase in energy levels, reduction of stress, improvement in the serotonin level to relieve depression and to enhance mood."

However, an FDA representative told *Family Circle* magazine, "There is no evidence of a biological basis for magnetic earrings affecting weight loss."

WebMD.com cited the Task Force on Weight Loss Abuse for the National Council against Health Fraud, which gave its "worst gimmick" prize in 2003 to MagnaSlim, a magnetized, acupressure product. It mentioned similar magnetized acupressure products, such as the earrings. The network wrote in its 2003 press release, "Combining the unproven theories of magnetic therapy and accupressure, MagnaSlim is a 'breakthrough in weight loss technology' that is said to control appetite and reduce stress and anxiety eating when worn at the wrist." Acupressure has been a favorite gimmick of weight loss promoters for years, usually zeroing in on a jazzy item that presses on so-called appetite centers on ears or wrists. Earrings or adhesives press beads, seeds, or other hard substances against these points. Or patches are soaked with herbal potions and attached in snake-oil-on-a-band-aid fashion. What's new here is that MagnaSlim contains '5 Proprietary blended magnets,' along with a "magnetized solution," that supposedly gives relief from hunger cravings. The magnetic field is claimed to penetrate every cell, realigning incorrectly positioned ions within the cells. Proper flow of "Chi" is restored by massage or heat at acupuncture points, which "polarizes Chi energy." Also sold as Magna 1.

See also: Slim Chance Awards.

FURTHER READING

Jibrin, Janis. "10 Diet Lies." *Family Circle*, November 1, 2010.
"Quick Weight Loss or Quackery." *Webmd.com*. http://www.webmd.com/diet/features/avoiding-quick-weight-loss-gimicks?page=2.
2003 Slim Chance Awards. Diet Scam Watch. http://www.dietscam.org/slim/2003.shtml.
www.aurislim.com.
www.earringtherapy.com.

Wheat Belly Diet

The Wheat Belly Diet gives followers a reason to reconsider the merits of their daily bread and to give it up in exchange for weight loss and good health. Dr. William Davis, a cardiologist, calls his diet a "radical wheat-ectomy" that will provide weight loss along with an end to many of the 21st-century problems that plague society including fatigue, arthritis, gastrointestinal distress, and obesity. Davis has lofty goals for his diet, a highly restrictive eating plan that moved to the top of the *New York Times* best-seller list following its release in 2011.

Davis links the growth of whole grain products with the growth of the national waistline. He points out that wheat is unlike other grains and its specific attributes make it destructive to human health. How did this long-standing staple of the American diet turn on us? Davis argues this is not the same grain our forebears baked into loaves. He describes how decades of genetic tinkering have created changes in the wheat protein structure. The changes were geared toward the goal of feeding a growing world population by creating wheat that would provide higher yields. Davis suggests Americans must eliminate wheat to have a healthy diet, a conclusion he says is supported by his own clinical studies and direct observation of patients who have made remarkable health improvements once they stopped eating wheat of any kind.

Davis assures dieters there is no problem or deficiency that develops from taking wheat out of a healthy diet and strongly urges followers to fill the gap with what he calls "real food," including vegetables, nuts, meats, eggs, olives, cheese, and avocados. He cautions against filling up on things like corn chips, energy bars, and fruit drinks. He encourages dieters to brace themselves against the pressure to eat "highly processed, herbicided, genetically modified, ready-to-eat, high-fructose corn syrup-filled, just-add-water food products" (Davis, p. 193) that come adorned with cartoon characters and clever marketing.

The author also takes an equally hardened approach to avoiding a long list of other foods in order to lose weight. He suggests that in addition to eliminating wheat, dieters should stop eating all cornstarch and cornmeal products like tacos, tortillas, and corn chips; snack foods from potato chips and rice cakes to popcorn; all desserts that include lots of sugar, such as pies, cakes, ice creams, and cupcakes; other grains such as quinoa, millet, oats, and buckwheat; dried fruits, especially cranberries, raisins, dates, and apricots; and all fruit juices and soft drinks because they cause spikes in blood sugar. He recommends severely limiting rice, both white and brown; potatoes, including white, red, sweet potatoes, and yams; legumes, especially black beans, kidney beans, chickpeas, and lentils; and gluten-free foods because they also cause quick blood sugar spikes.

Davis said he discovered the harmful effects of wheat in his own research. As a cardiologist, he was focused on controlling the risks of heart disease but found that wheat raises blood sugar, and, during digestion, one of the wheat proteins causes appetite stimulation, which then begins a cycle of cravings for more carbohydrates. He called this a prescription for weight gain and fat storage. Still, while critics approve of the general message of Davis's diet and its focus on fresh vegetables and less processed foods, they say that cutting out whole categories of foods is not sound nutrition. Instead, they recommend a diet that focuses on variety with all kinds of fruits and vegetables, whole grains, and lean proteins. Critics of the diet add that portion sizes are also important and more Americans would be better off if they just ate smaller servings of bread and pasta and other carbohydrate-laden foods rather than eliminating them altogether.

In his diet book, Davis lists safe foods. He advocates eating vegetables with breakfast, lunch, and dinner and cautions that some fruits, especially those high in sugar, such as bananas, pineapple, mango, and papaya, are okay but only in limited amounts. He calls raw nuts a healthy choice as long as they are not roasted in oils or processed in other ways. Oils can be used generously, as long as they are limited to what Davis describes as the healthy oils: olive oil, coconut oil, avocado oil, and cocoa butter. Oils to avoid include sunflower, safflower, canola, corn, and vegetable oils, and Davis welcomes plenty of meat and eggs as healthy alternative foods. He also encourages dieters to eat all kinds of cheeses but limit yogurt, milk, and butter consumption to a few servings per day. While soy products have become increasingly controversial, Davis recommends eating fermented forms of soy such as tofu, tempeh, and miso in limited portions. He admits vegetarians and vegans will have a tough time following his diet but suggests with careful planning it can be done.

Recognizing the difficulty of following his diet, Davis provides a week's worth of meal ideas in his book. Breakfast suggestions include hot coconut flaxseed cereal, different egg dishes, humus with sliced vegetables, a mozzarella and tomato salad, or an egg-and-pesto breakfast wrap. Lunch choices range from a spinach and mushroom salad, tuna-avocado salad, baked Portobello mushrooms with crabmeat and goat cheese, or a vegetable soup. Dinners might be a parmesan-crusted pork chop with roasted vegetables; a vegetable and mushroom stir fry, pecan-crusted baked chicken, or a baked wild salmon with steamed vegetables.

While Davis stands by his conclusions, it remains to be seen what further research by other nutritionists and physicians will uncover about modified and hybrid foods and how they impact human health. With the popularity of gluten-free foods, it is certain that the study of wheat consumption will be at the forefront of research for some time.

See also: Carbohydrates, Gluten-free, Obesity and Paleo Diet

FURTHER READING

Davis, William. *Wheat Belly: Lose the Wheat, Lose the Weight, and Find Your Path Back to Health.* New York: Rodale, Inc., 2011.

Palmer, Sharon. "Wheat: Friend or Foe? Some of Today's Hottest Diets Advise You to Say No to Wheat." *Environmental Nutrition* 36, no. 4 (April 2013): 1.

Tweed, Vera. "Grain of Truth: Stay Healthy and Trim, the Wheat-Free Way." *Better Nutrition* 74, no. 10 (October 2012): 60.

Xenical

Xenical is a weight-loss drug that was approved by the Food and Drug Administration (FDA) in May 1999. The drug works by blocking an enzyme needed to digest fat and prevents about 30 percent of ingested dietary fat from being absorbed by the body. That undigested fat accumulates in the intestines and is excreted in the stool. Side effects associated with Xenical include bloating, flatulence, oily stool, diarrhea, and fecal incontinence. Company officials say that maintaining a diet with no more than 30 percent of calories from fat can minimize these side effects.

Clinical trials also show that Xenical partially depletes fat-soluble vitamins A, D, E, and K and beta-carotene. Physicians advise patients taking the medication to also take a multivitamin. The drug is recommended only for patients considered clinically obese, with a BMI of 30 or higher, or those who suffer from other risk factors of obesity, including high blood pressure and diabetes. In a clinical study reported in the June 2001 edition of *Chemist & Druggist*, results showed more than 15,500 overweight men and women lost an average of 11 percent of body weight over a period of seven months while taking Xenical. The drug was taken in combination with a reduced-calorie diet. In 2007 the FDA approved the weight-loss pill, Alli, as an over-the-counter, lower-strength version of Xenical. This was the first nonprescription drug approved by the agency for dieters and sales of Alli were expected to be huge; however, the pill had not met projections and had been hampered by distribution problems and an issue with possible package tampering.

Xenical differs from weight control medications that work on brain chemistry to control appetite, like Redux and fen-phen. The FDA withdrew both Redux and fen-phen from the market in 1997, citing concerns over reported cases of heart-valve abnormalities in users. Diet industry analysts consider Xenical a competitor of the obesity drug Meridia, which was removed from the market in October 2010. Sales figures for Xenical's first full year in 2000 came to $225 million in U.S. retail sales. Sales in 2001 dropped to $157 million. By 2004, sales in America had dropped to $102 million; Hoffmann–La Roche officials, makers of the medication, had originally predicted annual sale of $1 billion. The company attributed the slower-than-expected sales to the failure of physicians to treat obesity with drug therapy and to patients' difficulties securing insurance reimbursements for Xenical. Those disappointing sales figures and the recall of all supplies of Alli in the United States and Puerto Rico in 2014 after reports of tampering were major blows to the manufacturer GlaxoSmithKline.

See also: Fen-Phen; Meridia.

FURTHER READING

Freeman, Miller. "Weight Loss Pill Offers Added Health Benefits." *Chemist & Druggist*, June 9, 2001, 10.

Gleick, Elizabeth. "Available from a Doctor Near You." *Time International*, October 25, 1999, 65.

Hirschler, Ben. "GSK Recalls Weight-Loss Drug Alli in U.S. on Tampering Concerns." *Reuters*, March 27, 2014. http://www.reuters.com/article/2014/03/27/us-gsk-alli-idUS BREA2Q12K20140327.

Morehouse, Macon. "Girth Control: Despite Nasty Side Effects, Americans Are Tripping over Their Scales to Get the New Diet Drug Xenical. Is It Safe?" *People Weekly*, June 7, 1999, 113–14.

Saul, Stephanie. "2 Approaches to the Nation's Obesity Epidemic Coming Up for Review." *The New York Times*, January 17, 2006, C2.

Wilhelm, Carolyn. "Growing the Market for Anti-Obesity Drugs." *Chemical Market Reporter* 256, no. 20 (May 15, 2000): 23.

Yo-Yo Dieting

Yo-yo dieting, also known as weight cycling, occurs when a person experiences cycles of weight loss and weight gain resembling the up and down of a yo-yo. The pattern begins with rapid weight loss normally associated with the use of fad diets or diet pills. However, once a goal weight is reached, dieters return to their original, poor eating habits. This causes the lost pounds to return, followed by extra weight gain. Each time yo-yo dieters lose weight through the use of pills, liquid diet drinks, or fads like a high-protein, high-fat, low-carbohydrate diet, like the Atkins diet, they lose mostly lean muscle and water but only a small amount of fat. However, when those pounds return, it is in the form of fat with very little muscle regained. The psychological effects of yo-yo dieting include depression and the erosion of confidence and self-esteem.

While research shows weight cycling may not benefit individuals who have only small amounts of weight to lose, doctors caution that severely obese individuals should not allow concerns about the hazards of weight cycling to deter them from efforts to control their body weight. Instead, individuals who undertake a weight-loss program should consult a doctor first. They should also expect to make lifelong changes in their eating, behavior, and physical activity. The National Task Force on the Prevention and Treatment of Obesity studies show that, for obese individuals, keeping off just 5 to 15 pounds permanently can have a positive impact on overall health.

See also: Atkins Nutritional Approach; Obesity.

FURTHER READING

O'Connor, Anahad. "The Claim: Repeated Dieting Slows Your Metabolism." *The New York Times*, May 17, 2005.

Reinberg, Steven. "Yo-Yo Dieting Can Hurt the Heart, Study Finds; Older Women Who Lose Weight and Then Regain It May Raise Their Risk of Cardiovascular Trouble." *Consumer Health News*, December 13, 2012, p: NA.

"Stop Yo-Yo Dieting for Good." *Prevention* 65, no. 4 (April 2013): 12.

The Zone

The Zone, published in 1995 by Barry Sears, is a one-man crusade against carbohydrates. The "Zone" is defined by its creator as a metabolic state in which the mind is relaxed and focused, and the body is strong and works at peak efficiency. As Sears explains, the Zone is not some mystical place but instead relates to keeping hormones, such as insulin, within specified ranges. To reach the "Zone," dieters must eat a ratio of 40 percent carbohydrates, 30 percent proteins, and 30 percent fat per meal. In other words, eat the butter, not the bread. And stay away from the "danger" zone foods like pasta, bagels, rice, potatoes, bananas, carrots, apple juice, and ketchup.

Sears calls the Zone diet a moderate-carbohydrate, moderate-protein, and moderate-fat program. A typical day's Zone menu includes protein in a percentage considerably above what the U.S. Department of Agriculture (USDA) suggests. The recommended dietary allowance (RDA) for a young man between the ages of 15 and 24 years is from 52 to 56 grams of protein per day, although intake often reaches as high as 90 grams per day. The RDA for a young woman in that same age range is from 40 to 46 grams per day, but the average woman in this category often eats up to 65 grams of protein per day. Sears maintains that the Zone diet is not high in protein because a typical day's menu is not over 100 grams of protein a day, which he says does not exceed the newest protein guidelines set by the American Heart Association (AHA). Those guidelines urge adults to eat between 10 and 35 percent of total daily calories in protein foods, depending on age, weight, and other factors. That recommendation means eating no more than 6 ounces (cooked) per day of lean meat, fish, or skinless poultry. The AHA also suggests that high-fiber plant foods and grains are an important part of a nutritionally balanced diet because they help lower cholesterol.

A Zone breakfast might include four scrambled egg whites with one ounce of low-fat cheese, a cup of strawberries, and a small cup of oatmeal. Lunch possibilities could be a chicken Caesar salad, two cups of vegetables, and a medium apple. Dinner might consist of six ounces of fish with slivered almonds, combined with four cups of vegetables, such as broccoli, onions, mushrooms, bell peppers, and tomatoes, with fresh fruit for dessert. The Zone allows an average person, defined by the American Dietetic Association (ADA) as a 154-pound active male, up to 1,500 calories per day. In contrast, the ADA suggests that same person eat a balanced diet of some 2,600 calories each day to maintain his or her current weight.

Sears claims a person in the "Zone" will experience permanent body-fat loss, optimal health, greater athletic performance, and improved mental productivity. Zoners will burn fat while they also fight heart disease, diabetes, premenstrual syndrome, chronic fatigue, depression, and cancer. The Zone literature suggests that when carbohydrate intake is controlled, the body burns fat faster and food cravings disappear. According to Sears, non-Zoners produce excess insulin from eating carbohydrates and this "excess" somehow creates food cravings, especially for more carbohydrates. The cycle of excess insulin production from complex carbohydrates, like pasta, breads, and bagels, is kept in motion by the resulting lowered blood sugar levels that the cravings produce. Sears says his theory is supported by published clinical research.

Critics argue that people develop excess insulin, a condition called insulin resistance, from being overweight and sedentary. When insulin resistance takes place, a person's cells won't absorb glucose unless an abnormally large amount of insulin is on hand. Nutrition and health critics maintain that this is not a consequence of eating too many carbohydrates and they say medical research has not linked insulin levels to weight gain in healthy people. Critics also point to studies showing that eating fat in the form of steak, cheese, or bacon can contribute to a number of health problems from high cholesterol levels to the development of cardiovascular disease.

Although The Zone contradicts decades of nutritional wisdom, scientists agree with one aspect of this diet: the body does turn carbohydrates into glucose. In fact, eating anything—whether it's carbohydrates, protein, or fat—causes blood-sugar levels to rise, which in turn stimulates insulin production. Critics say problems develop when a person loads up on protein and limits carbohydrates. Sears answers critics by saying the Zone cannot be considered a high-protein diet, since an individual who follows the program is eating more carbohydrates than protein. And the Zone doesn't forbid all carbohydrates; high-fiber fruits and vegetables are fine, but it discourages the more complex carbohydrates, which nutritionists say are important to a well-balanced diet.

The AHA cautions against what the association called high-protein weight-loss programs, listing the Atkins Diet, the Zone, Protein Power, and Sugar Busters! The report in the AHA journal Circulation cited a lack of credible scientific evidence of long-term weight loss for these programs and the possibility of increased risk for those with diabetes and heart disease.

Dieters following plans that limit specific categories of foods, like carbohydrates, will initially see pounds melt off due to water loss and because of a lowered total calorie intake. Although carbohydrates are essential for fueling muscles and the brain, the body can't store a very large amount. So when dieters eat fewer carbohydrates than their body needs, the body reacts as though it were starving and releases the water that's stored, along with its small supply of carbohydrates. In addition, the ongoing glucose shortages will cause the body to start burning fats for fuel, releasing fatty acids called ketones into the bloodstream. Doctors say abnormally high ketone levels lead to ketosis, and ketosis sets the stage for gout or kidney disease in susceptible people. Sears says it is impossible to develop ketosis on the Zone diet because it has more carbohydrates than protein, but critics maintain that the amount of carbohydrates eaten on the Zone diet still falls below daily intake requirements for a healthy diet.

Throughout The Zone, Sears cites his own studies, case histories, and testimonials as proof that this diet works. Critics point out none of his studies has been published in peer-reviewed journals where experts evaluate the articles before being accepted for publication. Sears says that investigators, including those from Harvard Medical School, have reconfirmed his data in peer-reviewed research. Many critics sarcastically suggest the real "zone" is actually a money zone, since there are over 2 million copies of his best seller in print and it has been translated into 14 languages. Sears followed *The Zone* with more titles: *Mastering the Zone*, which spent 11 weeks on the best-seller list; *The Anti-Aging Zone; The Soy Zone;* and *Zone Perfect Meals in Minutes.*

Although the Zone diet may provide short-term weight loss, its long-term effectiveness is still questionable. Skeptics include the AHA, whose Nutrition Committee reported as far back as 2001 that the initial, rapid weight loss often produced by high-protein diets is due mostly to a temporary fluid loss caused by eating fewer carbohydrates. The committee also noted that high-protein diets could compromise vitamin and mineral intake and cause heart, liver, and kidney abnormalities.

Representatives of the American Cancer Society (ACS) also had harsh words for what they called high-protein diets, which they charge can raise cholesterol levels, promote development of cardiovascular disease, and raise the risk of various cancers. In contrast, the ACS suggests a diet high in fruits and vegetables, low in fat, and lower in protein. Sears says his diet is in line with those recommendations because it is rich in fruits and vegetables. But the real answer to losing weight, according to nutritionists, is through hard work, changed eating habits, and increased exercise, a plan more commonly known as "eat less, exercise more."

See also: Dietary Guidelines for Americans; MyPlate; Sears, Barry; Sugar Busters!.

FURTHER READING

Goldstein, Joseph. "The New Age Cavemen and the City." *The New York Times,* January 8, 2010, ST1.

Kaufman, Frederick. "The Zone." *Harper's Magazine,* January 2000, 72.

Proulx, Lawrence G. "To Each His Zone: BestSelling Book Promises Amazing Rewards from Its Unorthodox Approach to Eating." *Washington Post,* February 4, 1997, Z16.

Ratnesar, Romesh. "Against the Grain: The Low-Carb Zone Diet Rises from Fad to Fixture." *Time,* December 15, 1997, 86.

Shaffer, Alyssa Lustigman. "The Great Nutrient Debate: Hollywood Loves 'the Zone' and Americans Love Their Pasta Bowls." *Weight Watchers Magazine,* March/April 1998, 39–42.

Squires, Sally. "Heart Association Skewers Atkins Diet; High Protein Plans Called Unproven, Risky." *Washington Post,* October 9, 2001, F01.

Timeline

1847	Physicians form the American Medical Association (AMA) with two goals: to draw up a code of moral ethics and to seek educational reform to raise the standards of medical training and establish uniform minimum requirements for medical degrees.
1850	The American Vegetarian Society is founded.
1863	William Banting writes what historians believe is the first diet book, *A Letter on Corpulence*. At his death in 1878, more than 58,000 copies of the book have been sold and "banting" is a popular term for dieting.
1879	Saccharin becomes the first sugar substitute. The discovery is the result of an accidental spill during research being done on food preservatives.
1894	The U.S. Department of Agriculture (USDA) develops the first food composition tables and dietary standards for Americans.
1906	Pure Food and Drug Act is enacted. This first federal food and drug law means manufacturers involved in interstate sales cannot make false statements on their product's label. However diet aids are exempt, since they are not considered drugs and obesity is not considered a disease.
1907	Yale scientists announce the results of a series of experiments proving that the strict diet and thorough mastication of food, practiced by Horace Fletcher and known as Fletcherism, has been an effective aid in treating obesity, gout, and dyspepsia. Researchers say the studies also prove that nerves play an important part

in digestion, agreeing with Fletcher that many emotions actually stop the flow of gastric juices. They agree with Fletcher's rule for eating: do not eat when you are mad or sad, only when you are glad.

1909   At a meeting of the Society of Internal Medicine in Paris, French doctor Marcel Labbé calls for an end to the medical treatment of obesity. He recommends that the best course of action is to reduce the intake of fats, bread, pastries, sweets, and salt and to exercise to lessen fat and increase muscular tissue.

1911   Dr. W. Wayne Babcock, a Philadelphia surgeon, announces the latest method of reducing stoutness, the surgical removal of abdominal fat. In his demonstration, he cut open the patient's abdomen, turned back the flesh, and removed superfluous fat. He cautions that great care must be taken to avoid severing any muscles. After the operation, Dr. Babcock reports that the woman is 12 pounds lighter.

1917   The U.S. government releases dietary recommendations in a publication titled *How to Select Foods,* and calls for five food groups: milk and meat; cereals; vegetables and fruits; fats and fat foods; and sugars and sugary foods.

1924   A scrub brush, slightly softer than a kitchen scrub brush, is introduced as a flesh reducer and weight-loss tool. For maximum results every part of the body is massaged four or five times a day. After rubbing, the dieter is told to take a cold shower. Promoters say dieters can expect a pound or so of "excess" fat to magically disappear each week. Dr. Lulu Hunt Peters, a popular diet-book author, publishes the first diet book for children, *Diet for Children (and adults) and the Kalorie Kids* (New York: Dodd, Mead and Company).

1925   Pennsylvania officials with the Delaware County Tuberculosis Association declare that survey results show local high school girls are "starving themselves" in an effort to maintain stylish silhouette figures and are "dangerously underweight." Weight-loss methods range from starvation diets to eating pickles and ice cream instead of regular meals. The association secretary claims the girls start dieting when they reach 15 years old, the flapper age.

1927   A noted British dietitian pronounces obesity the result of a state of mind. He suggests that the way to get thin is to adopt the correct attitude along with a correct diet and exercise.

1930   A slump in English potato sales is attributed to the "slim-figure craze" of English women. The Ulster Minister of Agriculture blames women who are no longer eating potatoes and announces that the government is searching for other markets.

1933   An overweight San Francisco physician dies from a violent fever generated by an overdose of the diet drug dinitrophenol, according to a report published in the *Lancet*. Dinitrophenol and the more powerful dinitro-ortho-cresol are both drugs that accelerate metabolism, and the report recommends that dieters seek medical guidance before taking either drug.

1934   Results of a scientifically supervised, 30-day diet of bananas and skim milk show that three women participants were able to lose a total of 32 pounds. Dr. Herman N. Bundesen, the Chicago Health Commissioner, supervised the diet and recommends it to anyone with excess pounds.

1935   The New York State Hairdressers and Cosmetologists Association calls for government legislation to ban dieting by women. They say "public health protection" is needed to stop the starvation mania endangering the health of its members.

1938   Congress passes the Food, Drug, and Cosmetic Act, requiring that products must be proven safe before they reach the market. Diet aids are covered by the Act for the first time.

1939   The Metropolitan Life Insurance Company reports a trend toward "fashionable thinness" among American women. The company compared average weights among insured women from the years 1922–1923 and 1932–1934 and noted a general 3- to 5-pound decline in average weight for each height and at every age.

1941   The Food and Nutrition Board of the National Academy of Sciences announces the development of its recommended daily allowances, or RDAs.

1942   The American Medical Association (AMA) issues a public statement disapproving of amphetamines for the treatment of obesity because of problems of dependence. The U.S. Department of Agriculture announces the "Basic Seven" food groups as part of its year-old recommended daily allowances. The seven food groups include green and yellow vegetables; oranges, tomatoes, and grapefruit; potatoes and other vegetables and fruit; milk and milk products; meat, poultry, fish, eggs, and dried peas and beans; bread, flour, and cereals; and butter and fortified margarine. The guide also suggests alternate choices in the event of wartime shortages.

1943   Overweight American women are compromising the nation's wartime food supply, according to the Metropolitan Life Insurance Company. Company officials release a new "ideal" weight table with three separate groups of women, those with slight, medium, and heavy builds. And company officials suggest wartime rationing of food can help with weight reduction programs.

1946   A U.S. Department of Agriculture bulletin advises overweight Americans to reduce their consumption of wheat and fats, pointing out that these are the foods most needed in Europe due to food rationing.

1947   A Cornell University doctor reports that nonglandular obesity in women should be regarded as a neurosis and must be treated with intensive psychotherapy.

1948   Milwaukee, Wisconsin, resident, Esther Manz, founds the organization Take Off Pounds Sensibly (TOPS), the first of the national dieting groups.

1950   The American Society of Bariatric Physicians begins as the National Obesity Society. After several name changes it becomes the ASBP with a shift in treatment of obesity away from glands toward appetite and exercise.

1952   Dietary experts with the U.S. Department of Health announce that New Yorkers lost 3.2 million pounds during a two-week heat wave. Director of the department's Bureau of Nutrition attributed the loss to the drop in appetite when temperatures soared. He calculated that 8 million New Yorkers ate 100 calories less each day, meaning an individual weekly loss of two-fifth of a pound during the early July record temperatures.

1954   A rounded plastic device to relieve hunger pangs is patented by the U.S. government. The device, invented by Dr. William S. Kroger of Evanston, Illinois, will abolish the hunger pangs that occur around mealtime, according to the doctor. He said pressing the device into the stomach just below the breastbone will produce a feeling of fullness. He blamed 98 percent of overweight on eating due to emotional tension. He believes his device will help in the national battle of the bulge.

1955   A patent is issued for a calorie counter, a small instrument to be carried in the pocket or handbag by dieters. The user records calories eaten during the day to gauge how much of a daily quota has been consumed. The patent is issued to Charles G. Hallowell of West Hartford, Connecticut.

1956   President Dwight D. Eisenhower establishes the President's Council on Physical Fitness to encourage American children to lead healthy, active, and physically fit lives. First named the President's Council on Youth Fitness by Eisenhower, the name was changed to the President's Council on Physical Fitness by President John F. Kennedy to reflect its expanded mandate to serve all Americans. The American Medical Association's Council on Foods and Nutrition warns against the indiscriminate use of new low-protein diets, also known as "Rockefeller" or "fabulous formula" diets. Based on experimental diets developed at the Rockefeller Institute of Medical Research, both plans call for lowered protein intake. One diet, the fabulous formula, is a liquid combination of corn oil, evaporated milk, and dextrose. The Rockefeller diet calls for low-protein foods. The council pointed to serious hazards not made clear in any publicity for the diets. The American Academy of Pediatrics, at its 25th and largest meeting, opens its session with a discussion of childhood obesity. The speakers caution American mothers who feed their babies on the "self-demand" regime that they may be overfeeding and subsequently setting their children up for a progression of problems with overweight. The U.S. Department of Agriculture "Basic Seven" food groups are condensed to the "Basic Four" in a publication titled *Essentials of an Adequate Diet*.

1957   The modern Christian dieting industry begins when Charlie Shedd, a minister who lost 100 pounds, publishes *Pray Your Weight Away*.

1958   Congress passes the Food Additives Amendment to the Food, Drug, and Cosmetic Act, which requires premarket approval from the Food and Drug Administration (FDA) for food additives developed after 1958.

1960   Overeaters Anonymous, a dieting group similar in style to Alcoholics Anonymous, is founded.

1961   Weight Watchers is established. The Food, Drug, and Cosmetic Act is revised to require that all new drugs and old drugs claiming new uses have to show that they are safe as well as effective.

1962   Findings released from the Hormone Research Laboratory of the University of California's Berkeley campus find the pituitary hormone ACTH has fat-dissolving activity and may greatly improve treatment of glandular obesity. Lab tests on rats and rabbits show a rapid breakdown of the solid form of fats into liquid fats that can be removed from the body by natural clearing mechanisms.

1963   The Federal Trade Commission (FTC) issues a complaint against the author and publisher of the former best-seller *Calories Don't Count*. The FTC charges that the book made false claims for the value of safflower oil in promoting improved health and weight loss. The commission files charges against Simon and Schuster, Inc., and the author, Dr. Herman Taller.

1964   The first time an advertising agency is indicted because of the ads it prepared for a client. A federal grand jury indicts a New York advertising agency on charges of writing fraudulent advertising copy for Regimen tablets, a weight-loss pill.

1965   The first time an advertising agency is convicted for promoting the product of a client. A federal jury finds the advertising agency of Kastor, Hilton, Chesley, Clifford & Atherton, Inc., guilty of promoting a fraudulent claim that Regimen tablets cause a substantial weight loss without dieting.

1967   The Oregon State Medical Examiner announces that six deaths have been linked to weight-reducing pills. Citing a two-year investigation into the pills by the State Crime Laboratory, he concludes that the pills depleted the dieters of potassium, leading to death. Although no brand name is released, the pills contained drugs that allegedly interacted to cause death, including amphetamines, Phenobarbital, digitalis, plain vegetable laxative, and a thiazide diuretic. The women who died ranged in age from 19 to 52.

1968   The Relaxacisor is promoted as a pleasant, effortless way to firm, tone, and tighten muscles without exercise. The handheld device delivers a mild electric shock to the skin, causing muscles to involuntarily contract. More than 400,000 Americans buy the machine before the FDA bans it as ineffective and dangerous.

1971   A group of New York doctors announces the first voluntary ban in the United States on prescribing amphetamines for use in treating obesity.

1972   The FDA announces a move to restrict unnecessary and potentially harmful use of diet pills and vitamins. The agency's action against diet pills is made public in testimony before a U.S. Senate subcommittee. Dr. Robert Atkins publishes *Dr. Atkin's' Diet Revolution*.

1973   The U.S. Senate Select Committee on Nutrition and Human Needs holds hearings devoted to people with "overnutrition," the estimated 30 percent of the U.S. population who are overweight. Dr. Robert Atkins appears before the committee to answer questions about the safety of his diet.

1974   The FDA announces that a drug produced from the urine of pregnant women must bear a label saying it is worthless for weight loss. The hormone human chorionic gonadotropin (HCG) has been used in antifat clinics around the country but the FDA declares that there is no evidence it is effective in treating obesity. The U.S. Postal Service bans "Slimmer Shake" or "Joe Weider's Weight Loss Formula XR-7" from the mail on the grounds of false advertising. The product promises a 14-pound weight loss in 14 days but the company only provides a 12-day supply. The advertising also claims there is no need to restrict caloric intake but the product arrives with instructions to eat only the "slimmer shake" plus one quart of milk per day and no other food.

1975   A New York man pleads guilty to mail fraud and false advertising for "Slim-Tabs Slenderizing tablets," a concoction allegedly designed to slim a dieter down 48 pounds in eight weeks. The company received $1.1 million in orders within a six-month period and promised that if customers were dissatisfied they would receive a $25 U.S. Savings Bond.

1977   The FDA proposes a ban on the artificial sweetener saccharin after evidence links its use to bladder tumors in experimental animals. Weight-watching groups lobby in Washington, D.C., and force Congress to place a moratorium on the FDA ban.

1978   The FDA reverses its earlier order calling for warning labels on all liquid protein diets. The new regulation requires warning labels only on protein products that provide more than 50 percent of a person's calories, if those products are promoted for weight loss or as a food supplement.

1979   Advertisements for an "electronic diet fork" explain that the eating utensil induces weight loss through behavior modification. The fork has lights in the handle: a green light tells dieters when to start eating; a red light tells them when to stop.

1980   Dr. Herman Tarnower, physician and author of the best-selling *Complete Scarsdale Medical Diet,* is shot and killed in the bedroom of his home. His longtime companion, Jean S. Harris, is tried and convicted of murder. The first Dietary Guidelines for Americans are released by the USDA and the Department of Health and Human Services, to be revised every five years.

1981   The *Beverly Hills Diet* is published, based on the notion that undigested food, stuck in the body, causes weight gain. During the first 10 days of the diet, only fruits are allowed. The book also claims that two-hour rests are needed between different food types so those different enzymes will not interfere with digestion. The *Journal of the American Medical Association* publishes a scathing criticism of the diet.

1982   The FDA orders starch blockers off the market after it receives reports of adverse reactions, including 30 cases requiring hospitalization and 1 death. Makers of starch blockers claim that enzymes extracted from beans can block digestion of significant amounts of dietary starch, causing weight loss.

1983   The first liposuction surgery to reduce subcutaneous body fat is performed in the United States. U.S. soft drink companies begin using NutraSweet artificial sweetener in diet beverages. Popular singer Karen Carpenter's death brings national attention to the serious consequences of anorexia nervosa and bulimia nervosa.

1984   A National Institutes of Health panel calls obesity a major killer in the United States.

1985   The Center for Science in the Public Interest (CSPI) indicts fast-food chains for deep-frying with beef fat rather than with oils lower in saturated fats.

1986   The FDA allows only two drugs to be used in nonprescription diet aids, phenylpropanolamine (PPA), an appetite suppressant, and benzocaine with caffeine, which numbs the tongue to reduce the sense of taste. The McDonalds Corporation announces that it will make a booklet available listing the ingredients of its fast foods following pressure from consumer groups to release that information. Coca-Cola announces that it is replacing its 99-year-old formula with a sweeter-tasting formula. Consumer protests convince the company to reintroduce the old formula as Coca-Cola Classic.

1987   The FDA approves Lovastatin, a cholesterol-lowering drug.

1988   A report published in the *Journal of the American Medical Association* concludes that 80 percent of middle-aged American men run a sizable risk of dying prematurely from heart disease due to high cholesterol levels in their blood.

1989   The FDA *Consumer* magazine issues a report listing questionable and unsafe diet remedies, including skin patches, herbal capsules, grapefruit diet pills, and Chinese magic weight-loss earrings.

1990   The Nutrition Labeling and Education Act of 1990 takes effect.

1991   The U.S. government introduces its Food Guide Pyramid, which encourages the consumption of grains, vegetables, and fruits, and recommends fewer servings each day of dairy and meat foods along with fats and sweets.

1992   Researchers speaking before the annual meeting of the New York Society of Behavioral Medicine in New York announce a newly defined eating disorder more common than anorexia or bulimia, called "binge eating disorder," marked by frequent, uncontrolled eating episodes. Unlike people with bulimia, those with binge eating disorder do not try to lose or purge extra calories; they simply gain weight. Experts say commercial weight-loss programs only increase the problem.

1994   The death of gymnast Christy Henrich due to anorexia nervosa and bulimia nervosa focuses attention on eating disorders among female athletes, especially in sports like gymnastics where thinness is stressed.

1995   The National Center for Health Statistics reports that the proportion of American children who are overweight has more than doubled in the last three decades, following its most recent study from 1988 to 1991.

1996   The American Cancer Society releases guidelines recommending that people lower their cancer risk by eating very little meat and consuming a higher proportion of plant foods. The FDA proposes new warning labels for over-the-counter diet pills containing phenylpropanolamine (PPA).

1997   The U.S. Surgeon General declares childhood obesity to be an epidemic in America. The FDA withdraws Redux and fen-phen diet drugs from the market, citing concerns over reported cases of heart-valve abnormalities in users.

1998   The National Institutes of Health estimates that 97 million adult Americans are overweight or obese. The newly released figures also show that 300,000 unnecessary deaths a year can be attributed to the disease of obesity. Obesity is defined by the federal government as excessive mass when compared to height. College student Jared Fogle creates his own weight-loss plan based on a daily diet of Subway sandwiches and little else. By 1999 he lost over 100 pounds and was well on his way to a total weight loss of 245 pounds and a career as a spokesperson for the chain restaurant.

1999   The FDA approves the obesity drug Xenical (Orlistat), a lipase inhibitor that decreases absorption of dietary fat by 30 percent.

2000   The U.S. Department of Agriculture Food Guide Pyramid is revised to reflect changing nutritional information. The USDA sponsors the Great Nutrition Debate, a discussion panel featuring popular diet-book authors as well as nutrition and weight-loss researchers. The FDA issues a public health warning cautioning consumers against taking products containing phenylpropanolamine. The FDA also asks manufacturers to voluntarily replace it with alternative active ingredients.

            French nutritionist Pierre Dukan publishes his first diet book to international acclaim. Dukan was convinced that overweight and obesity were due to eating too many carbohydrates. He joins the ranks of other high-protein advocates with his four-phase diet plan, which has been harshly criticized by his French medical peers.

2001   The Electronic Retailing Association, in collaboration with the Federal Trade Commission, is awarded one of the largest false advertising settlements in history—a $10 million judgment against

Enforma Natural Products for best-selling pills called Exercise in a Bottle and Fat Trapper. Fat Trapper was advertised as being able to "trap up to 120 grams of fat per day." Infomercials told consumers they "could eat what you want and never, ever, ever have to diet again."

Eating like the cavemen, or Paleolithic, nutrition gets a boost with the publication of *The Paleo Diet* by Loren Cordain. While the idea became popular with athletes and many struggling with autoimmune and other chronic health problems, the revised edition in 2010 would reach millions of dieters, thanks to the Internet and social media.

2002   The Internal Revenue Service recognizes obesity as a disease, clearing the way for taxpayers to claim weight-loss expenses as a medical deduction. To take the deduction, a person must participate in a weight-loss program for medical reasons. Only those who itemize and whose medical expenses total more than 7.5 percent of their adjusted gross income can take the deduction.

2003   Illinois becomes the first state to ban ephedra-based products.

The release of *The South Beach Diet* by cardiologist Dr. Arthur Agatston, an instant success, introduces millions of Americans to the concept of the glycemic index of foods. Agatston distinguished his diet from other carbohydrate-restrictive plans like the Atkins and Zone diets by also restricting the consumption of saturated fat.

2004   Reality television combines with the American dieting obsession to create *The Biggest Loser*, a program that chronicles the attempts of severely obese men and women as they struggle to lose weight through intensive fitness training, nutritional instruction, and behavior modification in front of the cameras.

The documentary film *Super Size Me* by director Morgan Spurlock is a critical success at the Sundance film festival. It follows Spurlock for 30 days as he eats only McDonalds food and supersizes his meals every time the option is offered. Supersized value meals are taken out of the McDonalds menu later that year.

2005   A program designed as an alternative to the classic gym workout sells millions of copies. The P90X by Tony Horton has been called the most successful fitness product in U.S. history with workouts based on the principles of variety, intensity, and consistency.

2006   Bananas are in short supply around the world with the release of the *Banana Diet*, an eating plan developed by a Japanese couple. The diet calls for bananas for breakfast along with a regular lunch and dinner plus other restrictions.

2007   The Food and Drug Administration (FDA) approves the first over-the-counter weight-loss pill. Orlistat, sold as "alli" by GlaxoSmithKline PLC, is the first nonprescription drug approved by the agency for dieters. The prescription version of the pill is Xenical.

2009   The First Lady, Michelle Obama, breaks ground on the White House Kitchen Garden in an effort to begin a national conversation about healthy nutrition. Although there have been other gardens on the White House lawn, this is the largest, most expansive to date.

            The Center for Science in the Public Interest issues a warning to U.S. consumers concerning free trials of acai diet products.

2010   The Let's Move campaign is announced by First Lady Michelle Obama as part of her goal to solve the national problem of childhood obesity within a generation of children. The program aims to unite public and private resources to mobilize families, communities, and schools to help kids become more active and eat better as a way to better health.

            The Food Safety Modernization Act is passed at the end of the year by Congress and signed by the president in an attempt to change the focus of government food safety systems. The law now allows the Food and Drug Administration to issue mandatory recalls when unsafe food is detected.

2011   MyPlate replaces the USDA MyPyramid as a reminder for Americans to think about healthy food choices. The MyPlate logo shows a plate with portions of grains, vegetables, fruits, lean protein foods, and a small serving of dairy products.

            The Healthy Eating Plate is released by nutritionists at the Harvard School of Public Health in partnership with editors at Harvard Health Publications to illustrate the flaws they suggest are in the USDA MyPlate program.

2012   Canadian officials approve stevia for use as a food additive and dietary supplement. The Food and Drug Administration still does not consider stevia to be an artificial sweetener. As a dietary supplement, it remains unregulated by the U.S. government.

2013   The DASH (Dietary Approaches to Stop Hypertension) diet is once again named the best diet overall by U.S. New & World Report based on a review by a panel of diet and nutrition experts. The diets were judged on safety, nutritional completeness, the likelihood that dieters would lose weight and whether the diet protected against health conditions such as heart disease and diabetes.

2014   Weight Watchers celebrity spokesperson Jennifer Hudson steps down after four years and an 80 pound weight loss. Calling the fours years a successful and rewarding partnership, company officials and Hudson are calling the decision mutual. Hudson is the only Weight Watchers spokesperson to date with a company center named in her honor.

Choosing a Safe and Successful Weight-Loss Program

INTRODUCTION

Do you need to lose weight? Have you been thinking about trying a weight-loss program? Diets and programs that promise to help you lose weight are advertised everywhere—through magazines and newspapers, radio, TV, and Web sites. Are these programs safe? Will they work for you?

This fact sheet provides tips on how to identify a weight-loss program that may help you lose weight safely and keep the weight off over time. It also suggests ways to talk to your health care provider about your weight. He or she may be able to help you control your weight by making changes to your eating and physical activity habits. If these changes are not enough, you may want to consider a weight-loss program or other types of treatment.

WHERE DO I START?

Talking to your health care provider about your weight is an important first step. Doctors do not always address issues such as healthy eating, physical activity, and weight control during general office visits. It is important for you to bring up these issues to get the help you need. Even if you feel uneasy talking about your weight with your doctor, remember that he or she is there to help you improve your health.

Prepare for the Visit:

- Write down your questions in advance.
- Bring pen and paper to take notes.

- Invite a family member or friend along for support if this will make you feel better.
- Talk to your doctor about safe and effective ways to control your weight. He or she can review any medical problems that you have and any drugs that you take to help you set goals for controlling your weight. Make sure you understand what your doctor is saying. Ask questions if you do not understand something.

You may want to ask your doctor to recommend a weight-loss program or specialist. If you do start a weight-loss program, discuss your choice of program with your doctor, especially if you have any health problems.

WHAT SHOULD I LOOK FOR IN A WEIGHT-LOSS PROGRAM?

Successful, long-term weight control must focus on your overall health, not just on what you eat. Changing your lifestyle is not easy, but adopting healthy habits may help you manage your weight in the long run.

Effective weight-loss programs include ways to keep the weight off for good. These programs promote healthy behaviors that help you lose weight and that you can stick with every day. Safe and effective weight-loss programs should include the following:

- A plan to keep the weight off over the long run
- Guidance on how to develop healthier eating and physical activity habits
- Ongoing feedback, monitoring, and support
- Slow and steady weight-loss goals—usually ½ to 2 pounds per week (though weight loss may be faster at the start of a program)
- Some weight-loss programs may use very low-calorie diets (up to 800 calories per day) to promote rapid weight loss among people who have a lot of excess weight. This type of diet requires close medical supervision through frequent office visits and medical tests.

WHAT IF THE PROGRAM IS OFFERED ONLINE?

Many weight-loss programs are now being offered online—either fully or partly. Not much is known about how well these programs work. However, experts suggest that online weight-loss programs should provide the following:

- Structured, weekly lessons offered online or by podcasts
- Support tailored to your personal goals
- Self-monitoring of eating and physical activity using handheld devices, such as cell phones or online journals

- Regular feedback from a counselor on goals, progress, and results, given by e-mail, phone, or text messages
- Social support from a group through bulletin boards, chat rooms, and/or online meetings

Whether the program is online or in person, you should get as much background as you can before deciding to join.

WHAT QUESTIONS SHOULD I ASK ABOUT THE PROGRAM?

Professionals working for weight-loss programs should be able to answer questions about the program's features, safety, costs, and results. The following are sample questions you may want to ask.

WHAT DOES THE WEIGHT-LOSS PROGRAM INCLUDE?

- Does the program offer group classes or one-on-one counseling that will help me develop healthier habits?
- Do I have to follow a specific meal plan or keep food records?
- Do I have to buy special meals or supplements?
- If the program requires special foods, can I make changes based on my likes, dislikes, and food allergies (if any)?
- Will the program help me be more physically active, follow a specific physical activity plan, or provide exercise guidelines?
- Will the program work with my lifestyle and cultural needs? Does the program provide ways to deal with such issues as social or holiday eating, changes to work schedules, lack of motivation, and injury or illness?
- Does the program include a plan to help me keep the weight off, once I've lost weight?

WHAT ARE THE STAFF CREDENTIALS?

- Who supervises the program?
- What type of weight-control certifications, education, experience, and training do the staff have?

DOES THE PRODUCT OR PROGRAM CARRY ANY RISKS?

- Could the program hurt me?
- Could the suggested drugs or supplements harm my health?
- Do the people involved in the program get to talk with a doctor?
- Does a doctor or other certified health professional run the program?

- Will the program's doctor or staff work with my health care provider if needed (e.g., to address how the program may affect an existing medical issue)?
- Is there ongoing input and follow-up from a health care provider to ensure my safety while I take part in the program?

HOW MUCH DOES THE PROGRAM COST?

- What is the total cost of the program?
- Are there other costs, such as membership fees, fees for weekly visits, and payments for food, meal replacements, supplements, or other products?
- Are there other fees for medical tests?
- Are there fees for a follow-up program after I lose weight?

WHAT RESULTS DO PEOPLE IN THE PROGRAM TYPICALLY HAVE?

- How much weight does the average person lose?
- How long does the average person keep the weight off?
- Do you have written information on these results?

IF IT SEEMS TOO GOOD TO BE TRUE . . . IT PROBABLY IS!

In choosing a weight-loss program, watch out for these false claims.

- Lose weight without diet or exercise.
- Lose weight while eating all of your favorite foods.
- Lose 30 pounds in 30 days.
- Lose weight in specific problem areas of your body.

Other warning signs include:

- Very small print
- Asterisks and footnotes
- Before-and-after photos that seem too good to be true

Source: Weight-control Information Network, National Institute of Diabetes and Digestive and Kidney Diseases.

APPENDIX C

What's on the Web?

AMERICAN CELIAC SOCIETY

Address: PO Box 23455, New Orleans, LA 70183-0455
Phone: 504-737-3293
Web address: www.americanceliacsociety.org.
Web site: The American Celiac Society is a nonprofit tax exempt organization that works to assist individuals who suffer from Celiac Sprue disease, dermatitis herpetiformis, Crohn's disease, lactose intolerance, wheat intolerance, different food allergies, and other dietary disorders. The organization provides education, supports research, and seeks funding to educate the public about problems facing its members. Membership is open to anyone with these problems as well as family and friends.

AMERICAN COUNCIL ON SCIENCE AND HEALTH (ACSH)

Address: 1995 Broadway, Second Floor, New York, NY 10023-5860
Phone: 212-362-7044
Fax: 212-362-4919
Web address: http://acsh.org/
Web site: The ACSH is a consumer education consortium made up of scientists, physicians, and policy advisers. The council tracks the accuracy of nutrition articles in the popular magazines and publishes its survey online. This site is geared for the general public and offers a useful, conservative interpretation of current health information, from product safety to food labeling to safety of "natural" products.

AMERICAN CULINARY FEDERATION, INC. (ACF)

Address: 10 San Bartula Drive, St. Augustine, FL 32086
Phone: 904-824-4468/800-624-9458
Fax: 904-825-4758
Web address: http://www.acfchefs.org/
Web site: The ACF, founded in New York City in 1929, is a professional not-for-profit organization for chefs working to promote a professional image of the American chef worldwide through education. The site includes a job bank, directories of accredited culinary programs, and apprenticeship programs plus information on receiving certification and a calendar of culinary events. The section titled "Chef and Child" provides a look at a culinary education program designed to teach nutrition and cooking to youngsters. The site also includes material appropriate for high school vocational educators.

AMERICAN DIABETES ASSOCIATION (ADA)

Address: 1701 North Beauregard Street, Alexandria, VA 22311
Phone: 800-342-2383
Web address: http://www.diabetes.org/
Web site: The ADA motto is to prevent and cure diabetes and to improve the lives of all people affected by diabetes. This easy-to-use Web site has information about the disease, risk factors, complications, and warning signs of diabetes. There are also sections on nutrition, exercise tips, and recipes, as well as general information. Users can request an information packet but the association cautions that representatives cannot make a diagnosis or recommend medical treatment. There are links to other Internet resources and to magazines and journals dealing with diabetes and related health issues.

AMERICAN DIETETIC ASSOCIATION (ADA)

Address: 216 West Jackson Boulevard, Chicago, IL 60606
Phone: 312-899-0040/800-366-1655
Web address: http://www.eatright.org/
Web site: The number-one feature of this attractive and easy-to-use site is its ability to help people "Find a dietitian," plus a toll-free hotline for professional advice on improving your diet. Users can also link to many other nutrition-related sites. Informational categories include consumer education and public policy, dietetic practice groups, medical and health professionals, and dietetic associations. This fact-filled site includes a "Tip of the day," as well as in-depth monthly features. Users can find information on the USDA Food Guide Pyramid, fact sheets, and a nutrition reading list, along with a link to the ADA's journal and other highly rated nutrition books.

AMERICAN HEART ASSOCIATION (AHA)

Address: 7272 Greenville Avenue, Dallas, TX 75231
Phone: 214-373-6300/800-242-8721
Web address: http://www.heart.org/HEARTORG/
Web site: This association Web site is colorful and user-friendly with an easy-to-use A to Z guide that provides clear, concise information on heart disease and stroke-related illness. There are sections dealing with nutrition, exercise, and professional publications, and a news bureau. Users can link to a special site for women who want heart health information or link to an additional site titled "Living with Heart Failure," designed for caregivers and patients. Visitors can send a message to Congress about various biomedical issues and other health care initiatives.

AMERICAN INSTITUTE FOR CANCER RESEARCH (AICR)

Address: 1759 R Street, NW, Washington, D.C. 20009
Phone: 202-328-7744/800-843-8114
Web address: http://www.aicr.org/
Web site: This national cancer charity has created a Web site that offers information on food, nutrition, the prevention of cancer, news updates, critiques of fad diets and diet books, plus a helpful resource that answers common questions posed by newly diagnosed cancer patients and their families. It features recipes as well as a nutrition hotline and kids' newsletter. Users can also link to other cancer and nutrition sites.

AMERICAN MEDICAL ASSOCIATION (AMA)

Address: 515 North State Street, Chicago, IL 60610
Phone: 312-464-5000
Web address: http://www.ama-assn.org/ama
Web site: While this site is clearly geared toward physicians, there are useful resources for the layperson, including a section on consumer health information. There is a members-only portion to this site with an AMA Staff Directory. Journals and the American Medical News are available, as well as JAMA (*Journal of the American Medical Association*) and its related links on HIV/AIDS, asthma, migraines, and women's health.

AMERICAN SOCIETY OF BARIATRIC PHYSICIANS

Address: 5600 South Quebec Street, Suite 109A, Englewood, CO 80111
Phone: 303-770-2526
Fax: 303-779-4834
Web address: http://www.asbp.org/

Web site: While there is a members-only section on this Web site, there
is also easy access for the general public to information about obesity and its
related surgical treatments. Other features include medical updates, related
links, and frequently asked questions, and the site offers assistance in finding
a bariatric physician. Bariatrics is the medical treatment of obesity and its associated problems, and is currently one of the fastest-growing specialties in
medicine.

ASK THE DIETITIAN

Web address: http://www.dietitian.com/
Web site: This site, developed by nutritionist Joanne Larsen, has a cool feature, the Healthy Body Calculator, found at http://www.dietitian.com/ibw/ibw
.html. Have a tape measure handy and know your weight. This interactive tool
creates a dietary recommendation as well as graphics to show where you fall in
the ideal health and body mass index ranges.

BIGGEST LOSER

Web address: http://www.biggestloser.com/
Web site: This site offers the interested dieter everything from nutrition advice
and tools to fitness equipment, video from weight-loss contestants and the opportunity to gain motivation from "Ambassadors" from previous shows. They also
link to Planet Fitness, a gym with locations around the country, a merchandizing
partnership that benefits the show and the health club by offering exercise classes
and fitness training with one click of the mouse.

BURGER KING CORPORATION

Address: 17777 Old Cutler Road, Miami, FL 33157-6347
Phone: 305-378-7011
Fax: 305-379-7262
Web address: http://www.bk.com/en/us/index.html
Web site: This colorful site is filled with feel-good information about Burger
King but also gets high marks for better-than-average nutritional information.
Unlike sites that bury their numbers on fats and calories, Burger King provides an
Interactive Nutritional Information Wizard, where users can select menu items,
theoretically eat a reasonable amount of calories, and limit their fat intake if they
choose. But advertising is still the most important part of this site, with entry to
a Kids Club filled with toys, games, and a clubhouse, plus a What's Hot section
that highlights the latest toy giveaway. Franchise locations as well as the company information are listed.

CENTER FOR FOOD SAFETY

Address: 666 Pennsylvania Avenue, SE, Suite 302, Washington, D.C., 20003
Phone: 202-547-9359
Fax: 202-547-9429
Web address: http://www.centerforfoodsafety.org/
Web site: The Center for Food Safety is a public interest and environmental advocacy organization addressing the impacts of the food production system on human health, animal welfare, and the environment. The site contains legislative alerts and information on food safety issues such as genetically modified organisms (bioengineered foods), irradiation, sludge, and methyl bromide. New is the True Food Network, a way for consumers to be updated on food safety issues and to receive suggestions on steps to take to "make a difference."

CENTER FOR SCIENCE IN THE PUBLIC INTEREST (CSPI)

Address: 1875 Connecticut Avenue, NW, Suite 300, Washington, D.C. 20009
Phone: 202-332-9110
Fax: 202-265-4954
Web address: https://www.cspinet.org/
Web site: The CSPI is a nonprofit education and advocacy organization working to improve the safety and nutritional quality of food. CSPI promotes health education about nutrition and alcohol and also represents the public's interests in the legislative, regulatory, and judicial arenas. The site offers excellent links to both private and government nutrition sources as well as access to CSPI's *Nutrition Action Healthletter*. An interesting nutrition quiz and a document library add to the wealth of information on this site. Special reports, such as "Liquid Candy: How Soft Drinks Are Harming America's Health," spell out the facts on soft drinks and health.

CENTERS FOR DISEASE CONTROL AND PREVENTION (CDC)

Address: 1600 Clifton Road, NE, Atlanta, GA 30333
Phone: 404-639-3311/800-311-3435
Web address: http://www.cdc.gov/
Web site: The CDC is an agency of the Department of Health and Human Services. The Web site is designed to answer a multitude of questions from the general public and Health Topics A–Z or frequently asked questions are filled with updated documents for that purpose. Categories of frequently asked questions range from Diabetes or *E. coli* to Hantavirus and Listeriosis. The site includes access to data and statistics, and training and employment information, as well as links to other sites. Geared for the general public, it is a useful first stop for anyone with concerns about a medical condition. But keep in mind that the

CDC strongly recommends against self-diagnosis or self-management without involvement of health care professionals.

COUNCIL FOR RESPONSIBLE NUTRITION (CRN)

Address: 1875 Eye Street, NW, Suite 400, Washington, D.C. 20006-5409
Phone: 202-872-1488
Fax: 202-872-9594
Web address: http://www.crnusa.org/
Web site: The CRN is a trade association representing companies that make nutritional supplements. This site offers comprehensive links to many government sites that deal with nutrition, legislation, and regulation of dietary supplements. Other useful information includes the section on scientific affairs with current scientific articles on dietary supplements.

DASH (DIETARY GUIDELINES FOR AMERICANS) EATING PLAN

U.S. Department of Health and Human Services; National Heart Lung and Blood Institute
Address: NHLBI Health Information Center, P.O. Box 30105, Bethesda, MD 20824-0105
Phone: 301-592-8573
Fax: 301-592-8563
Web address: https://www.nhlbi.nih.gov/health/health-topics/topics/dash/
Web site: Designed as a gateway to the DASH Eating Plan, this site offers a great deal of information from tips to getting started as well as menus, links to related topics, a list of benefits and commonsense information. Also links to several government health Web sites and offers information on clinical trials and how to find specific trials for different health issues.

FITDAY

Web address: http://www.fitday.com/
Web site: This attractive and colorful site offers users access to a food log for free. The interactive and informative food diary helps users lose weight and meet fitness and nutritional goals. For those who like to keep track of numbers and chart activities, this is a great place to get a handle on eating habits and food intake. There is also accurate weight loss and healthful eating advice as well as information on the USDA Food Guide Pyramid.

FOOD ALLERGY NETWORK

Address: 7925 Jones Branch Dr., Suite 1100, McLean, VA 22102
Phone: 800-929-4040/703-691-3179
Fax: 703-691-2713

Web address: http://www.foodallergy.org/

Web site: There is a measurable increase in Americans with identified food allergies; this helpful site offers facts on food allergies with sections that answer common questions, dispel myths, and offer the latest research on all types of food allergies. Users can also sign up for "Product Alerts," a free service via e-mail.

FOOD AND DRUG ADMINISTRATION (FDA)/U.S. DEPARTMENT OF HEALTH AND HUMAN SERVICES

Address: 10903 New Hampshire Ave., Silver Spring, MD 20993

Phone: 888-463-6332

Web address: http://www.fda.gov/

Web site: This FDA site is user-friendly government site and includes information on a wide range of topics from cosmetics to articles on acne, sports, asthma, and eating disorders. There are links to recall information, safety alerts, warning letters, and updates on food recalls. Everything from medical devices to tobacco products is listed in easy-to-find tabs.

FOOD AND NUTRITION BOARD (FNB)/INSTITUTE OF MEDICINE (IOM)

Address: 500 Fifth St., N.W., Washington, D.C. 20001

Phone: 202-334-2352

Fax: 202-334-1412

Web address: http://www.iom.edu/About-IOM/Leadership-Staff/Boards/Food-and-Nutrition-Board.aspx

Web site: The FNB is part of the National Academy of Sciences (NAS). The NAS is a private, nonprofit corporation created by Congress and is made up of biomedical scientists with expertise in nutrition and food science. The board makes recommendations to improve food quality and to promote public health and prevent diet-related diseases. This Web site provides access to ongoing FNB studies and upcoming events, plus links to related food and nutrition sites and to the Institute of Medicine (IOM) and NAS. Not for the casual user, this site is difficult to navigate because information is presented in highly technical terms.

HARVARD SCHOOL OF PUBLIC HEALTH

Address: 677 Huntington Ave. Boston, MA

Phone: 617-495-1000

Web address: http://www.hsph.harvard.edu/nutritionsource

Web site: Nutritionists at the Harvard School of Public Health have developed a guide to healthy eating and weight loss that they say addresses deficiencies in the government's MyPlate program. The Harvard program is called Healthy Eating Plate.

HEALTHFINDER/U.S. DEPARTMENT OF HEALTH AND HUMAN SERVICES

Address: 200 Independence Ave., S.W., Washington, D.C. 20201
Phone: 202-619-0257/877-696-6775
Web address: http://healthfinder.gov/
Web site: The Department of Health and Human Services' site covers everything from current topics like breastfeeding and folic acid to nutrition information from federal and state agencies. There are also a list of online medical journals, a database of toll-free numbers, a medical dictionary, a library locator, and information about support and self-help groups. There is a search engine for subject searches or for browsing by topics. This site is easy to navigate and is filled with understandable and useful information.

HEALTHY EATING PLATE

See Harvard School of Public Health

HEALTHY PEOPLE 2020

Web address: http://www.healthypeople.gov/2020/default.aspx
Web site: This site details the goals of the Healthy People 2020 initiative of the U.S. Department of Health and Human Services. It contains progress reports and reviews, links to community Healthy People initiatives, and information on how Americans' health compares with that of people in other countries. The 10 leading health indicators, for which there are updated statistics, are physical activity, overweight and obesity, tobacco use, substance abuse, responsible sexual behavior, mental health, injury and violence, environmental quality, immunization, and access to health care.

HEALTHY WEIGHT NETWORK

Address: 402 South 14th Street? Hettinger, ND 58639
Phone: 701-567-2646
Web address: www.healthyweight.net
Web site: Updated articles connecting readers to research and information on obesity, eating disorders, weight loss, and healthy living at any size. The organization hands out annual Slim Chance Awards to organizations that promote unhealthy, gimmicky, or unrealistic diet programs or products.

IEMILY

Address: 136 West Street, Suite 201, Northampton, MA, 01060
Phone: 413-587-0244
Web address: http://www.iemily.com/

Web site: This unique site was created for an underserved population—teenage girls. Look for solid and sensible nutrition information in the "Healthy Eating" section plus articles that explain topics like organic foods, food allergies, eating disorders, and strategies for fitness. Teens can also find information on vegetarianism, ethnic cuisine, sport-specific nutrition, and how to develop a basic healthy, active, and realistic lifestyle. The attractive site continues to change and grow, like the audience it serves.

INTERNATIONAL FOOD INFORMATION COUNCIL (IFIC)

Address: 1100 Connecticut Avenue, NW, Suite 430, Washington, D.C. 20036
Phone: 202-296-6540/202-296-6547
Web address: http://www.ific.us/
Web site: The IFIC collects and disseminates scientific information on food safety and nutritional health to nutritional professionals and educators, plus government officials, journalists, and consumers. The IFIC was founded in 1985 and is a nonprofit organization. Information for educators is included, along with sections on general nutrition facts, current nutrition developments, and additional resources. A lengthy glossary, plus the variety of food safety and nutritional information, makes this site better than average.

MAYO CLINIC NEWSWISE

Address: 200 First Street, SW, Rochester, MN 55905
Phone: 507-266-4057
Web address: http://www.newswise.com/institutions/newsroom/275/
Web site: Presented by the famous Mayo Health Clinic, this site is rated among the best by the Tufts University Nutrition Navigator. The format is user-friendly and offers information on anything from past articles concerning nutritional topics to podcasts and videos showing healthful cooking and food safety. Ask the Mayo Dietitian is in a question-and-answer format, and there are quizzes and tests, some interactive, so users can test their nutrition knowledge.

MCDONALDS CORPORATION

Address: 1 McDonalds Plaza, Oak Brook, IL 60523-1928
Phone: 630-623-3000
Web address: http://www.mcdonalds.com/us/en/home.html
Web site: An attractive and easy-to-use site; business comes first as it features all the promotional products McDonalds has to offer consumers. However, there is good nutritional information to be had if you click on menu tabs like Nutrition Choices. Consumers can find the breakdown on all McDonalds food products as well as fat grams and calories of each. The information gives interested

consumers the opportunity for informed menu selections, something that other fast-food chains lack.

MEALS FOR YOU

Phone: 630-983-1506

Web address: http://www.mealsforyou.com/

Web site: Welcome to a Web site that is free, fast, and easy to use, where it's possible to find thousands of recipes by type, ingredients, or nutrient content. This site is operated by Proco Marketing, Inc., operating since 1996 with recipes, meal plans, nutritional information, shopping lists, and other nutrition content. Users can search by categories of menus for diabetics, vegetarians, and dieters. The site offers menu plans, complete with nutrient analysis and a shopping list, and has been highly rated by Tufts University School of Nutrition Science and Policy as "Among the Best" Web sites offering nutrient analysis and information.

MYPLATE/U.S. DEPARTMENT OF AGRICULTURE

Address: USDA Center for Nutrition Policy and Promotion, 3101 Park Center Dr., Alexandria, VA 22302-1594

Web address: http://www.choosemyplate.gov/index.html

Web site: This site features the government's newest tool for understanding nutrition. The MyPlate graphic is designed to promote healthy eating and uses the concept of a plate to show portion sizes and combinations of food groups to achieve good nutrition. Features include videos, information about eating on a budget, nutrition tips, sample menus and recipes, and daily food plans. Information is targeted to different age groups from preschoolers and kids to pregnant women and college students. There are also calorie tools and weight management for consumers.

NATIONAL ACADEMY OF SCIENCES (INSTITUTE OF MEDICINE/FOOD AND NUTRITION BOARD)

Address: Institute of Medicine, 500 Fifth St., NW, Washington, D.C. 20001

Phone: 202-334-2352

Fax: 202-334-1412

Web address: http://www.iom.edu/About-IOM/Leadership-Staff/Boards/Food-and-Nutrition-Board.aspx

Web site: The NAS is a private, nonprofit corporation made up of biomedical scientists with expertise in nutrition, food science, food safety, and other areas. They provide independent advice on scientific issues to government. The site sections include news, current projects, publications, reports, books, articles, and a subject index for searching. This site offers important information but is difficult for the casual browser to navigate.

NATIONAL ASSOCIATION OF ANOREXIA NERVOSA AND ASSOCIATED DISORDERS (ANAD)

Address: 750 E. Diehl Road #127, Naperville, IL 60563
Phone: (Helpline) 630-577-1330/Business: 630-577-1333
Web address: http://www.anad.org/
Web site: The ANAD was founded in 1976 and is among the oldest national nonprofit organizations helping eating disorder victims and their families. The site offers access to free hotline counseling, an international network of support groups for sufferers and their families, and referrals to health care professionals. There are sections on insurance discrimination and legislative news. The association also provides educational speakers, programs, and presentations for schools, colleges, public health agencies, and community groups. There is an online form to request information or to volunteer.

NATIONAL CENTER FOR HEALTH STATISTICS (NCHS)

Address1600 Clifton Rd., Atlanta, GA 30333.
Phone: 800-232-4636
Web address: http://www.cdc.gov/nchs/
Web site: This center is affiliated with the Centers for Disease Control and Prevention (CDC), under the U.S. Department of Health and Human Services. Health Topics A–Z is a list of disease and health subjects found on the CDC Web site. Those are divided by categories from teens to environmental health and women's health. This site links to vital records for the entire United States and also links to the U.S. State Department.

NATIONAL COALITION FOR PROMOTING PHYSICAL ACTIVITY (NCPPA)

Address: 805 15th Street, NW, Suite 650, Washington, D.C. 20005
Phone: 202-449-8372
Fax: 202-466-9666
Web address: http://www.ncppa.org/
Web site: The NCPPA is a national network of public, private, and industry organizations working to improve access and knowledge of physical activity through physical fitness, sports, education, and worksite health promotion. Founded by the American College of Sports Medicine, the American Heart Association, and the American Alliance for Health, Physical Education, Recreation,

and Dance, it now includes over 150 organizations working to promote fitness on the local, state, and national levels. The site contains a wealth of information and includes a direct link to the Healthy People 2010 site as well as a list of state coalitions and a national calendar of events.

NATIONAL COUNCIL AGAINST HEALTH FRAUD (NCAHF)

Phone: 919-533-6009
Web address: http://www.ncahf.org/
Web site: The NCAHF is a nonprofit voluntary health agency focused on health fraud, misinformation, and quackery as public health problems. This straightforward format is user-friendly and contains hundreds of articles to educate consumers and health professionals about fraud and quackery. The site also supports sound consumer health laws and will assist with legal actions against fraudulent products or product claims.

NATIONAL INSTITUTES OF HEALTH (NIH)/U.S. DEPARTMENT OF HEALTH AND HUMAN SERVICES

Address: 31 Center Dr., Bethesda, MD 20892-0148
Phone: 301-496-4000
Web address: http://www.nih.gov/
Web site: This government site offers a very comprehensive list of hotline resources on any imaginable health problem from A to Z. There are sections about the NIH, news and events, scientific resources from journals to research labs, and health information in the form of publications as well as access to resources like MedlinePlus. Information is also provided in Spanish. The NIH is part of the U.S. Department of Health and Human Services.

NEW YORK ONLINE ACCESS TO HEALTH (NOAH)

Web address: www.noah.cuny.edu/wellness.nutrition/nutrition.html
Web site: NOAH is a consumer health Web site of quality filtered materials in English or Spanish. The volunteer staff receives the information from medical librarians working in academic, special, hospital, and public libraries throughout New York. Page editors organize and arrange the full-text consumer information, which is available through an effective keyword search.

OBESITY SOCIETY

Address: 8758 Georgia Ave., Suite 1320, Silver Spring, MD 20910
Phone: 800-974-3084/301-563-6526
Fax: 301-563-6595
Web address: http://www.obesity.org/

Web site: The focus of this site is information about obesity and its treatment, and includes helpful resources for understanding insurance issues as well as a body mass index. There are links to other sites like the American Heart Association. They offer a health newsletter as well as a news section, links to education, and events plus career information for health professionals.

PHYSICIANS COMMITTEE FOR RESPONSIBLE MEDICINE (PCRM)

Address: 5100 Wisconsin Avenue, NW, Suite 400, Washington, D.C. 20016
Phone: 202-686-2210
Web address: http://www.pcrm.org/
Web site: PCRM, a nonprofit organization, promotes preventive medicine and a nutrition program, which focuses on a vegan diet. It supports research into diabetes, cancer, and other health care issues, and has also developed a program for healthful eating for businesses, hospitals, and schools, called the Gold Plan. A keyword search can locate topics like restaurant reviews and physician referrals, and there are special resources available for medical students and educators. Dr. Neal Barnard founded PCRM in 1985 to promote preventive medicine through the use of diet and exercise.

PRESIDENT'S COUNCIL ON FOOD SAFETY

Address: 200 Independence Avenue, SW, Washington, D.C. 20201
Phone: 888-SAFEFOOD
Web address: http://www.foodsafety.gov/
Web site: The President's Council on Food Safety was established in August 1998 to coordinate the nation's food safety policy and resources. This site is a gateway to government food safety information and is jointly sponsored by the Department of Commerce, the Environmental Protection Agency, the U.S. Department of Health and Human Services, and the U.S. Department of Agriculture and is maintained by the FDA's Center for Food Safety and Applied Nutrition. Sections include Consumer Advice; Kids, Teens, and Educators; Report Illnesses; and Product Complaints. There is also quick access to current government publications on safety topics, to current food recalls and links to federal and state government agencies.

PRESIDENT'S COUNCIL ON PHYSICAL FITNESS AND SPORTS

Address: 1101 Wootton Parkway, Suite 560, Rockville, MD 20852
Phone: 240-276-9567
Fax: 240-276-9860
Web address: http://www.fitness.gov/

Web site: This government site, part of the U.S. Department of Health and Human Services, has information about the history of the Council as well as links to other federal agencies and health organizations. There are exercise and nutrition tips aimed at youngsters and information about health and exercise plus a resource link for coaches, teachers, and fitness professionals. This site links to a huge index of government health publications and gives information about the Presidential Sports Award.

PREVENTIVE MEDICINE RESEARCH INSTITUTE (PMRI)

See WebMDHealth.

QUACKWATCH

Web address: http://www.quackwatch.com/

Web site: Quackwatch is a nonprofit corporation designed to combat health-related frauds, fads, and faulty products and is closely linked to the National Council Against Health Fraud. Founded by Dr. Stephen Barrett in 1969 as the Lehigh Valley Committee Against Health Fraud, it assumed its current name following the launching of its Web site in 1997. This no-frills site provides access to health-related articles. Quackwatch has also sponsored research projects to look at dubious advertising and questionable methods used by advertisers as well as several other projects. The site launched Nutriwatch in 2000 as a monitor of sensible nutrition and any quackery associated with diet, nutrition, or diet products.

SHAPE UP AMERICA

Address: 6707 Democracy Boulevard, Suite 306, Bethesda, MD 20817
Web address: http://www.shapeup.org/

Web site: Shape Up America is a national initiative to promote healthy weight and nutrition, and increased physical activity across America. Made up of a large coalition of industry, physical fitness, medical, health, and nutritional experts, Shape Up America works to promote the importance of a healthy weight; works to educate people about ways to achieve appropriate body weight; and cooperates with other organizations to advance a healthy lifestyle. The site offers a support center for practical tips on weight loss, an interactive weight-loss program, a cyber kitchen, and a center to determine your body mass index (BMI).

SNACK FOOD ASSOCIATION

Address: 1600 Wilson Blvd., Suite 650, Arlington, VA 22209
Phone: 703-836-4500
Web address: http://www.sfa.org/

Web site: Ever thought of snacking across America? This site provides regional recipes using every possible snack food from chocolate-covered potato chips to spicy Santa Fe trail mix. The association was founded in 1937 and continues to grow just as the industry it supports does. Users can find information on the state of the snack food industry and on consumer snacking behavior, various industry publications, and an interesting timeline and a history of snack foods. If you wanted to know who invented the potato chip, the information is easily available.

SOCIETY FOR NUTRITION EDUCATION (SNE)

Address: 9100 Purdue Road, Suite 200, Indianapolis, IN 46268
Phone: 317-328-4627/800-235-6690
Fax: 317-280-8527
Web address: http://www.sneb.org/contact.html
Web site: The Society for Nutrition Education is an international community of professionals involved in nutritional education and health promotion. While the Web site is geared for nutrition educators, it provides access to the society's official publication, the *Journal of Nutrition Education and Behavior* (JNEB), a great resource on the history of and up-to-date developments in nutrition education.

SUBWAY

Address: 325 Bic Drive, Milford, CT 06461-3059
Phone: 203-877-4281/800-888-4848
Web address: http://www.subway.com/subwayroot/default.aspx
Web site: This colorful, interactive site covers every aspect of Subway from its menu and nutritional content to catering, career opportunities, and celebrity endorsements including Jared Fogle, the man who lost over 200 pounds following his own Subway diet. There are monthly featured foods and new menu items along with information for those who want to open their own franchise.

TACO BELL/TRIGON GLOBAL RESTAURANTS

Address: 1 Glen Bell Way, Irvine, CA 92618
Phone: 949-863-3915
Web address: http://www.tacobell.com/
Web site: This fast-food restaurant site offers easy-to-find nutritional information plus the usual company information about franchise locations, employment, and even an online gift shop. The nutrition section deals with facts, ingredients, as well as food allergies and even a diabetic exchange. Though not as interactive as the McDonalds or Subway sites, this is still a colorful and informative tool.

Also links to Kentucky Fried Chicken (KFC) and Pizza Hut, both under the Trigon corporate umbrella.

USDA FOOD AND NUTRITION INFORMATION CENTER

Address: 10301 Baltimore Avenue, Beltsville, MD 20705-2351
Phone: 301-504-5414/fax; 301-504-6409
Web address: https://fnic.nal.usda.gov/
Web site: Sponsored by the USDA National Agricultural Library, this site connects users to the resources of the National Agricultural Library, which contains educational materials, research briefs, and food-composition data. There are links to the Dietary Guidelines for Americans as well as a list of frequently asked questions. This site is geared toward professionals looking for technical information. However, there is some information aimed at consumers.

U.S. DEPARTMENT OF AGRICULTURE (USDA)

Address: 1400 Independence Avenue, SW, Washington, D.C. 20250
Phone: 202-720-2791
Web address: http://www.usda.gov/wps/portal/usda/usdahome /, http://www.cnpp.usda.gov/, http://www.cnpp.usda.gov/
Web site: The USDA site has a wealth of government information, starting with a message from the secretary, and including a history of American agriculture. One cool feature is the interactive Healthy Eating Index. Plug in what you've eaten in recent days and the site produces a score on how healthy your overall diet is. There is also access to the Code of Federal Regulations for agriculture, animals, and forests, and a link to the USDA Fraud Hotline. The site also links to the USDA Center for Nutrition Policy and Promotion. That site offers professionals who work on nutrition and hunger issues access to USDA documents but it is not for the casual browser. The documents include a healthy eating index and resources for nutrition educators.

U.S. DEPARTMENT OF HEALTH AND
HUMAN SERVICES (HHS)

Address: 200 Independence Avenue, SW, Washington, D.C. 20201
Phone: 202-619-0257/877-696-6775
Web address: http://www.hhs.gov/
Web site: The Department of Health and Human Services is the U.S. government's principal agency overseeing all aspects of American health, with more than 300 programs on everything from food and drug safety to Medicare and Medicaid. The site offers a healthy eating link on its home page as well as links to other HHS agencies and sponsored sites, such as News and Public Affairs, What's

New, and a calendar of events and health observances. It also links to YouthInfo, a Web site developed to provide the latest information about America's adolescents. That site contains a profile of youth, resources for parents, and speeches on topics of interest to youth. The department also sponsors and links to Healthy People 2020 as a way to promote physical activity across the nation.

VEGETARIAN RESOURCE GROUP (VRG)

Address: P.O. Box 1463, Baltimore, MD 21203
Phone: 410-366-VEGE
Web address: https://www.vrg.org/
Web site: The VRG is a nonprofit organization that works to educate the public on vegetarian and related issues such as health, ecology, world hunger, and nutrition. Financial support comes largely from membership, contributions, and book sales. The site provides news, recipes, and a huge list of nutrition and related links. There is a lengthy section on vegetarian nutrition, geared for anyone interested in meatless eating. Although developed for students and consumers, health care professionals may find useful information as well.

WAKE FOREST UNIVERSITY—BAPTIST MEDICAL CENTER

Address: School of Medicine, 1 Medical Center Boulevard, Winston-Salem, NC 27103
Phone: 336-716-2011
Web address: http://www.wakehealth.edu/
Web site: Run by Wake Forest University's Bowman Gray School of Medicine and its Center for Research on Human Nutrition and Chronic Disease Prevention, this site gives a nutritional breakdown of common foods, including fast food via its Drive thru Diet section. The school's research center devised this site to promote preventive health care. It also offers a calorie calculator in its Interactive Tools section to estimate calories, fat, cholesterol, and sodium levels in a variety of common foods and beverages.

WEBMD HEALTH

Address: 111 8th Ave, 7th Floor, New York, NY 10011
Phone: 212-624-3700
Web address: http://www.webmd.com/
Web site: This site features an enormous amount of medical information, from nutrition to pregnancy, sports fitness to news on drugs and supplements. Special features include live health events on the Web, interactive tools, health news, and the latest medical reference content. There are also a great deal of information and tools for those wanting to lose weight or improve their diet. The site

reminds users that it is not a substitute for seeing a doctor or other health care professional, and it provides links to other health-related web pages.

WEIGHT-CONTROL INFORMATION NETWORK

Address: 1 Win Way, Bethesda, MD 20896-3665
Phone: 202-828-1025/877-946-4627
Fax: 202-828-1028
Web address: http://win.niddk.nih.gov/
Web site: This site is sponsored by the National Institute of Diabetes and Digestive and Kidney (NIDDK) Diseases, part of the National Institutes of Health. The site offers information for health professionals as well as consumers on weight control, obesity, and nutritional disorders. With access to thousands of articles, books, and educational materials, this site is very helpful for consumers as well as professionals. It also features *WIN Notes*, a quarterly newsletter published by NIDDK.

WEIGHT WATCHERS

Phone: 800-651-6000
Web address: https://www.weightwatchers.com/
Web site: Like the Web pages of other diet programs, this site features everything from frequently asked questions to information about the program and its new points system to tips from spokesperson Jessica Simpson. There are recipes and weight-loss articles plus access to Weight Watchers' products and a history of the organization. The presentation uses bright, bold colors and appealing photographs to showcase everything from food and recipes to success stories. The site is very user-friendly.

YALE RUDD CENTER FOR FOOD POLICY AND OBESITY

Address: Yale University, 309 Edwards Street, New Haven, CT 06511
Phone: 203-432-6700/Fax: 203-432-9674
Web address: http://www.yaleruddcenter.org/
Web site: This no-nonsense Web site is clear and concise. The home page includes a short introduction to the center, including its services and location. There is a wealth of information on everything from food and addiction to how foods are marketed to youngsters, public policies, and weight bias and stigma associated with obesity. The articles and information are detailed and to the point. This is a very useful tool for students, consumers, and health care professionals.

Myths and Facts about Weight Loss

Myth: Fad diets work for permanent weight loss.

Fact: Fad diets are not the best ways to lose weight and keep it off. These eating plans often promise to help you lose a lot of weight quickly, or tell you to cut certain foods out of your diet to lose weight. Although you may lose weight at first while on these kinds of diets, they can be unhealthy because they often keep you from getting all the nutrients that your body needs. Fad diets may seriously limit or prohibit certain types of food, so most people quickly get tired of them and regain the lost weight.

Research suggests that losing half to two pounds a week by eating better and exercising more is the best way to lose weight and keep it off. By improving your eating and exercise habits, you will develop a healthier lifestyle and control your weight. You will also reduce your chances of developing heart disease, high blood pressure, and diabetes.

Myth: Skipping meals is a good way to lose weight.

Fact: Your body needs a certain amount of calories and nutrients each day in order to work properly. If you skip meals during the day, you will be more likely to make up for those missing calories by snacking or eating more at the next meal. Studies show that people who skip breakfast tend to be heavier than those who eat a nutritious breakfast. A healthier way to lose weight is to eat many small meals throughout the day that include a variety of nutritious, low-fat, and low-calorie foods.

Myth: I can lose weight while eating anything I want.

Fact: This statement is not always true. It is possible to eat any kind of food you want and lose weight. But you still need to limit the number of calories that you eat every day, usually by eating smaller amounts of food. When trying to lose weight, you can eat your favorite foods—as long as you pay attention to the total amount of food that you eat. You need to use more calories than you eat to lose weight.

Myth: Eating after 8 P.M. causes weight gain.

Fact: It doesn't matter what time of day you eat—it is how much you eat during the whole day and how much exercise you get that make you gain or lose weight. No matter when you eat your meals, your body will store extra calories as fat. If you want to have a snack before bedtime, make sure that you first think about how many calories you have already eaten that day.

Try not to snack while doing other things, like watching television, playing video games, or using the computer. If you eat meals and snacks in the kitchen or dining room, you are less likely to be distracted and more likely to be aware of what and how much you are eating. (If you want to snack while watching TV, take a small amount of food with you, like a handful of pretzels or a couple of cookies—not the whole bag.)

Myth: Certain foods, like grapefruit, celery, or cabbage soup, can burn fat and make you lose weight.

Fact: No foods can burn fat. Some foods with caffeine may speed up your metabolism (the way your body uses energy or calories) for a short time, but they do not cause weight loss. The best way to lose weight is to cut back on the number of calories you eat and be more physically active.

Myth: Natural or herbal weight-loss products are safe and effective.

Fact: A product that claims to be "natural" or "herbal" is not necessarily safe. These products are not usually tested scientifically to prove that they are safe or that they work.

Some herbal or other natural products may be unsafe to use with other drugs or may hurt people with certain medical conditions. Check with your doctor or other qualified health professional before using any herbal or natural weight-loss product.

Myth: Nuts are fattening and you shouldn't eat them if you want to lose weight.

Fact: Although high in calories and fat, most (but not all) types of nuts have low amounts of saturated fat. Saturated fat is the kind of fat that can lead to high blood cholesterol levels and increase the risk of heart disease.

Nuts are a good source of protein and fiber, and they do not have any cholesterol. In small amounts, nuts can be part of a healthy weight-loss program.

Myth: Eating red meat is bad for your health and will make it harder to lose weight.

Fact: Red meat, pork, chicken, and fish contain some saturated fat and cholesterol. But they also have nutrients, like protein, iron, and zinc, that are important for good health.

Eating lean meat (meat without a lot of visible fat) in small amounts can be part of a healthy weight-loss plan. A serving size is two to three ounces of cooked meat, which is about the size of a deck of cards. Choose cuts of meat that are lower in fat, such as beef eye of the round, top round, or pork tenderloin, and trim any extra fat before cooking. The "select" grade of meat is lower in fat than "choice" and "prime" grades.

Myth: Fresh fruits and vegetables are more nutritious than frozen or canned.

Fact: Most fruits and vegetables (produce) are naturally low in fat and calories. Frozen and canned fruits and vegetables can be just as nutritious as fresh. Frozen or canned produce is often packaged right after it has been picked, which helps keep most of its nutrients. Fresh produce can sometimes lose nutrients after being exposed to light or air.

Myth: Starches are fattening and should be limited when trying to lose weight.

Fact: Potatoes, rice, pasta, bread, beans, and some vegetables (like squash, yams, sweet potatoes, turnips, beets, and carrots) are rich in complex carbohydrates (also called starch). Starch is an important source of energy for your body.

Foods high in starch can be low in fat and calories. They become high in fat and calories when you eat them in large amounts, or if they are made with rich sauces, oils, or other high-fat toppings like butter, sour cream, or mayonnaise. Try to avoid high-fat toppings and choose starchy foods that are high in fiber, like whole grains, beans, and peas.

The Dietary Guidelines for Americans recommend 6 to 11 servings a day from the bread, cereal, rice, and pasta group, even when trying to lose weight. A serving size can be 1 slice of bread, 1 ounce of ready-to-eat cereal, or 1/2 cup of pasta, rice, or cooked cereal.

Myth: Fast foods are always an unhealthy choice and you should not eat them when dieting.

Fact: Fast foods can be part of a healthy weight-loss program with a little bit of know-how. Choose salads and grilled foods instead of fried foods, which are high in fat and calories. Use high-fat, high-calorie toppings, like full-fat mayonnaise and salad dressings, only in small amounts.

Eating fried fast food (like French fries) or other high-fat foods like chocolate once in a while as a special treat is fine—but try to split an order with a friend or order a small portion. In small amounts, these foods can still be part of a healthy eating plan.

Myth: Fish has no fat or cholesterol.

Fact: Although all fish has some fat and cholesterol, most fish is lower in saturated fat and cholesterol than beef, pork, chicken, and turkey. Fish is a good source of protein. Types of fish that are higher in fat (like salmon, mackerel, sardines, herring, and anchovies) are rich in omega-3 fatty acids. These fatty acids are being studied because they may be linked to a lower risk for heart disease.

Grilled, baked, or broiled fish (instead of fried) can be part of a healthy weight-loss plan.

Myth: High-protein/low-carbohydrate diets are a healthy way to lose weight.

Fact: A high-protein/low-carbohydrate diet provides most of your calories each day from protein foods (like meat, eggs, and cheese) and few calories from carbohydrate foods (like breads, pasta, potatoes, fruits, and vegetables). People on these diets often get bored because they crave the plant-based foods they are not allowed to have or can have only in very small amounts. These diets often lack key nutrients found in carbohydrate foods.

Many of these diets allow a lot of food high in fat, like bacon and cheese. High-fat diets can raise blood cholesterol levels, which increases a person's risk for heart disease and certain cancers.

High-protein/low-carbohydrate diets may cause rapid weight loss—but most of it is water weight and lean muscle mass—not fat. You lose water because your kidneys try to get rid of the excess waste products of protein and fat, called ketones, that your body produces.

This is not a healthy way to lose weight! It overworks your kidneys, and can cause dehydration, headaches, and bad breath. It can also make you feel nauseous, tired, weak, and dizzy. A buildup of ketones in your blood (called ketosis) can cause your body to produce high levels of uric acid, which is a risk factor for gout (a painful swelling of the joints) and kidney stones. Ketosis can be very risky for pregnant women and people with diabetes.

By following a reduced-calorie diet that is well balanced between carbohydrates, proteins, and fats, you will still lose weight—without hurting your body. You will also be more likely to keep the weight off.

Myth: Dairy products are fattening and unhealthy.

Fact: Dairy products have many nutrients your body needs. They have calcium to help children develop strong bones and to keep adult bones strong and healthy. They also have vitamin D to help your body use calcium, and protein to build muscles and to help organs work properly.

Low-fat and nonfat dairy products are as nutritious as whole-milk dairy products, but they are lower in fat and calories. Choose low-fat or nonfat milk, cheese, yogurt (frozen or regular), and reduced-fat ice cream.

For people who can't digest lactose (a type of sugar found in milk and other dairy products), lactose-free dairy products can be used. These are also good sources of protein and calcium. If you are sensitive to some dairy foods, you may still be able to eat others, like yogurt, hard cheese, evaporated skim milk, and buttermilk. Other good sources of calcium are dark leafy vegetables (like spinach), calcium-fortified juice, bread, soy products (like tofu), and canned fish with soft bones (like salmon).

Many people are worried about eating butter and margarine. Eating a lot of foods high in saturated fat (like butter) has been linked to high blood cholesterol levels and a greater risk of heart disease. Some research suggests that high amounts of trans fat can also cause high blood cholesterol levels. Trans fat is found in margarine, and in crackers, cookies, and other snack foods made with hydrogenated vegetable shortening or oil. Trans fat is formed when vegetable oil is hardened to become margarine or shortening, a process called "hydrogenation." More research is needed to find out how trans fat affects the risk of heart disease. Foods high in fat, like butter and margarine, should be used in small amounts.

Myth: Low-fat or no fat means no calories.

Fact: Remember that most fruits and vegetables are naturally low in fat and calories. Other low-fat or nonfat foods may still have a lot of calories. Often these foods will have extra sugar, flour, or starch thickeners to make them taste better. These ingredients can add calories, which can lead to weight gain.

A low-fat or nonfat food is usually lower in calories than the same size portion of the full-fat product. The number of calories depends on the amount of carbohydrate, protein, and fat in the food. Carbohydrate and protein have about 4 calories per gram, and fat has more than twice that amount (9 calories per gram).

Myth: "Going vegetarian" means you are sure to lose weight and be healthier.

Fact: Vegetarian diets can be healthy because they are often lower in saturated fat and cholesterol and higher in fiber. Choosing a vegetarian diet with a low-fat content can be helpful for weight loss. But vegetarians—like nonvegetarians—can also make poor food choices, like eating large amounts of junk (nutritionally empty) foods. Candy, chips, and other high-fat, vegetarian foods should be eaten in small amounts.

Vegetarian diets need to be as carefully planned as nonvegetarian diets to make sure they are nutritious. Vegetarian diets can provide the recommended daily amount of all the key nutrients if you choose foods carefully. Plants, especially fruits and vegetables, are the main source of nutrients in vegetarian diets. Some types of vegetarian diets (like those that include eggs and dairy foods) contain animal sources, while another type (the vegan diet) incorporates no animal foods. Nutrients normally found in animal products that are not always found in a vegetarian diet are iron, calcium, vitamin D, vitamin B_{12}, and zinc. Here are some foods that have these nutrients:

Iron: cashews, tomato juice, rice, tofu, lentils, and garbanzo beans (chick peas).

Calcium: dairy products, fortified soymilk, fortified orange juice, tofu, kale, and broccoli.

Vitamin D: fortified milk and soymilk, and fortified cereals (or a small amount of sunlight).

Vitamin B_{12}: eggs, dairy products, and fortified soy milk, cereals, tempeh, and miso. (Tempeh and miso are foods made from soybeans. They are low in calories and fat, and high in protein.)

Zinc: whole grains (especially the germ and bran of the grain), eggs, dairy products, nuts, tofu, leafy vegetables (lettuce, spinach, cabbage), and root vegetables (onions, potatoes, carrots, celery, radishes).

Vegetarians must eat a variety of plant foods over the course of a day to get enough protein. Those plant foods that have the most protein are lentils, tofu, nuts, seeds, tempeh, miso, and peas.

CLAIMS THAT RAISE A CAUTION FLAG

http://www.ftc.gov/bcp/conline/pubs/alerts/paunch.html

Paunch Lines: Weight Loss Claims Are No Joke for Dieters

Are you one of the estimated 50 million Americans who will go on a diet this year? If so, you may be tempted by advertisements for products promising easy, quick ways to lose weight. You should know that, when it comes to losing weight, gimmicks usually don't deliver on their promises.

While some dieters succeed in taking off weight, perhaps as few as 5 percent manage to keep it off in the long run. Most experts agree that the best way to lose weight is to eat fewer calories and burn more energy by increasing physical activity. Experts suggest aiming for a goal loss of about a pound a week. This usually means cutting about 500 calories a day from your diet, eating healthy, low-fat foods, finding a regular exercise activity you enjoy, and sticking to it.

When it comes to evaluating claims for weight loss products, the Federal Trade Commission recommends a healthy portion of skepticism. Before you spend money on products or programs that promise fast or easy weight loss, weigh the claims and consider these tips:

"**Lose 30 Pounds in Just 30 Days.**" As a rule, the faster you lose weight, the more likely you are to gain it back. Also, fast weight loss could harm your health. Unless your doctor advises it, don't look for programs that promise quick weight loss.

"**Lose All the Weight You Can for Just $39.99.**" Some weight loss programs have hidden costs. For example, some don't advertise the fact that you must buy their prepackaged meals that cost more than the program fees. Before you sign up for any weight-loss program, ask for a rundown of all the costs. Get them in writing.

"**Lose Weight While You Sleep.**" Claims for diet products and programs that promise weight loss without effort are phony.

"**Lose Weight and Keep It Off for Good.**" Be suspicious about products promising long-term or permanent weight loss. To lose weight and keep it off, you must change how you eat and how much you exercise.

"*John Doe Lost 84 Pounds in Six Weeks.*" Don't be misled by someone else's weight loss claims. Even if the claims are true, someone else's success may have little relation to your own chances of success.

"*Scientific Breakthrough . . . Medical Miracle.*" There are no miracle weight loss products. To lose weight, you have to reduce your intake of calories and increase your physical activity. Be skeptical about exaggerated claims.

Source: The Weight Control Information Network of the National Institute of Diabetes & Digestive & Kidney Diseases of the National Institutes of Health, posted December 2000. URL: http://www.niddk.nih.gov/health/nutrit/pubs/myths/index.htm.

Index

About the Authors

MARJOLIJN BIJLEFELD is a freelance writer and editor. She is the author of *The Gun Control Debate: A Documentary History* (Greenwood, 1997), *Teen Guide to Personal Financial Management* (Greenwood, 2000), and *Food and You: A Guide to Healthy Habits for Teens* (Greenwood, 2001).

SHARON K. ZOUMBARIS is a professional librarian, freelance writer, and storyteller. She is author of *Teen Guide to Personal Financial Management* (Greenwood, 2000) along with *Food and You: A Guide to Healthy Habits for Teens* (Greenwood, 2001), *Nutrition: Health & Medical Issues Today* (2009), and *The Encyclopedia of Wellness* (2012).